ECG in Medical Practice

Concerned mainly with basic concepts, abnormalities in cardiac disease and 151 tracings of ECG for practice

ECG in Medical Practice

FIFTH EDITION

ABM Abdullah MRCP (UK) FRCP (Edin)
UGC Professor
University Grants Commission Bangladesh
Bangabandhu Sheikh Mujib Medical University
Dhaka, Bangladesh

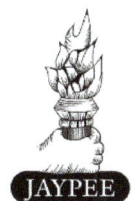

JAYPEE
JAYPEE BROTHERS MEDICAL PUBLISHERS
The Health Sciences Publisher
New Delhi | London

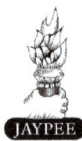

Jaypee Brothers Medical Publishers (P) Ltd

Headquarters
EMCA House
23/23-B, Ansari Road, Daryaganj
New Delhi 110 002, India
Landline: +91-11-23272143,
+91-11-23272703
+91-11-23282021, +91-11-23245672
E-mail: jaypee@jaypeebrothers.com

Overseas Office
JP Medical Ltd.
83, Victoria Street, London
SW1H 0HW (UK)
Phone: +44-20 3170 8910
E-mail: info@jpmedpub.com

Corporate Office
Jaypee Brothers Medical Publishers (P) Ltd.
4838/24, Ansari Road, Daryaganj
New Delhi 110 002, India
Phone: +91-11-43574357
Fax: +91-11-43574314
E-mail: jaypee@jaypeebrothers.com

EU GPSR Authorised Representative
Logos Europe, 9 rue Nicolas Poussin
17000, La Rochelle, France
Phone: +33 (0) 6 67 93 73 78
E-mail: Contact@logoseurope.eu

Website: www.jaypeebrothers.com
Website: www.jaypeedigital.com

© 2020, Jaypee Brothers Medical Publishers

The views and opinions expressed in this book are solely those of the original contributor(s)/author(s) and do not necessarily represent those of editor(s) of the book.

All rights reserved. No part of this publication may be reproduced, stored or transmitted in any form or by any means, electronic, mechanical, photocopying, recording or otherwise, without the prior permission in writing of the publishers.

All brand names and product names used in this book are trade names, service marks, trademarks or registered trademarks of their respective owners. The publisher is not associated with any product or vendor mentioned in this book.

Medical knowledge and practice change constantly. This book is designed to provide accurate, authoritative information about the subject matter in question. However, readers are advised to check the most current information available on procedures included and check information from the manufacturer of each product to be administered, to verify the recommended dose, formula, method and duration of administration, adverse effects and contraindications. It is the responsibility of the practitioner to take all appropriate safety precautions. Neither the publisher nor the author(s)/editor(s) assume any liability for any injury and/or damage to persons or property arising from or related to use of material in this book.

This book is sold on the understanding that the publisher is not engaged in providing professional medical services. If such advice or services are required, the services of a competent medical professional should be sought.

Every effort has been made where necessary to contact holders of copyright to obtain permission to reproduce copyright material. If any have been inadvertently overlooked, the publisher will be pleased to make the necessary arrangements at the irst opportunity. The **CD/DVD-ROM** (if any) provided in the sealed envelope with this book is complimentary and free of cost. **Not meant for sale.**

Inquiries for bulk sales may be solicited at: jaypee@jaypeebrothers.com

ECG in Medical Practice / ABM Abdullah

First Edition: 2004
Fifth Edition: 2020, Reprint: **2025**

ISBN: 978-93-89587-25-8

Dedicated to

Professor Taimur AK Mahmud MCPS FCPS
Ex-professor of Medicine
Bangabandhu Sheikh Mujib Medical University
Dhaka, Bangladesh

My beloved colleague, well-wisher and a source of inspiration

"The value of experience is not in seeing much but in seeing wisely"
— **Sir William Osler**

Preface to the Fifth Edition

By the good grace of Almighty Allah and encouragement of my family members and well-wishers, I am pleased to prepare the fifth edition of *ECG in Medical Practice*. This book was first published in 2004. Since its publication, immense popularity and wide acceptability of the previous editions among the medical students and doctors have encouraged me to prepare this new one.

Even with the development of sophisticated technology in cardiology, ECG is still a valuable and unparallel initial investigation in any cardiac disease. So, the basic concept of ECG and its diagnostic value still remain unchanged.

I am highly pleased to present the 5th edition, in which numerous new informations, latest investigations, and management have been added. Those who had the opportunity to read the previous edition, will find that in this new edition, some new ECG strips have been incorporated and new explanations have been re-written in the light of recent updates in cardiology.

Since 2004 of its first edition, this fifth edition will probably a pleasant one and hopefully will be acceptable by the respected valued readers. I also hope this edition will help the students to prepare for both undergraduate and postgraduate examination and to develop their clinical competence and confidence in cardiology.

In spite of my sincere best efforts, I believe there is still some scope of further improvement of this book and make it even more better. Any constructive comments and criticisms will be highly welcomed and appreciated, which will reinforce to understand ECG in an easy way.

For better practice, I have added 151 ECG tracings with answers which are provided in the last part. I would advise the reader to see the tracing first, then make your own interpretation and finally compare with the given diagnosis written at the end of the chapter.

ABM Abdullah

Preface to the First Edition

Despite the advent of many high-tech diagnostic procedures, ECG still remains one of the most basic, useful and easily available tools for the early diagnosis and evaluation of many cardiac problems.

In spite of a lot of books on this topic, I have written another new book, which is simple, concise, easy and a practical one that will help any physician, especially the beginners with little knowledge or experience on ECG.

The aim of this book is to guide the students and doctors about the basic concepts in ECG, its interpretation and recognition of cardiac abnormalities. It is also my intention to include common abnormalities in ECG and common cardiac problems that will help the students in any specialty of medicine, especially those who will appear in any examination.

To simplify and also to practice, I have arranged this book in three chapters:
- Chapter 1—contains the basic principles of ECG along with normal ECG pattern and the abnormalities.
- Chapter 2—contains the ECG abnormalities in different cardiac and extra-cardiac diseases.
- Chapter 3—contains 100 ECG tracings of varying difficulty (from simple to more complex) for self-practice. Interpretation of these ECG are written in the last few pages (I would advise first to interpret the ECG by yourself, then compare the findings).

Whenever you are going through an ECG, always proceed systematically. Never leave anything to chance and never assume anything. Always describe the basic things and finally look for any abnormality.

Being an internist, I have prepared this book after going through dozens of different ECG books and have tried my best to fill up the gaps, I have noticed in those during my long teaching experience. It is my students and doctor colleagues who have constantly inspired and insisted me to prepare such a book so that they can have a complete and easy grasp over the topic in a short-time. I believe, this book will not only fulfil their demand but also be of great help for those who are willing to self-learn the basic concepts of ECG.

I was always careful not to overburden the busy clinicians and practitioners with the unnecessary details.

I would like to emphasize that efficiency, skill and fluency in interpreting ECG will only be achieved by going through the ECG tracings repeatedly and reviewing the topics frequently.

I would always appreciate and welcome constructive criticism from the valued readers about this book.

ABM Abdullah

Acknowledgments

I would like to take the opportunity to extend my sincere gratitude to Professor Kanak Kanti Barua, Vice Chancellor, Bangabandhu Sheikh Mujib Medical University, Dhaka, Bangladesh for his encouragement and valuable suggestions in preparing this book. Also, I would like to acknowledge Professor Shohael Mahmud Arafat FCPS (Medicine) MRCP (UK) FRCPE FICP (Hon), Chairman, Department of Medicine, Bangabandhu Sheikh Mujib Medical University, Dhaka, Bangladesh for his encouragement and valuable suggestions to enrich the book.

I am also highly grateful to Dr Mustasin Haider Sami, Dr Abhishek Bhadra, and Dr Hasanul Karim for graphical presentations and computer composing of the entire book. They have also gone through the whole manuscript and made necessary corrections and modifications. I can, without any hesitation, mention that they have worked as the co-authors.

I must acknowledge the contributions of my colleagues, doctors, and students who were kind enough to help me in writing such a book of its kind. They are always a source of my inspiration and encouragement.

- Professor MU Kabir Chowdhury FRCP (Glasgow) DDV
- Professor Sunil Kumar Biswas MCPS (Medicine) MD (Internal Medicine)
- Professor Md Gofranul Hoque FCPS
- Professor Tahmida Hassan DDV MD
- Dr Shahnoor Sarmin MCPS FCPS MD (Cardiology)
- Dr Ayesha Rafiq Chowdhury FCPS (Medicine) MD (Cardio) MRCP (UK)
- Dr Md Abul Kalam Azad FCPS MD (Rheumatology)
- Dr Md Razibul Alam MBBS MD (Gastroenterology)
- Dr Samprity Islam MBBS MD (Pulmonology)
- Dr Tazin Afrose Shah MBBS FCPS
- Dr Ahmed-Al-Muntasir-Niloy MD internist (USA)
- Dr Sadi Abdullah MBBS DTCD MRCP (UK)
- Dr Imtiaz Ahmed MBBS MRCP (UK) FCPS (Medicine)
- Dr Sadia Sabah MBBS MD (Resident)
- Dr Md Shakhawat Hossain Rokan MBBS
- Dr Abhijit Chowdhury MBBS Internist (Australia)
- Dr Parvin Akhter MBBS MD (Internal Medicine)
- Dr Nazma Azim Daizy MBBS MD (Resident)
- Dr Nuzhat Nadia MBBS
- Dr Nazia Hasin MBBS
- Dr Israt Rubaiya MBBS
- Dr Sumayia Sultana MBBS
- Dr Nazmun Nahar MBBS
- Dr Dolon Sarkar MBBS
- Dr Aminul Kibria MBBS

My special thanks to Mr Jitendar P Vij for his constant support and encouragement and his associates particularly to, Mr MS Mani, Mr Shashi Kumar Shamboo, Dr Richa Saxena, Kamakshi Khanna and the team of M/s Jaypee Brothers Medical Publishers (P), Ltd, New Delhi, for their untiring endeavor and hard work, which made it possible for the "painless delivery" of this book. They have also notably enhanced the physical quality of the book making it beautiful and attractive. I must be grateful to my students who were repeatedly encouraging and demanding to write such a book.

Last, but not the least, I would like to express my gratitude to my wife, whose untiring support and sacrifice has made it possible to bring out such a nice book. I am also grateful to my daughter Dr Sadia Sabah and my son Dr Sadi Abdullah for their encouragement and inspiration in preparing such a book.

ABM Abdullah

Contents

Chapter 1: Basic Concepts of ECG 1
- Specialized Conductive System of The Heart *3*
- Anatomy of Conductive Tissue *4*
- Coronary Circulation *5*
- Properties of Cardiac Muscles *6*
- Nerve Supply of The Heart *6*
- Electrocardiogram *7*
- Before Interpretation of Electrocardiogram *10*
- Brief Discussion About Electrocardiogram Paper *11*
- Normal Electrocardiogram *14*
- Intervals In Electrocardiogram *16*
- Brief Discussion of Waves and Intervals in Electrocardiogram *17*
- Rhythm of Heart *32*
- Calculation of Heart Rate *33*
- Cardiac Axis *34*
- Normal Variants In Electrocardiogram *37*
- Exercise Electrocardiogram (Exercise Tolerance Test or ETT) *38*
- Holter Monitoring (Ambulatory Electrocardiogram) *40*

Chapter 2: ECG Changes in Different Diseases 41
- Left Ventricular Hypertrophy *43*
- Right Ventricular Hypertrophy *46*
- Biventricular Hypertrophy (Combined Left Ventricular Hypertrophy and Right Ventricular Hypertrophy) *49*
- Left Atrial Hypertrophy *50*
- Right Atrial Hypertrophy *51*
- Combined Left and Right Atrial Hypertrophy (Biatrial Hypertrophy) *53*
- Sinus Arrhythmia *54*
- Sinus Tachycardia *55*
- Sinus Bradycardia *58*
- Supraventricular Tachycardia *60*
- Atrial Tachycardia *64*
- Nodal Rhythm (Junctional Rhythm) *66*
- Wandering Pacemaker *68*
- Atrial Fibrillation *70*
- Ashman Phenomenon (Ashman Beats) *74*
- Atrial Flutter *75*
- Ectopic Beat *77*
- Atrial Ectopic *79*
- Ventricular Ectopic *80*
- Ventricular Bigeminy *84*
- Ventricular Trigeminy *86*

- Ventricular Quadrigeminy 86
- Ventricular Pentageminy 87
- Ventricular Hexageminy 87
- Ventricular Tachycardia 88
- Torsades De Pointes 91
- Ventricular Fibrillation 93
- Ventricular Flutter 94
- Heart Block 95
- SA Block 98
- Sick Sinus Syndrome 100
- Atrioventricular Block (AV Block) 102
- First-Degree AV Block 102
- Second-Degree AV Block 103
- Complete Heart Block (3rd Degree) 105
- Atrioventricular Dissociation 108
- Bundle Branch Block 110
- Fascicular Block (Hemiblock) 112
- Left Bundle Branch Block 115
- Myocardial Infarction 117
- Myocardial Ischemia 128
- Ventricular Aneurysm 131
- Acute Pericarditis 133
- Pericardial Effusion 135
- Wolff–Parkinson–White Syndrome 137
- Lown–Ganong–Levine Syndrome 141
- Pacemaker 142
- Digoxin Effect 147
- Hypokalemia 150
- Hyperkalemia 152
- Hypermagnesemia 155
- Hypomagnesemia 156
- Hypocalcemia 157
- Hypercalcemia 159
- Pulmonary Embolism 161
- Dextrocardia 164
- Hypothermia 166
- Chronic Obstructive Pulmonary Disease 167
- Atrial Septal Defect 168
- Hypothyroidism 170
- Hyperthyroidism 171
- Pulseless Electrical Activity or Electromechanical Dissociation 172
- Raised Intracranial Pressure 173

Chapter 3: 151 Tracings of ECG 174
- Findings of ECG Tracings 327

Suggested Reading 345

Index 347

CHAPTER 1

Basic Concepts of ECG

"Workout the best method for examination and practice it until it is a second nature to you"

ECG in Medical Practice

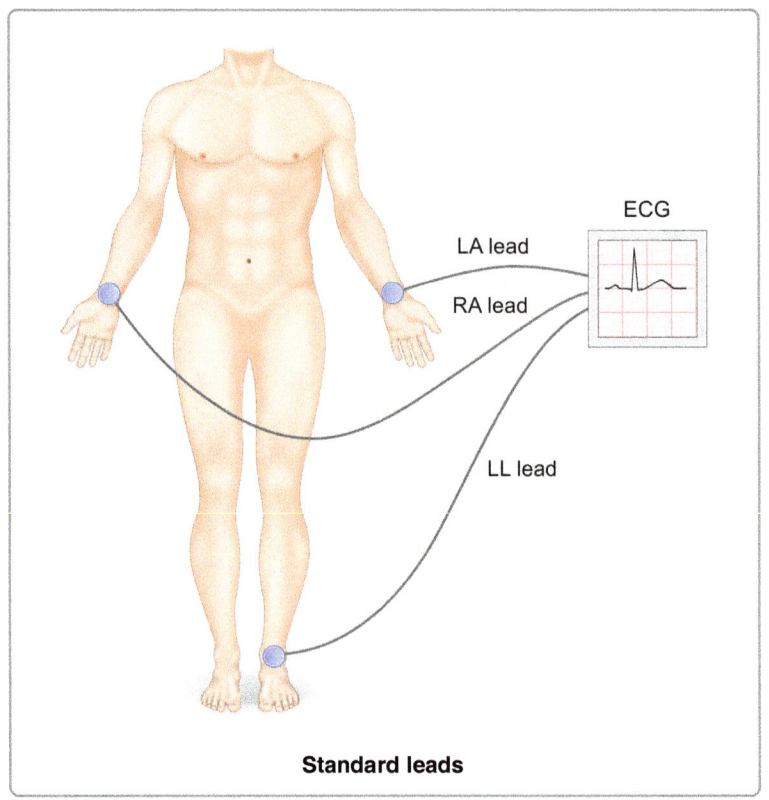

Standard leads

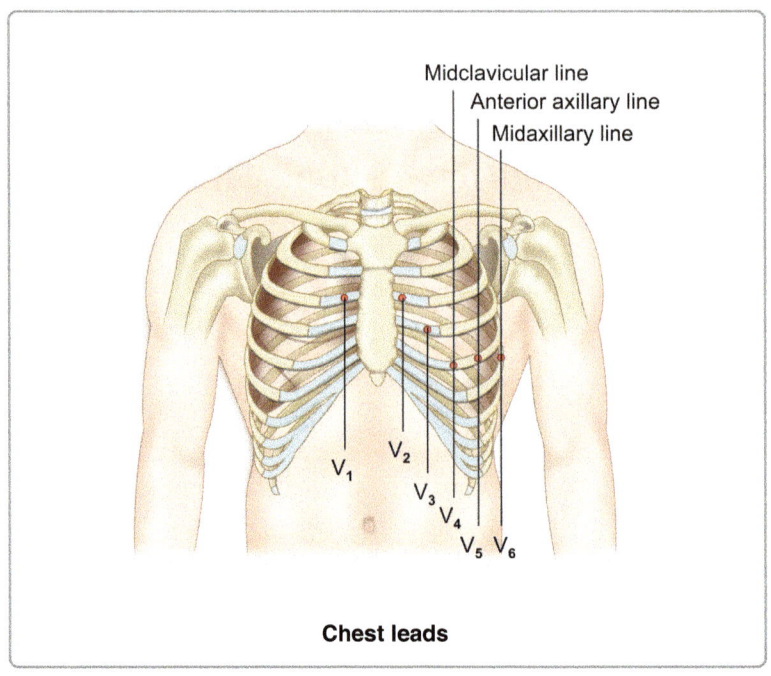

Chest leads

SPECIALIZED CONDUCTIVE SYSTEM OF THE HEART

There are five specialized tissues which are called conductive system of the heart. These are:
- Sinoatrial (SA) node
- Atrioventricular (AV) node
- Bundle of His
- Right bundle branch (RBB) and left bundle branch (LBB)
- Purkinje fibers

These specialized conductive pathways allow the heart to be electrically activated in a predictable manner (see the sequence below).

The electrical activity or the impulse of the heart starts in the SA node (which is called primary pacemaker), then spreads across the atria (by three internodal pathways and Bachmann's bundle), causing depolarization of both atria. From the atria, the impulse reaches the AV node, where there is some delay, which allows atria to contract and pump blood into the ventricles. The impulse then spreads along the bundle of His, then along the LBB and RBB, finally into the ventricular muscles through Purkinje fibers, causing ventricular depolarization.

Initially, the ventricular septum is depolarized and moves from left to right, then depolarization is of body of the left ventricle, and finally the right ventricle.

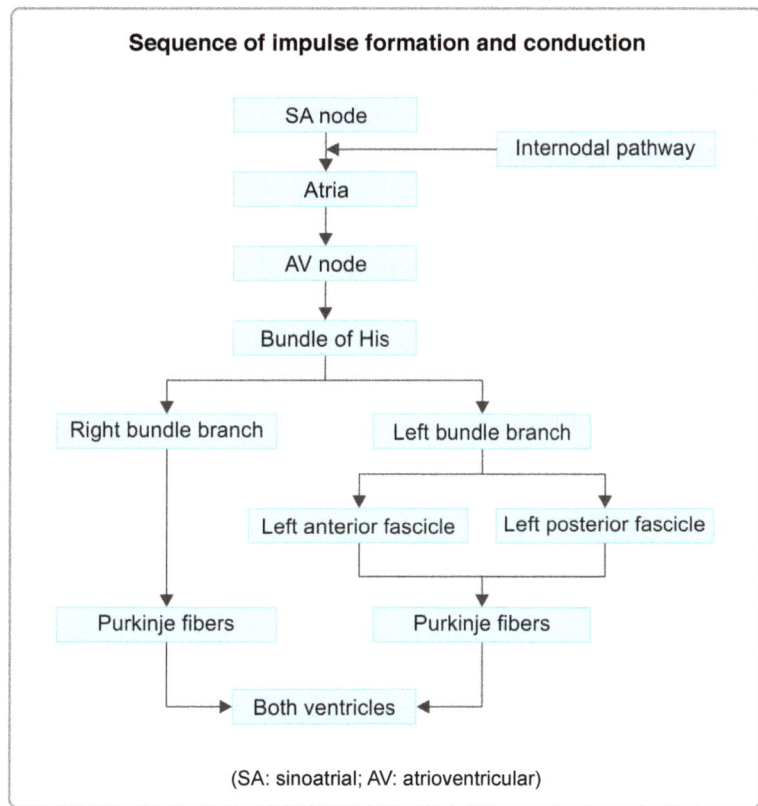

This is the normal sequence of stimulation of the specialized tissue. Normal rhythm is called sinus rhythm. The way electrical impulse flows through the heart is called conduction. If abnormalities of electrical activity of the heart or if any disturbance of this sequence occur, there is rhythm disturbance, which is called arrhythmia, or if there is any abnormality of conduction, it is called heart block. Any changes of normal flow of electricity through the heart can be detected by electrocardiogram (ECG) tracing and may indicate damaged cardiac muscle or any abnormality.

Sinoatrial node is the dominant pacemaker. Other pacemaker sites in the heart are atria, AV node, and ventricles. All these are dormant, but can initiate impulse at a slow rate when SA node fails.

ANATOMY OF CONDUCTIVE TISSUE

1. *SA node*: It is located in the superior and right side of right atrium, near the root of superior vena cava. Normally, the impulse arises in the SA node, called sinus rhythm. From the SA node, the impulse spreads along three internodal pathways (anterior, middle, and posterior) into both right and left atria. Finally, these three internodal pathways enter into the AV node. There is an additional internodal pathway, called Bachmann's bundle, which transmits impulse to the left atrium.
Normal rate in SA node is 60-100/min.
2. *AV node*: The AV node is smaller than the SA node. It is located in the subendocardial surface of right side of right atrium, at the posterior part of interatrial septum, near the opening of coronary sinus, just above the tricuspid valve. If the SA node is blocked or fails, the AV node can initiate cardiac impulse and perform as a pacemaker. Normal rate of the AV node is 40-60/min. According to the electrical response, the AV node is divided into three parts:
   - High nodal (AN region)
   - Mid nodal (N region)
   - Low nodal (NH region)

   In ECG, these three regions can be detected by looking at the configuration of "P" wave (see details on page no. 17).
3. *Bundle of His*: It is the extension of the tail of the AV node that extends downward and to the left, then enter into the interventricular septum, near the junction of muscles and fibrous part of ventricular septum. Then, it is divided into two branches: Right and left bundle branches.
   When there is AV block, bundle of His can initiate cardiac impulse and perform as a pacemaker. Normal rate of bundle of His is 20-40/min.
4. *Right bundle branch*: It extends on the right side of interventricular septum and spreads into the right ventricle through Purkinje fibers.
5. *Left bundle branch:* It divides into anterior and posterior fascicles. Anterior fascicle spreads into the anterosuperior part of the left ventricle. Posterior fascicle spreads into the posteroinferior part of the left ventricle, through Purkinje fibers.
6. *Purkinje fibers*: These are the terminal network of fibers, diffusely spread into the ventricular muscles in subendocardial and subepicardial myocardium. Normal intrinsic rate of Purkinje fibers is 15-40/min.

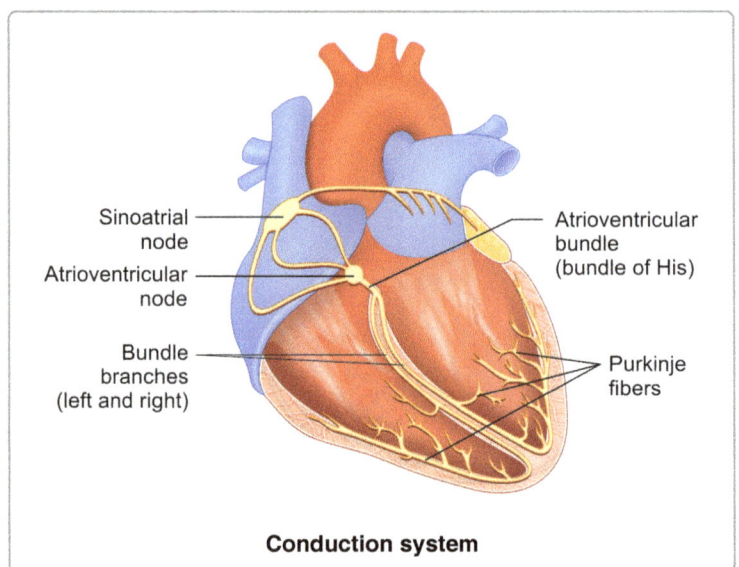

Conduction system

NB: Most specialized cardiac fibers contain large number of automatic cells. But atrial and ventricular muscles fibers, under normal condition, have no automatic activity.

CORONARY CIRCULATION

There are two major coronary arteries: (1) Right and (2) left.

1. Right Coronary Artery

It arises from the right coronary sinus of Valsalva, runs along the right AV groove, and gives marginal branch that supplies right atrium and right ventricle. It continues as posterior descending artery, which runs in the posterior interventricular groove and spreads into the posterior part of interventricular septum and inferoposterior aspect of the left ventricular wall.

Right coronary artery supplies the following parts:
- *SA node*: 60% cases
- *AV node*: 90% cases
- Right atrium and right ventricle
- Inferoposterior aspect of left ventricle

So, the occlusion of right coronary artery results in sinus bradycardia, AV block, infarction of inferior part of left ventricle, and occasionally of right ventricle.

2. Left Coronary Artery

It arises from the left coronary sinus of valsalva. Within 2.5 cm of its origin, left main coronary artery divides into two branches: (1) Left anterior descending artery and (2) Circumflex artery.
- *Left anterior descending artery*: It runs in the anterior interventricular groove and gives branches to supply the anterior part of interventricular septum, anterior wall, and apex of the left ventricle.
- *Circumflex artery*: It runs posteriorly in the left AV groove and supplies the marginal branch to the left atrium, also lateral and posteroinferior part of the left ventricle.

Left coronary artery also supplies:
- SA node in 40% cases
- AV node in 10% cases
- Bundle of His
- Right and left bundle branches

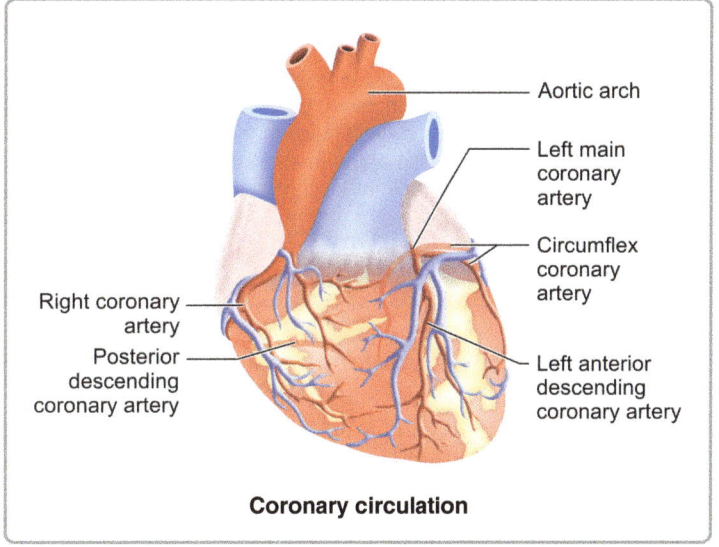

Coronary circulation

Occlusion of the left anterior descending artery and the circumflex artery causes infarction of the corresponding territories of left ventricle. Occlusion of the left main coronary artery causes extensive damage and is usually fatal.

Venous system mainly follows coronary arteries, but drains to the coronary sinus in the AV groove, then to the right atrium.

Coronary vessels receive sympathetic and parasympathetic innervations. Stimulation of α-receptor causes vasoconstriction and $β_2$ causes vasodilatation. Sympathetic stimulation of coronary artery causes dilatation and parasympathetic stimulation also causes mild dilatation of normal coronary artery. Healthy coronary endothelium releases nitric oxide, which promotes vasodilatation. Systemic hormones, neuropeptides, and endothelin also influence arterial tone and coronary flow.

PROPERTIES OF CARDIAC MUSCLES

Cardiac muscles have some special properties:
- *Automaticity*: Without external stimulus, heart muscle can initiate normal cardiac impulse by the SA node.
- *Autorhythmicity*: Cardiac muscle can contract after a regular interval called autorhythmicity.
- *Excitability*: Cardiac muscle can be excited by adequate external stimulus.
- *Conductivity*: Cardiac muscle has the ability to conduct impulse from one muscle cell to another cell.
- *Contractility*: Ability to contract after depolarization.
- *Refractory period*: It is a period during which activated muscle fibers do not respond to further stimulus. It is of two types: (1) Absolute refractory period and (2) Relative refractory period.
  - Absolute refractory period: During this period, muscle fibers do not respond to any stimulus.
  - Relative refractory period: With very strong stimulus, muscle fibers may respond.
- *All-or-none law*: If external stimulus is too little, no cardiac impulse is initiated. But with adequate stimulus, all muscle fibers contract with its best ability.
- *Functional syncytium*: Cardiac muscle fibers are electrically connected with one another by a gap junction. When one muscle fiber is excited, the action potential spreads to whole cardiac muscle fibers, because of the presence of intercalated disc. It is called syncytium.

NB: Remember the following points:
- Purkinje fibers transmit impulse faster than any tissue of the heart, at the rate of 4,000 mm/s.
- Atrial muscles transmit impulse at the rate of 800–1,000 mm/s.
- Ventricular muscles transmit impulse at the rate of 400 mm/s.
- AV node transmit impulse at the rate of 200 mm/s (slowest). This slow conduction in the AV node is a protective mechanism. It prevents to transmit rapid atrial contraction or impulse.

NERVE SUPPLY OF THE HEART

The heart is supplied by both sympathetic and parasympathetic (in cardiac plexus).
- Sympathetic (adrenergic) supplies both atria and ventricular muscle, and also conductive specialized tissue.
- Parasympathetic preganglionic fibers and sensory fibers reach the heart through vagus nerves. Cholinergic nerves supply the SA node and the AV node via muscarinic (M_2) receptors.

Nerve supply is mainly through β_1 and β_2 receptors.
- β_1 receptor is predominant in heart, having both inotropic and chronotropic effect.
- β_2 receptor is predominant in vascular muscles and causes vasodilatation.

Under basal condition, predominant effect is parasympathetic through vagus nerve over sympathetic, resulting in slow heart rate. So during sleep, the heart rate is slow. Also in athlete, there is predominant vagal effect (so heart rate may show bradycardia).

Heart consists of three types of cells:
- *Pacemaker cells*: They generate the impulse.
- *Electricity conducting cells*: They transmit the impulse.
- *Myocardial cells*: They maintain the contractile functions of the heart.

ELECTROCARDIOGRAM

Definition

It is the graphical representation of electrical potentials produced when the electric current passes through the heart. Electrical activity is the basic characteristic of heart and is the stimulus for cardiac contraction.

Electrical activity is detected by electrodes attached to the skin. Normal electrical conduction of the heart allows the impulse that is generated by the SA node, to be propagated to and stimulate the cardiac muscle, which contracts after stimulation. It is the ordered, rhythmic stimulation of the myocardium during the cardiac cycle that allows efficient contraction of the heart, thereby allowing blood to be pumped throughout the body. Disturbance of electrical function is common in heart disease.

Electrocardiogram records the electrical impulse on ECG paper by electrodes placed on the body surface, called waves or deflections. Waves that appear on ECG paper represent the electrical activities of the myocardial cells. The following points of waves are observed recorded on ECG paper:
- *Duration*: It is measured in horizontal direction.
- *Height or amplitude*: It is measured in vertical direction.
- *Configuration*: It indicates the shape and appearance of particular wave.

One heartbeat is recorded as a grouping of waves which are designed by P-QRS-T and U.
- P wave — It represents atrial depolarization
- PR interval — It represents the time taken for the cardiac impulse to spread over the atrium
- QRS complex — It represents ventricular depolarization
- T wave — It represents ventricular repolarization
- U wave — It represents repolarization of interventricular septum

In a normal ECG recording, there are 12 leads, which are different view parts of heart's electrical activity.
- Three bipolar limb leads
- Three unipolar limb leads
- Six chest leads

Bipolar Limb Leads

These are also called limb leads, which are designated as L_I, L_{II}, and L_{III}.

- L_I — Difference of potential between left arm and right arm (LA and RA).
- L_{II} — Difference of potential between right arm and left leg (RA and LL).
- L_{III} — Difference of potential between left arm and left leg (LA and LL).

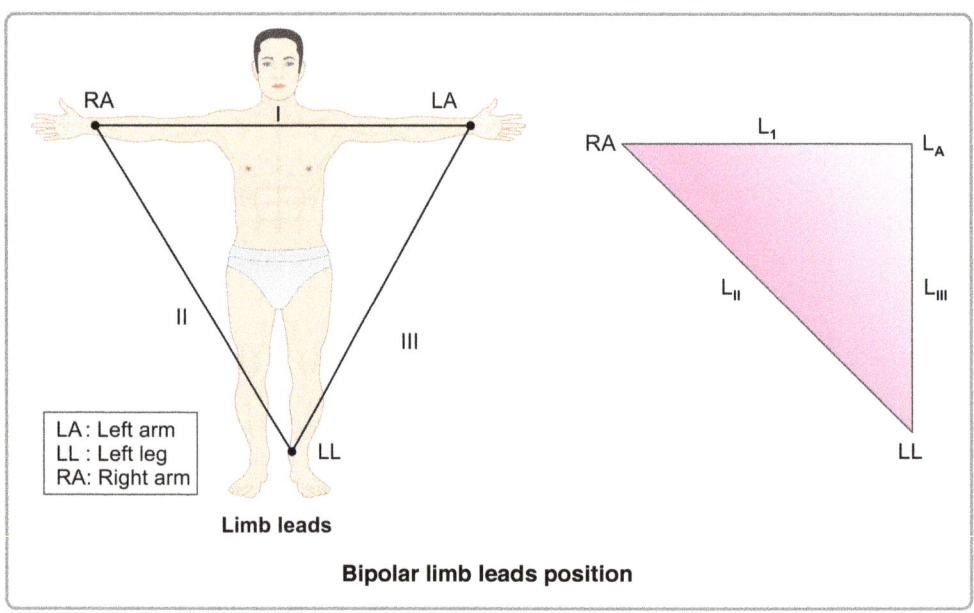

Bipolar limb leads position

Unipolar Limb Leads

These are also called augmented limb leads, which are designated as aVR, aVL, and aVF (which means augmented vector right, augmented vector left, and augmented vector foot, respectively). Three unipolar leads have very low voltage, which cannot be recorded satisfactorily. For this reason, recordings of these leads are increased in amplitude. For this reason, they are called augmented unipolar leads, which are represented as aVR, aVL, and aVF.

- aVR — augmented unipolar RA lead. It records the changes of potential occurring in the part of heart facing toward the right shoulder. Position of the lead on body is in the right wrist.
- aVL — augmented unipolar LA lead. It records the changes of potential of heart facing toward the left shoulder. Position of the lead on body is in the left wrist.
- aVF — augmented unipolar LL lead. It records the changes of potential of heart facing toward the left hip. Position of the lead on body is in the left foot.

Chest Leads (Unipolar)

Designated by "V".
Electrodes are placed in the following places on the chest wall **(See figure on page 2)**.
- V_1—4th intercostal space at right sternal border.
- V_2—4th intercostal space at left sternal border.
- V_3—midway between V_2 and V_4 on left side.
- V_4—5th intercostal space in left midclavicular line.
- V_5—5th intercostal space in left anterior axillary line.
- V_6—5th intercostal space in left midaxillary line.

NB: Before application of the electrode, skin preparation by a special jelly should be ensured which improves the quality of ECG. Limb lead electrodes are attached at the wrists and ankle, with the patient in a supine position and a pillow under the head.

Chapter 1: Basic Concepts of ECG

View of the Heart in All Leads

By looking the following leads, the site and surface of heart lesion are identified.

- L_I, aVL, V_5, and V_6 — reflects lateral (or anterolateral aspect of heart).
- L_{II}, L_{III}, and aVF — reflects inferior aspect of heart.
- V_1 and V_2 — reflects right ventricle.
- V_3 and V_4 — reflects interventricular septum.
- V_5 and V_6 — reflects left ventricle.
- V_1 to V_6 — reflects anterior aspect of heart.
- L_I, aVL, and V_1 to V_6 — reflects extensive anterior aspect of heart or anterolateral.
- L_I and aVL — high lateral
- L_{II}, L_{III}, aVF, L_I, aVL, V_5, and V_6 — inferolateral

NB: Remember the following points:

- There is no lead which represents posterior wall of the heart (it is seen in V_1 and V_2).
- Additional leads can be taken from V_3R and V_4R, sites on the right side of chest equivalent to V_3 and V_4. It is helpful for the diagnosis of right ventricular infarction (usually associated with inferior infarction).
- aVR and V_1 are oriented toward the cavity of heart.

BEFORE INTERPRETATION OF ELECTROCARDIOGRAM

Before interpreting an ECG, one must know the details about the ECG paper, standardization, and different waves in ECG. It is a matter of good exposure, experience, and understanding of the pattern interpretation, which requires a method of systematic ECG analysis.

So, everyone must have some basic knowledge about the ECG paper, normal ECG tracing, different waves, limits of normal value, duration and rhythm, etc.

During interpretation: Look at the following points carefully:
1. Standardization (see in the beginning)—like this ⊓, which is 10 mm (1 mV), normally.
2. Paper speed—25 mm/s.
3. Rhythm—by looking at RR interval (L_{II} is usually called rhythm lead), see whether it is regular or irregular.
4. Count the heart rate (per minute).
5. *Different waves and segments*: Important points to be seen are as follows:
    - P—Whether normal, small or tall, inverted, wide, notched, bifid, variable configuration
    - PR—Normal or prolonged or short
    - Q—Normal or pathological
    - R—Normal or tall or short, notched or M pattern
    - QRS—Normal or wide, high or low voltage, variable or change of shape
    - ST segment—Normal or elevated or depressed
    - T—Normal or tall or small or inverted
    - U wave—Normal or small
    - QT—Short or prolonged
6. Axis—whether normal or right or left axis deviation (LAD).
7. Abnormalities—any arrhythmia, infarction, hypertrophy, etc.

Ques. What is rhythm?
Ans. It is the interval between two successive RR waves.

Ques. What are the diseases diagnosed by looking at an ECG?
Ans.
- Tachycardia or bradycardia
  - Chamber enlargement (right or left atrial or both and right or left ventricular or both)
  - Myocardial infarction (acute or old)
  - Myocardial ischemia
  - Arrhythmias (such as atrial fibrillation or flutter, ventricular tachycardia or fibrillation or ectopics, etc.)
  - Pericardial disease such as acute pericarditis and pericardial effusion.
  - Block (first degree block, SA block, AV block, and bundle branch block)
  - Drug effect (such as digoxin)
  - Extracardiac abnormalities—electrolyte imbalance (such as hypokalemia or hyperkalemia), hypocalcemia or hypercalcemia, low-voltage tracing (in myxedema, hypothermia, and emphysema). Pulmonary disease such as pulmonary embolism and cor pulmonale.
  - Exercise ECG to see coronary artery disease.
  - Also, Holter monitoring ECG to detect arrhythmia and conduction defect.

Systematic approach in ECG interpretation: Look at the following points chronologically-
- Rate—what is the rate?
- Rhythm—regular or irregular, regularly followed by occasional irregular.
- Characters of individual waves (P, PR, Q, R, QRS, ST, T, and U).
- Specific pathological changes.

Chapter 1: Basic Concepts of ECG

BRIEF DISCUSSION ABOUT ELECTROCARDIOGRAM PAPER

Electrocardiogram paper shows small and large squares. In each small square, thin horizontal and vertical lines are present in 1 mm interval. A heavier thick line is present in every 5 mm interval (five small squares). Time is measured horizontally and voltage height is measured vertically.

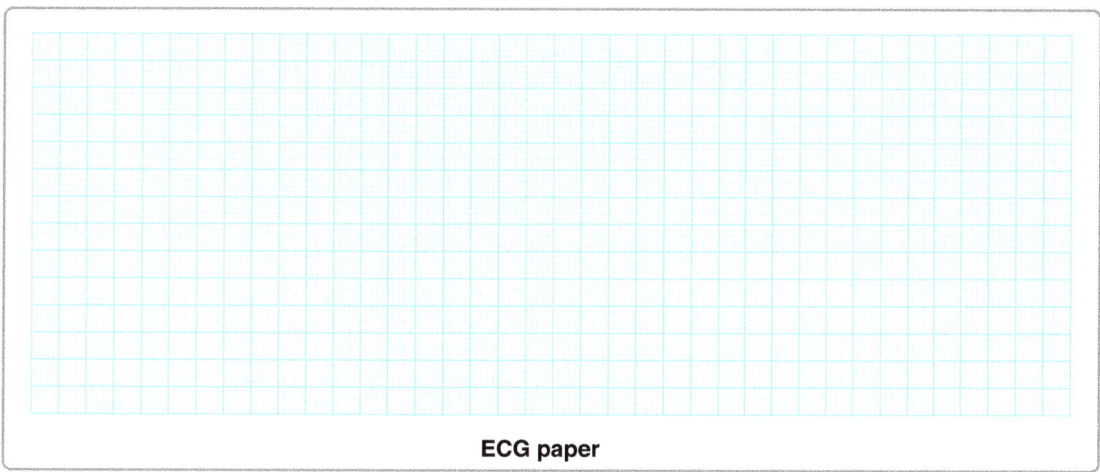

ECG paper

1. *One small square*:
   - Height = 1 mm
   - Horizontal (in time) = 0.04 second
2. *One big square (five small squares)*:
   - Height = 5 mm
   - Horizontal (in time) = 0.04 × 5 second = 0.2 second
   So, 0.2 second = 5 mm
   1 second = 5/0.2 = 25 mm
   So, recording speed is 25 mm/s (i.e., 1,500 mm/min).
   A faster recording speed (50 mm/s) is occasionally used to visualize wave deflection.
3. *Isoelectric line*: It is the baseline in ECG paper.
4. Different waves or deflections in ECG tracings are measured. If the wave is above the baseline, it is called positive deflection and if it is below the baseline, it is called negative deflection.
5. Positive deflection means the stimulus spreads toward the electrode, and negative deflection means stimulus spreads away from the electrode.

NB: Remember the following points:

Standardization of ECG
- Normally, 1 mV current — 10 mm height (10 small squares)
- Half strength — 5 mm
- Double strength — 20 mm
- Recording speed — 25 mm/s (i.e., 1,500 mm/min)

ECG in Medical Practice

During Interpretation of any ECG

- Before telling low voltage or high voltage, always see whether the normal standardization is correct or not (i.e., it should be 10 mm in height).
- Arm leads are properly placed or not.
- Be careful about artifact.

Criteria of Low-voltage Tracing

- In standard limb leads—QRS <5 mm (mainly R wave in L_I, L_{II}, and L_{III})
- In chest leads—QRS <10 mm (mainly R wave in V_1 to V_6)

Causes of Low-voltage ECG Tracing

- Incorrect standardization (i.e., if <10 mm)
- Obesity
- Pericardial effusion
- Chronic constrictive pericarditis
- Myxedema
- Emphysema
- Hypothermia
- Pneumothorax
- Plural effusion
- Previous massive myocardial infarction
- Dilated cardiomyopathy

Causes of High-voltage ECG Tracing

- Incorrect standardization (i.e., if >10 mm)
- Hypertrophy of left or right ventricle

Summary of ECG Conventions and Intervals

- Depolarization toward the electrode	—	Positive deflection (above the isoelectric line)
- Depolarization away from the electrode	—	Negative deflection (below the isoelectric line)
- Sensitivity	—	10 mm = 1 mV
- Paper speed	—	25 mm/s
- Each large (5 mm) square	—	0.2 second
- Each small (1 mm) square	—	0.04 second
- Normal standardization	—	10 mm
- Rhythm	—	Interval between two successive RR waves

Chapter 1: Basic Concepts of ECG

Ques. What is depolarization and repolarization?
Ans.
- *Depolarization*: It means initial spread of stimulus through the muscle, causing activation or contraction.
- *Repolarization*: It means the return of stimulated muscle to the resting state (recovery from activation or contraction).

Artifact in ECG

Sometimes in an ECG tracing, there may be unexplained abnormal waves which are due to electrical current interference or muscle tremor or spasm. These are actually artifacts.

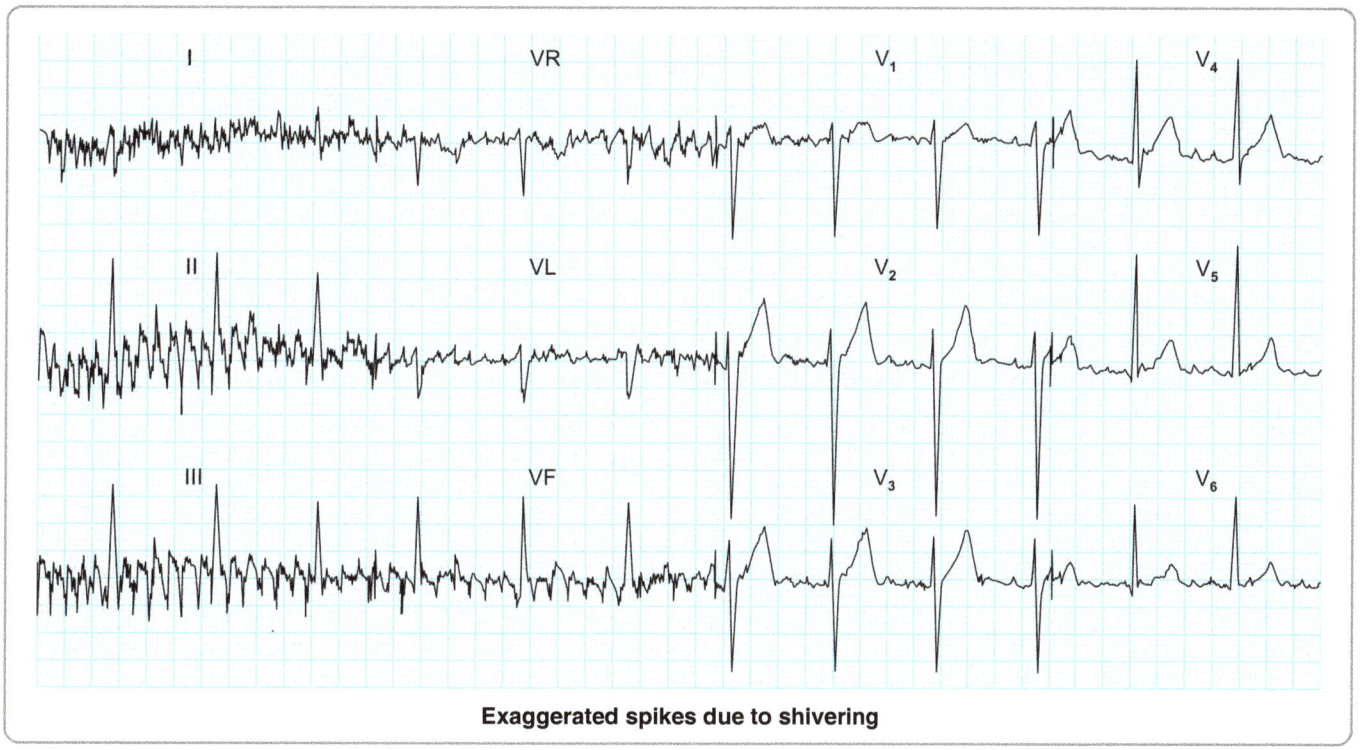

Exaggerated spikes due to shivering

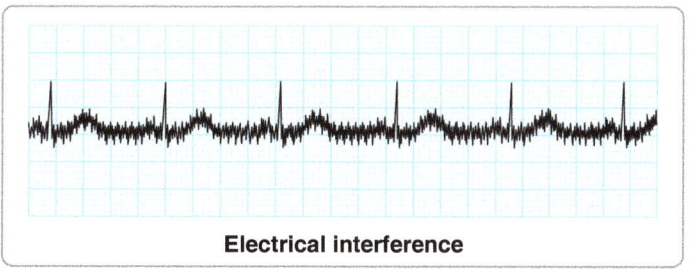

Electrical interference

NORMAL ELECTROCARDIOGRAM

Characters of Normal ECG

- Normal ECG recording consists of P wave (atrial beat), followed by QRS, ST, and T waves (ventricular beat).
- Capital letters P, Q, R, S, and T indicates large wave (>5 mm).
- Small letters p, q, r, s, and t indicates small wave (<5 mm).

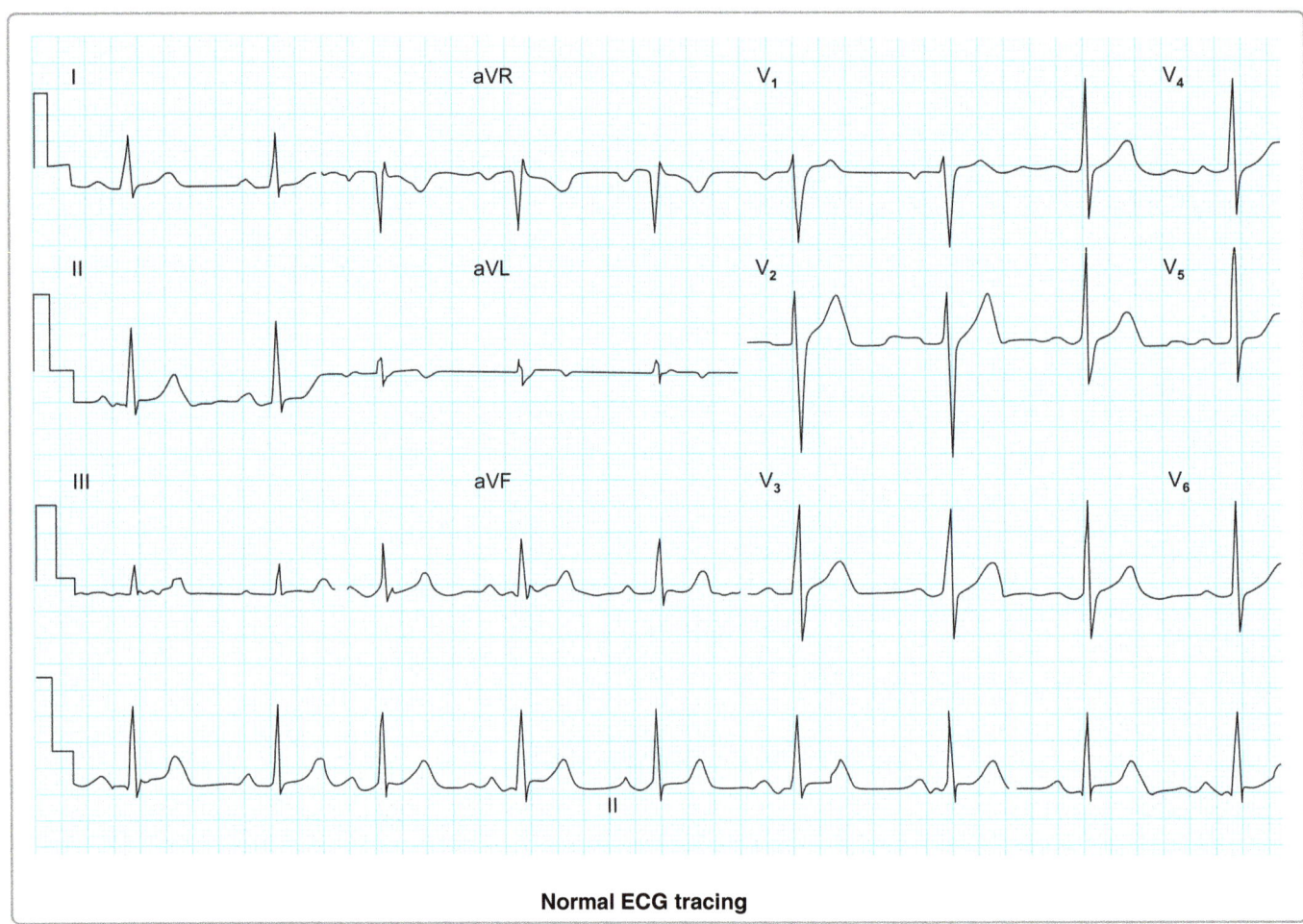

Normal ECG tracing

Types of Waves in ECG

- P — It is the deflection produced by atrial depolarization
- QRS — It is the deflection produced by ventricular depolarization
- Q (q) — It is the first negative deflection produced by ventricular depolarization. It precedes the R wave
- R (r) — It is the first positive deflection produced by ventricular depolarization
- S (s) — It is the negative deflection after R wave produced by ventricular depolarization
- T — It indicates ventricular repolarization

Other Waves

- J point—seen at the beginning of ST segment. J point is the junction between the termination of QRS complex and beginning of ST segment. J (junction) point indicates the end of QRS complex. It is often situated above the baseline, particularly in healthy young males.
- U wave—not always seen. When present, it follows the T wave, preceding the next P wave. It indicates the repolarization of interventricular septum or slow repolarization of the ventricles.

Electrocardiogram of Reversed Arm Leads

If the limb electrodes are wrongly attached (right one on the left and left one on the right), there will be inverted P in L_1. Also, abnormal QRS complex and T wave in L_1. It is called "technical dextrocardia." QRS is normal in chest leads.

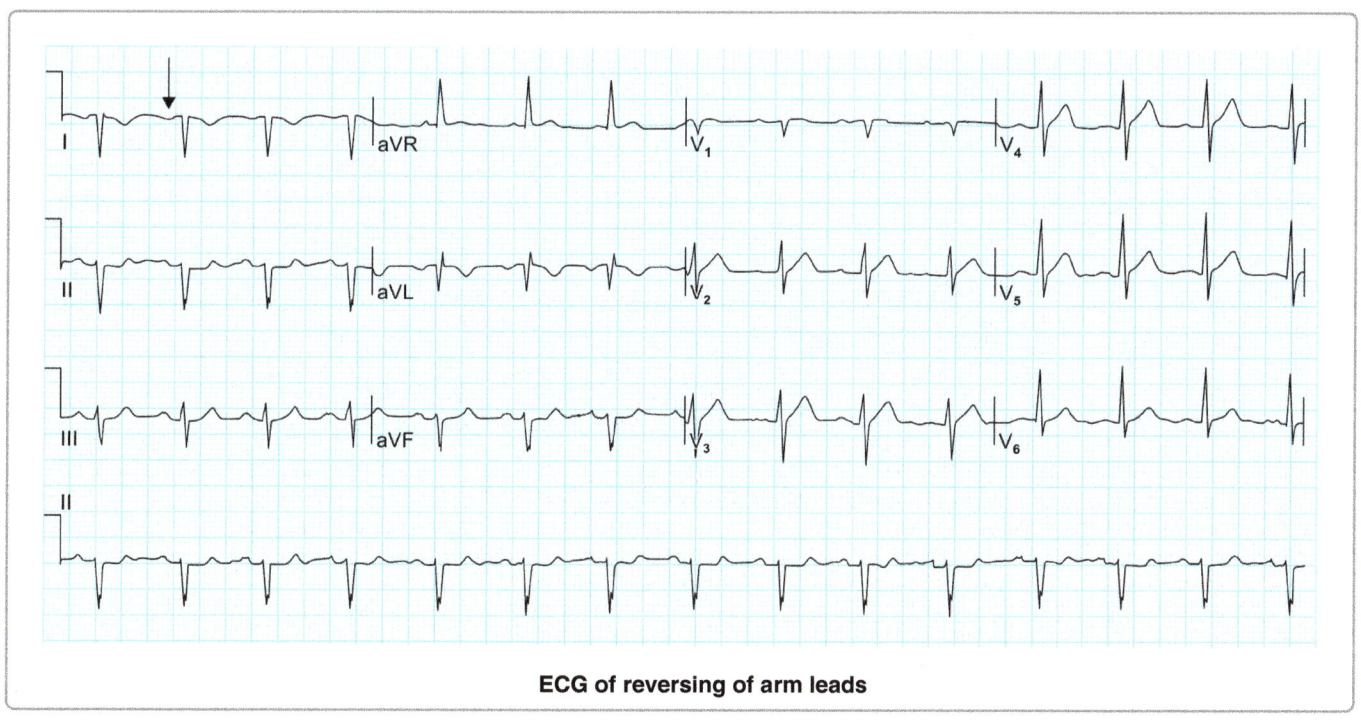

ECG of reversing of arm leads

INTERVALS IN ELECTROCARDIOGRAM

In any ECG, there are different waves and intervals described as follows:
- *PR interval*: It is the distance between the beginning of P to beginning of QRS (or Q). Ideally, it is called PQ interval.
- *PP interval*: It is the distance between two successive P waves. In sinus rhythm, P-P interval is regular.
- *RR interval*: It is the distance between two successive R waves. In sinus rhythm, R-R interval is regular.
- *QT interval*: It is the distance between the beginning of Q wave and the end of T wave.

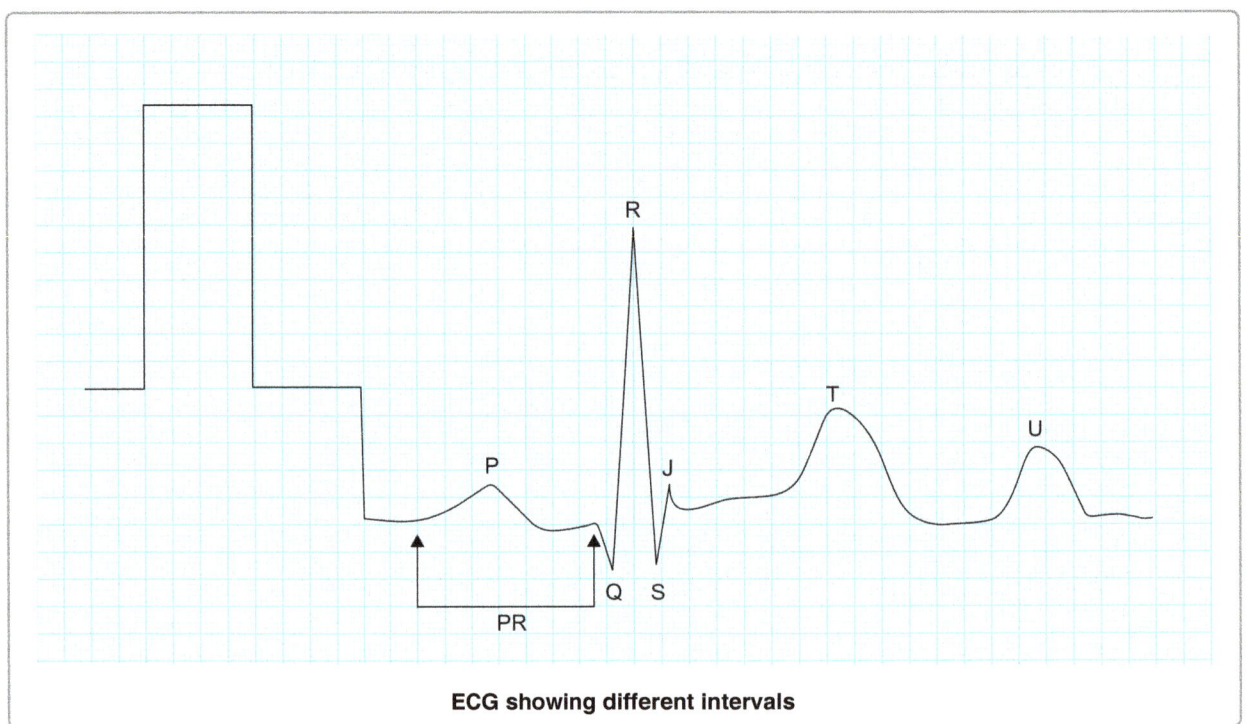

ECG showing different intervals

Segment in ECG

The portion of the baseline is called the isoelectric line.
- *ST segment*: It is the distance from the end of QRS complex to the beginning of T wave. It indicates the beginning of ventricular repolarization. Normally, it is in isoelectric line, but may vary from –0.5 to +2 mm in chest leads.
- *PR segment*: It is the distance between the termination of P wave and the onset of QRS complex. Normally, it is at the isoelectric line.

NB: Remember the following points:
- Ventricles contain majority of the heart muscles (left ventricle contains more than the right). So, QRS complex is larger than P wave.
- Atrial repolarization is small and is buried in QRS complex. So, it is not seen in ECG (no wave is seen due to atrial repolarization in ECG).

Chapter 1: Basic Concepts of ECG

BRIEF DISCUSSION OF WAVES AND INTERVALS IN ELECTROCARDIOGRAM

P Wave

Characters of Normal P Wave

- P wave results from spread of electrical activity through the atria.
- *Width or duration (in time, horizontally)*: 0.10 second (2.5 small squares).
- *Height*: 2.5 mm (2.5 small squares). Height × Duration = 2.5 × 2.5 small squares.
- P wave is better seen in L_{II}, as atrial depolarization is toward L_{II} (also seen in V_1), because the impulse spreads from the right atrium to the left atrium.
- P wave is upright in all leads, mainly L_I, L_{II}, and aVF (except aVR). P is inverted in aVR and occasionally in aVL.
- *P wave in V_1 may be biphasic*: Equal upward and downward deflection, notched, and wide. Activation of the right atrium produces positive component and activation of the left atrium produces negative component.
- Normal P is rounded, neither peaked nor notched.

Abnormalities of P Wave

P wave may be:
- Absent, or fibrillary or saw-toothed
- Tall or small
- Wide, notched, and biphasic
- Inverted
- Variable and multiple

Causes of absent P wave:
- Atrial fibrillation (P is absent or replaced by fibrillary *f* wave)
- Atrial flutter (P is replaced by flutter wave, which shows saw-tooth appearance)
- SA block or sinus arrest
- Nodal rhythm (usually absent in mid nodal)
- Ventricular ectopic and ventricular tachycardia
- Supraventricular tachycardia (SVT) (P is hidden within QRS, due to tachycardia)
- Hyperkalemia (may be small or absent)
- Idioventricular rhythm

Causes of tall P wave:
- Tall P is called P pulmonale (height >2.5 mm, i.e., >2.5 small squares).
- It is due to right atrial hypertrophy or enlargement [due to cor pulmonale and chronic obstructive pulmonary disease (COPD)].

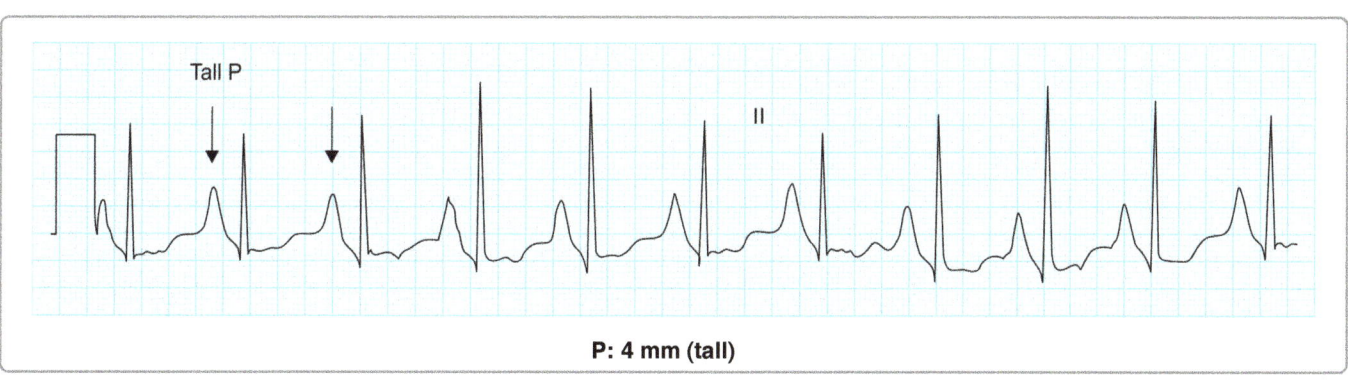

P: 4 mm (tall)

Causes of small P wave:
- Atrial tachycardia
- Atrial ectopic
- Nodal rhythm (high nodal)
- Nodal ectopic (high nodal)
- Hyperkalemia

Causes of wide P wave:
- It is broad and notched P is called P mitrale (duration >0.11 second, or >2.5 small squares). It is found in mitral stenosis.
- It is due to left atrial hypertrophy or enlargement.
- In V_1, P wave may be biphasic with a small positive wave preceding a deep and broad negative wave (indicates left atrial enlargement or hypertrophy).

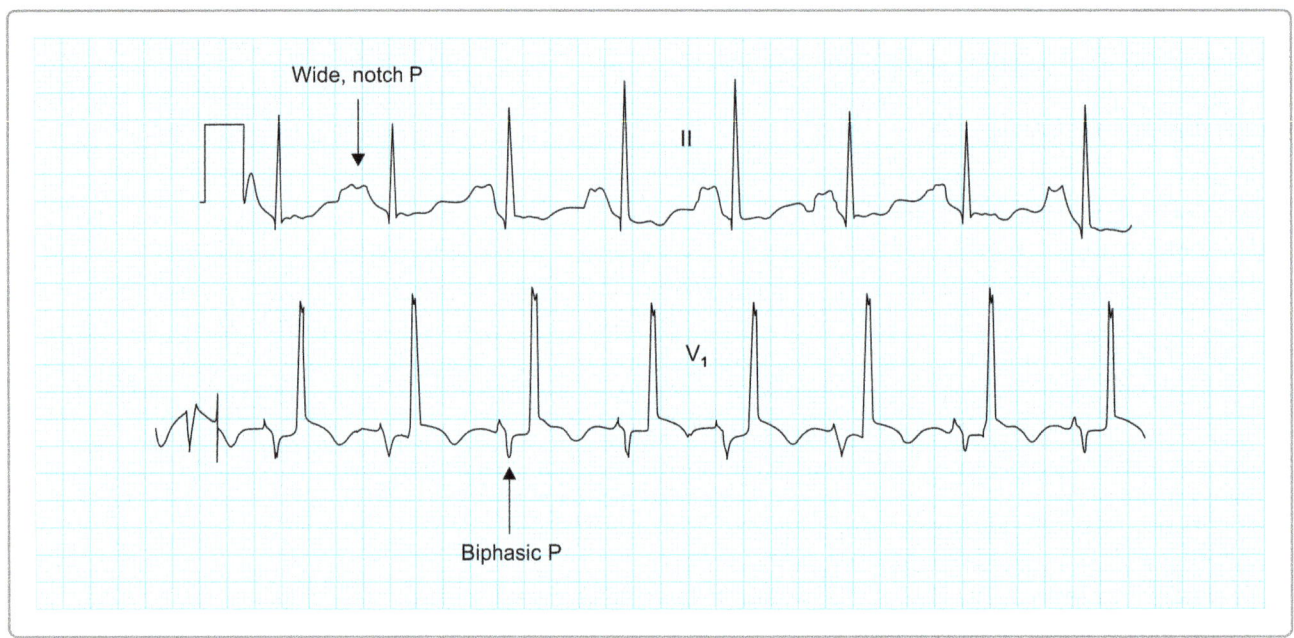

Causes of inverted P wave (negative in L_I, L_{II}, and aVF):
- Incorrectly placed leads (reversed arm electrodes)
- Dextrocardia
- Nodal rhythm with retrograde conduction
- Low atrial and high nodal ectopic beats

Causes of variable P wave:
- Presence of variable P waves indicates wandering pacemaker (P may be inverted, some small, and some upright).

Causes of multiple P waves (consecutive two or more):
- AV block (either partial or complete heart block)
- SVT with AV block

P-R Interval

Characters of Normal P-R Interval

- It is the distance between the onset of P wave to the beginning of Q wave (if Q wave is absent, then measure up to the onset of R wave).
- It is the time required for the impulse to travel from the SA node to the ventricular muscle. The impulse is transmitted to the ventricle via the AV node.
- P-R interval varies with age and heart rate.
- P-R interval is short, if the heart rate is increased, and long, if the heart rate is decreased.
- Normal PR interval—0.12–0.20 second (maximum five small squares):
  - In children, upper limit is 0.16 second.
  - In adolescent, upper limit is 0.18 second.
  - In adult, upper limit is 0.20 second.
- P-R is short, if it is <0.10 second and long, if it is >0.20 second.

Abnormalities of P-R Interval

PR interval may be:
- Prolonged
- Short
- Variable

Prolonged P-R interval (>0.2 second)
It is due to first degree heart block. Causes are as follows:
- Ischemic heart disease (occasionally, inferior myocardial infarction)
- Acute rheumatic carditis
- Myocarditis (due to any cause)
- Atrial dilatation or hypertrophy
- Hypokalemia
- Hypomagnesemia
- Drugs—digitalis toxicity, quinidine, occasionally β-blocker, and calcium channel blocker (e.g., verapamil)

Short P-R interval (<0.12 second)
Causes are as follows:
- Normal variant
- Wolff-Parkinson-White (WPW) syndrome. In this case, there is delta wave.
- Lown-Ganong-Levine (LGL) syndrome. In this case, there is no delta wave.
- Nodal rhythm
- Nodal ectopic (high nodal)
- Occasionally, if dissociated beat is present and also in infant, steroid therapy

Variable P-R interval
Causes are as follows:
- *Wenckebach phenomenon (Mobitz type I)*: In such case, there is progressive lengthening of P-R interval followed by a drop beat.
- *Partial heart block (Mobitz type II)*: P-R interval is fixed and normal, but sometimes P is not followed by QRS.
- *2:1 AV block*: In which, alternate P wave is not followed by QRS.
- *Complete AV block*: There is no relation between P and QRS.
- *Wandering pacemaker*: There is variable configuration of P.

QRS Complex

Characters of Normal QRS Complex

- QRS complex represents the depolarization of ventricular muscles.
- It consist of three waves: Q, R, and S.
- First downward deflection is called Q wave.
- Upward deflection after Q is R wave.
- Downward deflection after R is S wave.
- Depolarization of the left ventricle contributes to main QRS (as the mass of the left ventricle is two to three times more than the mass of right ventricle).
- QRS is predominantly positive in leads that look at the heart from the left side—L_1, aVL, V_5, and V_6.
- It is negative in leads that look at the heart from the right side—aVR, V_1, and V_2.
- In V_1, S is greater than R.
- In V_5 and V_6, R is tall.
- QRS appears biphasic (part above and part below the base line) in V_3 and V_4.
- Normal duration of QRS is 0.08–0.11 second (<3 small squares) and height <25 mm.

Various Forms and Components of QRS Complex

- *Q wave*: Initial downward deflection.
- *R wave*: Initial upward deflection.
- *S wave*: Downward deflection after R wave.
- *rS complex*: Small initial r wave, followed by large S wave.
- *RS complex*: A complex with R and S waves of equal amplitude.
- *Rs complex*: A large R wave followed by a small s wave.
- *qRS complex*: Small initial downward deflection, followed by a tall R, which is followed by a large S.
- *Qr complex*: Large Q, followed by a small r.
- *QS complex*: Complex with complete negative deflection (no separate Q and S).
- *rSr complex*: Small r, then deep S, followed by small r.
- *RSR complex*: Tall R, then deep S, followed by tall R.
- *RR complex*: When deflection is completely positive and notched (M pattern).

Abnormalities of QRS Complex

QRS may be:
- High voltage
- Low voltage
- Wide
- Change in shape
- Variable

Causes of high-voltage QRS

- Incorrect calibration
- Thin chest wall
- Ventricular hypertrophy (right or left or both)
- WPW syndrome
- True posterior myocardial infarction (in V_1 and V_2)

Chapter 1: Basic Concepts of ECG

Causes of low-voltage QRS (<5 mm in L_I, L_{II}, L_{III}, and <10 mm in chest leads)
- Incorrect calibration
- Thick chest wall or obesity
- Hypothyroidism
- Pericardial effusion
- Emphysema
- Chronic constrictive pericarditis
- Hypothermia

Causes of wide QRS (>0.12 second, three small squares)
If it is >0.12 second, it is called wide QRS.
- Bundle branch block [left bundle branch block (LBBB) or right bundle branch block (RBBB)]
- Ventricular ectopics
- Ventricular tachycardia
- Idioventricular rhythm
- Ventricular hypertrophy
- Hyperkalemia
- WPW syndrome
- Pacemaker (looks like LBBB with spike)
- Drugs (quinidine, procainamide, phenothiazine, and tricyclic antidepressants)

Causes of changes in shape of QRS
- Right or left bundle branch block (slurred or M pattern)
- Ventricular tachycardia
- Ventricular fibrillation
- Hyperkalemia
- WPW syndrome

Causes of variable QRS
- Multifocal ventricular ectopics
- Torsades de pointes
- Ventricular fibrillation

Alternative QRS voltage (alternate large and small QRS complex)
Normally, voltage of all QRS complex is same. But, if the voltage of QRS complex alternates between high and low in successive beats, it is called electrical alternans. Causes are as follows:
- Moderate-to-severe pericardial effusion (due to malignant, tubercular, or postsurgical). It may indicate cardiac tamponade or impending tamponade.
- Organic heart disease such as ischemic cardiomyopathy and diffuse myocarditis.

NB: Electrical alternans of QRS may be clinically associated with cardiomegaly, gallop rhythm, and signs of left ventricular failure.

Q Wave

Characters of Normal Q Wave

- Q wave is usually absent in most of the leads. However, small q wave may be present in I, II, aVL, V_5, and V_6. This is due to septal depolarization.
- Small q may be present in L_{III} (which disappears with inspiration).
- Depth—<2 mm (two small squares).
- Width—one small square.
- It is 25% or less in amplitude of the following R wave in the same lead (one-fourth of the R wave).

Characters of Pathological Q Wave

- Deep >2 mm (two small squares)
- Wide >0.04 second or more (>1 mm or one small square)
- Should be present in more than one lead (if present in one lead, it is not pathological).
- Associated with loss of height of R wave.
- Q wave should be >25% of the following R wave of the same lead.

Causes of Pathological Q Wave

- Myocardial infarction (the most common cause)
- Ventricular hypertrophy (left or right)
- Cardiomyopathy
- LBBB
- Emphysema (due to axis change or cardiac rotation)
- Q only in L_{III} is associated with pulmonary embolism (S_I, Q_{III}, and T_{III} pattern).

NB: Remember the following points:

- Q wave in V_1, V_2, and V_3 may be seen in left ventricular hypertrophy (LVH) and may be mistaken as old myocardial infarction.
- Abnormal Q wave in L_{III} may be found in pulmonary embolism.
- Abnormal Q wave in L_{III} and aVF may be found in WPW syndrome (confuses with old inferior myocardial infarction).

R Wave

Characters of Normal R Wave

- It is the first positive (upward) deflection, due to ventricular depolarization.
- Duration <0.01 second.
- R wave usually small (<1 mm) in V_1 and V_2. It increases progressively in height in V_3 to V_6 (tall in V_5 and V_6), i.e., R is small in V_1 and V_2, tall in V_5 and V_6.

Normal Height of R Wave

- In aVL <13 mm
- In aVF <20 mm
- In V_5 and V_6 <25 mm
  (If R wave is >25 mm, it is always pathological).

Abnormalities of R Wave

R wave may be:
- Tall
- Small
- Poor progression

Causes of tall R wave
- Left ventricular hypertrophy (in V_5 or V_6 >25 mm, aVL >13 mm, aVF >20 mm).
- In V_1, tall R may be due to:
  - Normal variant
  - Right ventricular hypertrophy (RVH)
  - True posterior myocardial infarction
  - WPW syndrome (type A)
  - Right bundle branch block
  - Dextrocardia

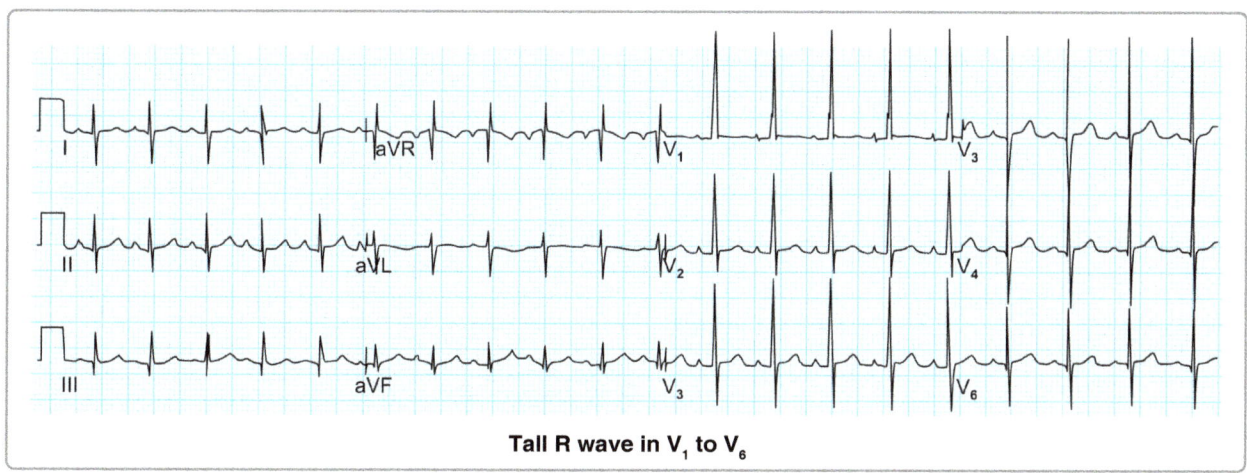

Tall R wave in V_1 to V_6

Causes of small R wave

Looks like low-voltage tracing.
- Incorrect ECG calibration (standardization)
- Obesity
- Emphysema
- Pericardial effusion
- Hypothyroidism
- Hypothermia

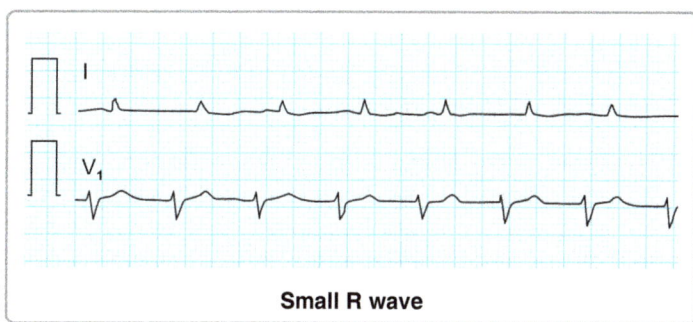

Small R wave

R wave progression

The height of R wave gradually increases from V_1 to V_6. This phenomenon is called R wave progression.

Poor progression of R wave:
Normally, amplitude of R wave is tall in V_5 and V_6. In poor R wave progression, amplitude of R wave is progressively reduced in V_5 and V_6. Causes are as follows:
- Anterior or anteroseptal myocardial infarction
- Left bundle branch block
- Left ventricular hypertrophy (though R is tall in most cases)
- Dextrocardia
- Cardiomyopathy
- COPD
- Left-sided pneumothorax
- Left-sided pleural effusion (massive)
- Marked clockwise rotation
- Chest electrodes placed incorrectly
- Deformity of the chest wall
- Normal variation

ECG in Medical Practice

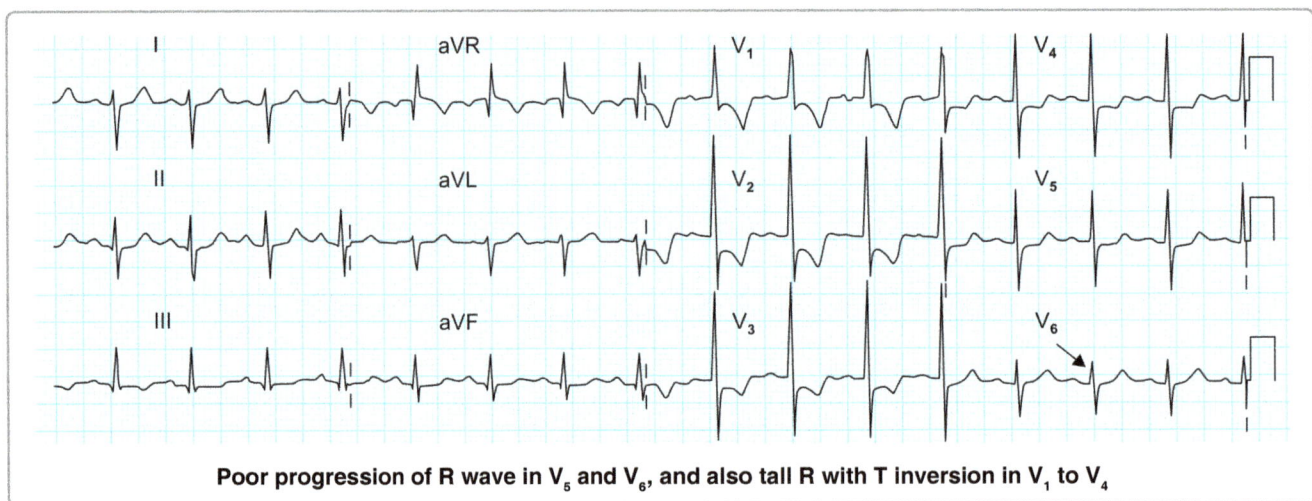

Poor progression of R wave in V₅ and V₆, and also tall R with T inversion in V₁ to V₄

S Wave

Characters of Normal S Wave

- It is the negative deflection after R wave (normally one-third of R wave).
- Normally, deep in V_1 and V_2, as the impulse is going to the muscles of the left ventricle and then to the right ventricle.
- It is progressively diminished from V_1 to V_6 (small S wave may be present in V_5 and V_6).
- In V_3, R and S waves are almost equal (corresponds with interventricular septum).

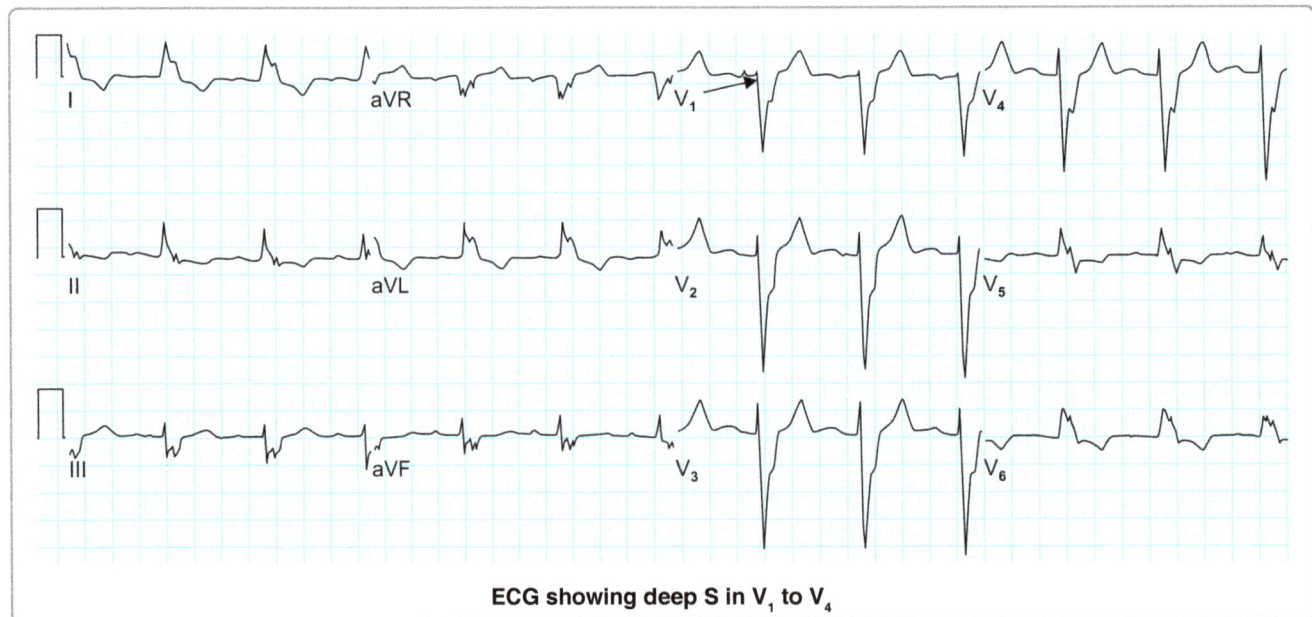

ECG showing deep S in V₁ to V₄

ST Segment

Characters of Normal ST Segment

- Measured from the end of S to the beginning of T wave. It represents beginning of ventricular repolarization.
- Normally, it is in isoelectric line (lies at same level of ECG baseline).
- ST elevation is normal up to 1 mm in limb leads and 2 mm in chest leads (mainly V_1 to V_3).
- In Negroes, ST elevation of 4 mm may be normal, which disappears on exercise.
- Normally, ST segment may be depressed, <1 mm.

Abnormalities of ST Segment

ST segment may be:
- Elevated
- Depressed

Causes of ST elevation (>2 mm)
- Acute myocardial infarction (ST elevation with convexity upward)
- Acute pericarditis (ST elevation with concavity upward, chair-shaped or saddle-shaped)
- Prinzmetal's angina, also called vasospasm angina (ST elevation with tall T).
- Ventricular aneurysm (persistent ST elevation)
- Early repolarization (high take-off)
- Normal variant in Africans and Asians.
- May be in hyperkalemia.

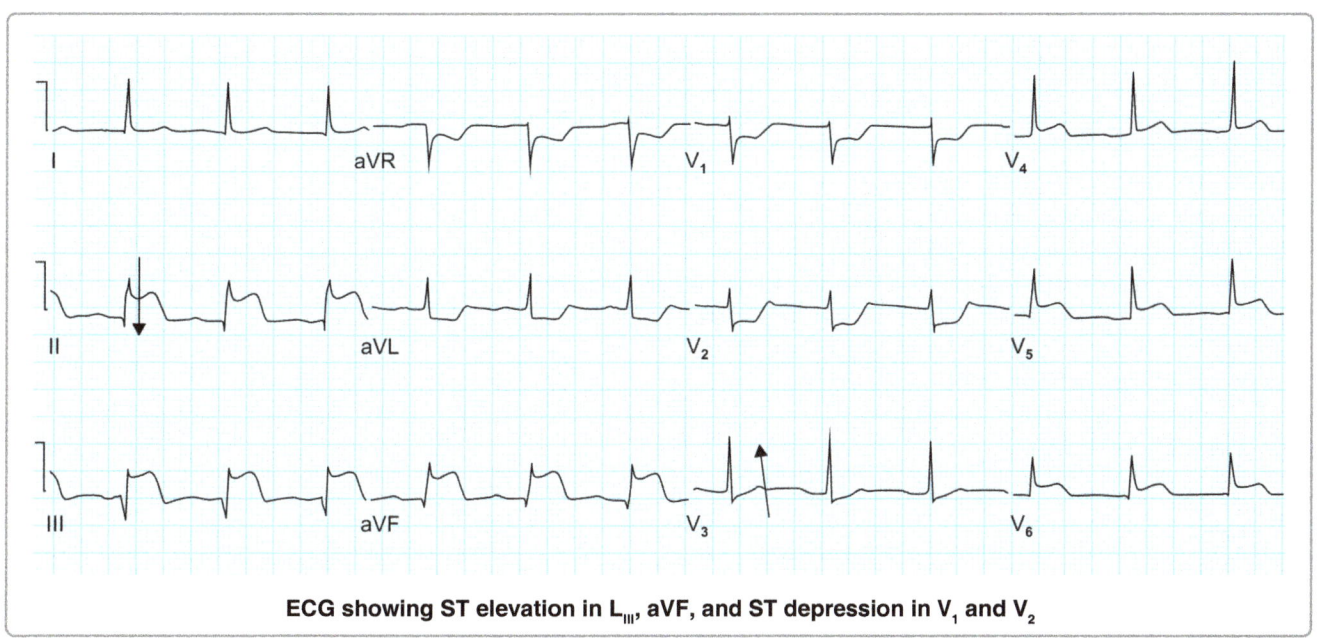

ECG showing ST elevation in L_{III}, aVF, and ST depression in V_1 and V_2

Causes of ST depression (below the isoelectric line)
- Acute myocardial ischemia (horizontal or down slope ST depression with sharp angle ST-T junction)
- Ventricular hypertrophy with strain (ST depression with convexity upward and asymmetric T inversion).
- Digoxin toxicity (sagging of ST depression—like thumb impression, also called reverse tick).
- Acute true posterior myocardial infarction (in V_1 and V_2), associated with dominant R and tall upright T wave.
- Reciprocal change in STEMI (ST-elevation myocardial infarction).

Early repolarization (high take-off)
- It is a benign, normal finding in young healthy person, more in black males.
- It is seen in chest leads, commonly V_4 to V_6 (rarely, in other chest lead).
- ST elevation is usually associated with J point elevation.
- It is not associated with inversion of T wave or abnormal Q wave.

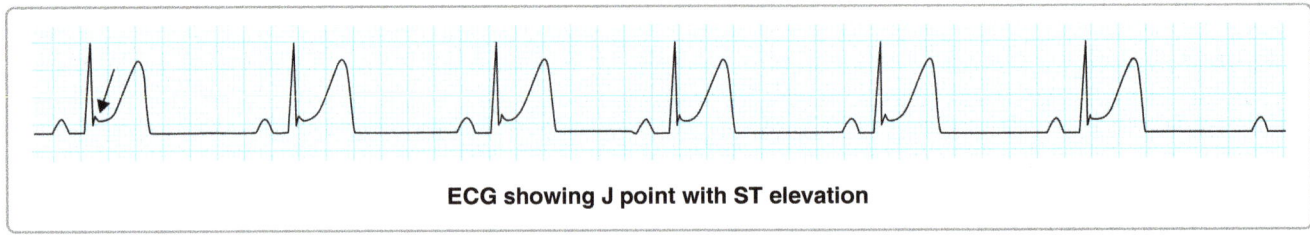

ECG showing J point with ST elevation

NB: Remember the following points:
- Early repolarization syndrome confuses with acute myocardial infarction and acute pericarditis.
- To differentiate from these, detail history, serial ECG tracing (that shows no change), and comparison with old ECG are helpful.

T Wave

Characters of Normal T Wave

- It indicates ventricular repolarization.
- It follows S wave and ST segment.
- It is upright in all leads, except aVR.
- Usually, it is >2 mm in height. It may be normally inverted in V_1 and V_2.
- Normally, it is not >5 mm in standard leads and 10 mm in chest leads.
- It is minimum one-fourth of R wave of the same lead.
- The tip of T is smooth (rounded).

Abnormalities of T Wave

T wave may be:
- Inverted
- Tall peaked and tented
- Small
- Biphasic

Causes of T inversion
- Myocardial ischemia and infarction
- Subendocardial myocardial infarction (non-Q wave myocardial infarction)
- Ventricular ectopics
- Ventricular hypertrophy with strain

- Acute pericarditis
- Cardiomyopathy
- Myxedema
- Bundle branch block
- Drugs (digoxin and phenothiazine)
- *Physiological*: Nonspecific (smoking, anxiety, anorexia, exercise, after heavy meal, or glucose)

Causes of tall peaked T wave
- Hyperkalemia (tall, tented, or peaked)
- Hyperacute myocardial infarction (tall T wave)
- Acute true posterior myocardial infarction (tall T in V_1 to V_2)
- Prinzmetal's angina
- It may be normal in some Africans and Asians.

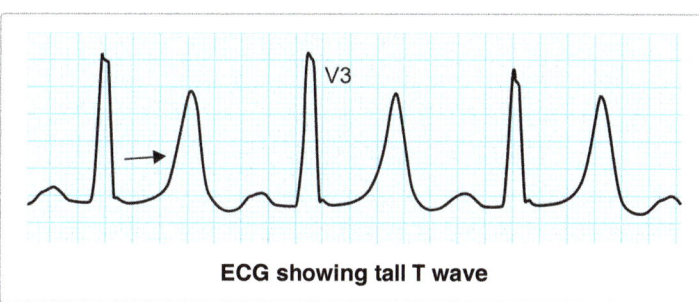

ECG showing tall T wave

Ques. How to differentiate between tall T due to hyperkalemia from hyperacute myocardial infarction?
Ans. As follows:
- *In hyperkalemia*: T is tall, tented, narrow-based, and symmetrically peaked. QT interval is short.
- *In hyperacute myocardial infarction*: T is broad, not tented, and asymmetrical. QT interval is prolonged.

Ques. What is the other causes of tall, peaked T?
Ans. Prinzmetal's angina (also called vasospasm angina).

Ques. How to differentiate between hyperacute myocardial infarction and Prinzmetal's angina?
Ans. Tall-peaked T wave may also be found in Prinzmetal's angina, confused with hyperacute myocardial infarction. To differentiate it from myocardial infarction, in Prinzmetal's angina, serial ECG shows fall down of T wave, Q wave never appears and enzymes are not raised.

Causes of small T wave:
- Hypokalemia
- Hypothyroidism
- Pericardial effusion

Biphasic T wave:
It means part of T is above isoelectric line and part below the isoelectric line. Causes are as follows:
- Myocardial ischemia
- Hypokalemia

To differentiate between these two, morphology of T is as follows:
- *In myocardial ischemia*: T wave goes up and then down (**Fig. A**).
- *In hypokalemia*: T wave goes down then up (**Fig. B**).

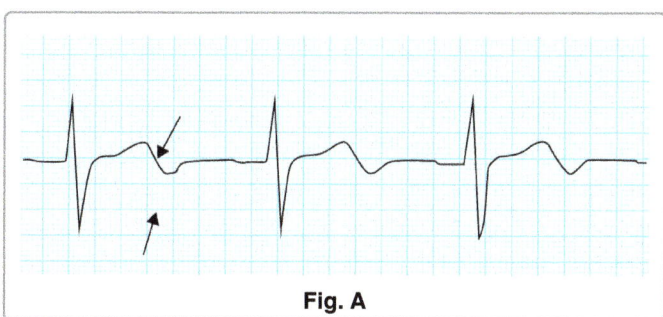

Fig. A

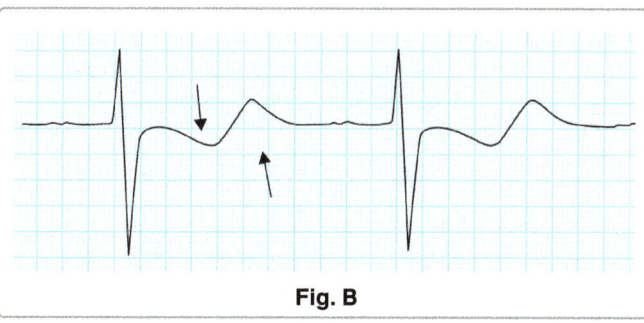

Fig. B

Ques. What is juvenile T wave pattern?

Ans. It is a disorder in which T is inverted in V_1 to V_3 (rarely V_4 to V_6). T inversion is neither symmetrical nor deep. It is common in children and young adults, more in female <40 years. Frequently, it is associated with sinus arrhythmia and high left ventricular voltage.

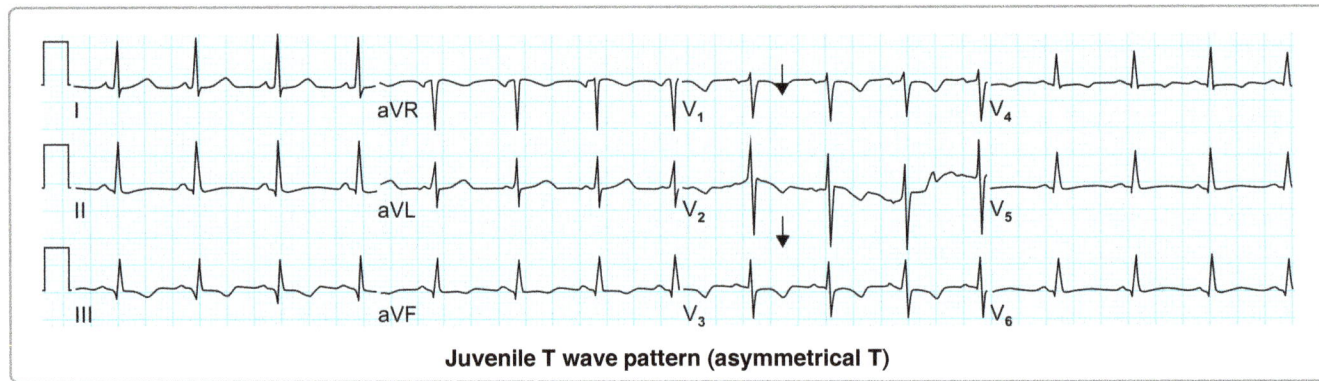

Juvenile T wave pattern (asymmetrical T)

Camel hump T waves:
Camel hump T waves have a double peak. Causes are as follows:
- Prominent U waves fused to the end of the T wave (as seen in severe hypokalemia).
- Hidden P waves embedded in the T wave, as seen in sinus tachycardia and various types of heart block.

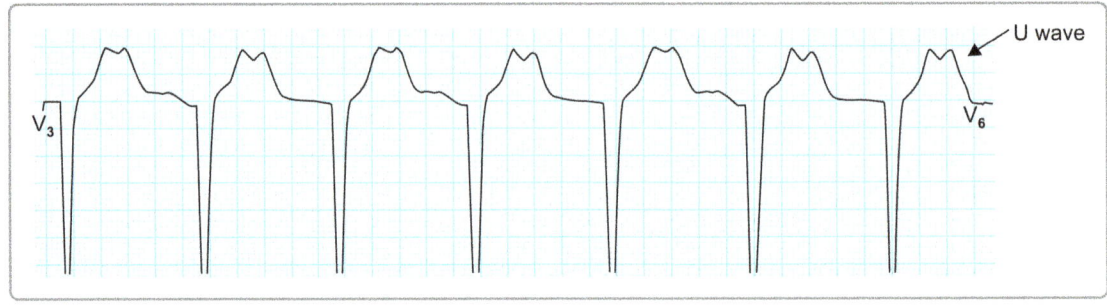

Flattened T waves:
Flattened T waves are usually considered as a nonspecific finding. However, flattened T wave may be due to the following causes:
- Ischemia
- Hypocalcemia

See the ECG on the next page.

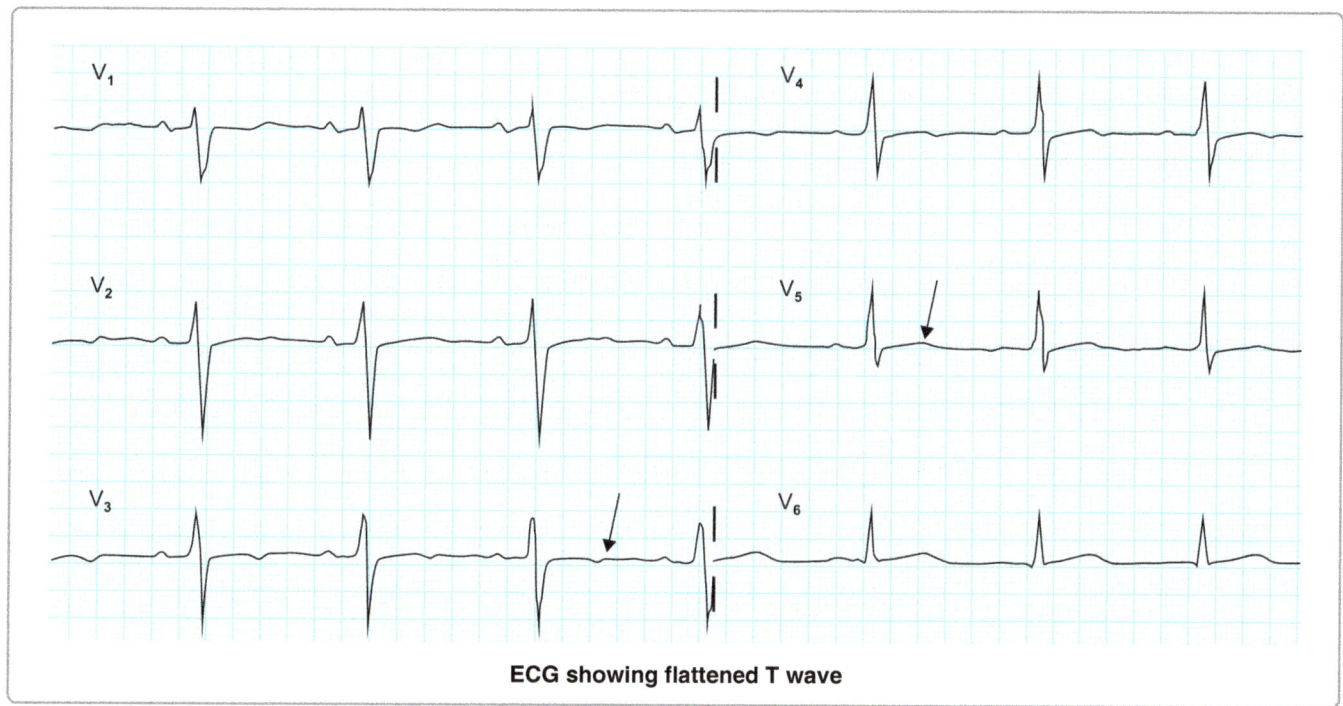

ECG showing flattened T wave

U Wave

Characters of Normal U Wave

- U wave is seen after T wave.
- It may be present in normal ECG, usually smaller and in the same direction of the preceding T wave.
- It represents slow repolarization of interventricular Purkinje fibers and also papillary muscles (but actual genesis of U wave is still controversial).
- Better seen in chest leads (V_2 to V_4).
- Normal amplitude is 1 mm (2 mm in athlete).
- U wave is easily visible when QT interval is short and heart rate is slow.

Abnormalities of U Wave

U wave may be:
- Inverted
- Prominent

Causes of inverted U wave
- Ischemic heart disease
- Left ventricular hypertrophy with strain (hypertensive heart disease).

Causes of prominent U wave
- May be normally present in young athlete (usually small).
- Hypokalemia (the most common)
- Bradycardia
- Ventricular hypertrophy
- Hyperthyroidism

- Hypercalcemia
- Drugs (phenothiazine, quinidine, and digoxin)
- Congenital long QT syndrome

Ques. What is the significance of large U wave?
Ans. The patient is prone to develop torsades de pointes tachycardia.

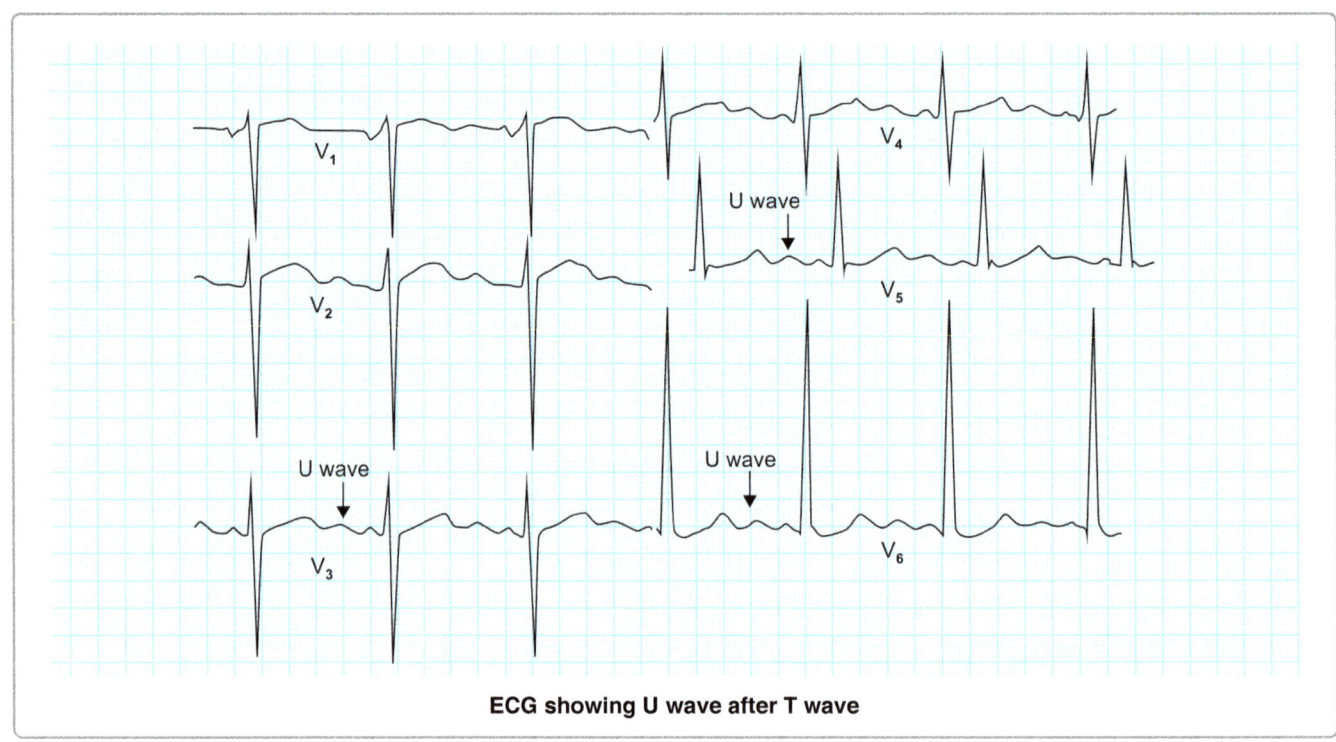

ECG showing U wave after T wave

QT Interval

Characters of Normal QT Interval

- It is the distance from the beginning of Q wave (or R wave, if there is no Q wave) to the end of T wave.
- It represents the total time required for both depolarization and repolarization of the ventricles.
- Normal QT interval is 0.35–0.43 seconds. It is better seen in aVL (because there is no U wave).
- Its duration varies with heart rate, becoming shorter as the heart rate increases and longer as the heart rate decreases. In general, QT interval at heart rate between 60 and 90/min does not exceed in duration, half the preceding RR interval.
- Corrected formula for real QT is:

$$QTc = \frac{QT}{\sqrt{RR}}$$

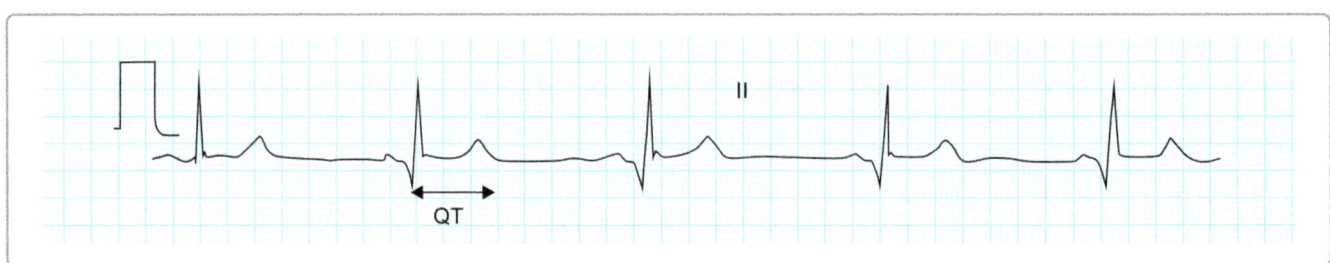

Abnormalities of QT Interval

QT interval may be:
- Short
- Long

Causes of short QT interval
- Digoxin effect
- Hypercalcemia
- Hyperthermia
- Tachycardia
- Hyperkalemia
- Acidosis

Causes of long QT interval
- Hypocalcemia
- Hypokalemia
- Hypomagnesemia
- Bradycardia
- Acute myocarditis
- Acute myocardial infarction
- Hypothermia
- Drug (quinidine, procainamide, flecainide, amiodarone, tricyclic antidepressant, disopyramide, and pentamidine)
- Cerebral injury (head injury and intracerebral hemorrhage)
- Hypertrophic cardiomyopathy
- During sleep
- Congenital long QT syndrome
- *Hereditary syndrome*:
    - Jervell and Lange-Nielsen syndrome (congenital deafness, syncope and sudden death)
    - Romano–Ward syndrome (same as above except deafness)

Ques. What are the clinical importance of prolongation of QT interval?

Ans. Prolonged QT interval may be detected in an asymptomatic individual. It may be associated with ventricular arrhythmia. Rarely, it can cause torsades de pointes tachycardia and sudden death.

ECG in Medical Practice

RHYTHM OF HEART

To see the rhythm—successive RR interval should be seen.
- If the RR interval is equal, it is called regular rhythm.
- If the RR interval is irregular, then it is called irregular rhythm.

NB: Remember the following points:
- Irregularity of heart rhythm indicates arrhythmia or heart block.
- To see any rhythm disturbance, preferably long rhythm strip (L_{II}) should be taken.
- When strong suspicion of arrhythmia, ambulatory ECG (Holter monitor ECG) should be taken.

Causes of Irregular Rhythm

- *Physiological*: Usually found in sinus arrhythmia
- *Pathological*:
  - Atrial fibrillation
  - Atrial flutter
  - SA block or sinus arrest
  - Atrial tachycardia with block
  - Second-degree heart block
  - Ventricular fibrillation

Ques. What are the causes of regularly irregular rhythm?
Ans. Causes of regularly irregular rhythm are:
- *Physiological*: Common in sinus arrhythmia
- *Pathological*: Ectopic beat, second-degree heart block (e.g., 2:1 or 3:1 block), SA block or sinus arrest

Ques. What are the causes of irregularly irregular rhythm?
Ans. Causes of irregularly irregular rhythm are:
- Atrial fibrillation
- Atrial flutter
- Multiple ectopics
- Atrial tachycardia with block
- Ventricular fibrillation

Characters of Sinus Rhythm

Sinus rhythm shows the following five characters:
- P wave is of sinus origin (means characters of normal P wave).
- P waves and QRS complexes are regular (that means P-P and R-R interval should be constant and identical).
- Constant P wave configuration in a given lead.
- P-R interval and QRS interval should be within normal limit.
- Rate should be between 60 beats/min and 100 beats/min (atrial and ventricular rates are identical).

NB: Remember the following points:
- Sinus rhythm means that impulse is arising from SA node.
- PP interval (atrial) and RR interval (ventricular) are equal in sinus rhythm, but varies if the rhythm is irregular.
- To see rhythm, look RR interval.
- Always count atrial and ventricular rate separately (especially important in complete heart block).

Ques. What is arrhythmia?
Ans. It is the abnormality in initiation or propagation of cardiac impulse.

CALCULATION OF HEART RATE

In any ECG, heart rate should be calculated. Methods vary according to the cardiac rhythm, whether regular or irregular. Standard speed in ECG paper is 25 mm/s. Heart rate is the number of beats per minute. It is calculated by looking at the ECG tracing in the following way:

In the ECG paper:
- 0.04 second = 1 small square
- 0.2 second = 5 small squares or 1 large square
- So, 1 second = 25 small squares or 5 large squares
- So, 1 minute = 25 × 60 = 1,500 small squares or 5 × 60 = 300 large squares

Heart rate is determined in the following way:
1. *When the cardiac rhythm is regular*:
   - Calculate R-R or P-P interval in small squares or large squares (if rhythm is sinus, R-R or P-P interval is same).
   - If small square is calculated:

$$\text{Then the heart rate is} = \frac{1500}{\text{Small squares between R} - \text{R or P} - \text{P}}$$

   - If large square is calculated:

$$\text{Then the heart rate is} = \frac{300}{\text{Large squares between R} - \text{R or P} - \text{P}}$$

Examples:
- Suppose, the number of small squares between R-R and P-P is 15.

$$\text{So the heart rate is } \frac{1500}{15} = 100 \text{ beats/min}$$

- Suppose, the number of large squares between R-R is 5.

$$\text{So the heart rate is } \frac{300}{5} = 60 \text{ beats/min}$$

2. *When the rhythm is irregular*:

In irregular rhythm, the above method is not valid. In such case, QRS complex is counted in 6 seconds (30 small square) in rhythm strip, multliplied by 10.

Proceed in the following way:
- Count the number of R in 30 large squares (it is equivalent to 6 seconds).
- Then, simply multiply this by 10 (it becomes rate in 1 minute).

Example:
- Suppose, the number of R in 30 large squares is 12.
- So, the heart rate is 12 × 10 = 120 beats/min.

NB: In ECG, PP interval indicates atrial rate and RR interval indicates ventricular rate. Normally, PP and RR intervals are same. But in some arrhythmia, atrial and ventricular rates are different. These should be counted separately. Examples are atrial fibrillation, atrial flutter, complete heart block, ventricular fibrillation, etc.

CARDIAC AXIS

Definition

It is the sum of all the depolarization waves as they spread through the ventricles as seen from the front. Axis is the direction of the ECG waveform in frontal plane measured in degrees. The axis of ECG is the major deflection of the overall electrical activity of the heart. It may be normal, LAD, right axis deviation (RAD), or indeterminate. QRS complex is the most important to determine the axis, usually limb leads are examined (not precordial leads).

Axis Determination

- Axis can be derived most easily from the amplitude of QRS complex in L_I, L_{II}, and aVF.
- The greatest amplitude of R wave in L_I or L_{II} or aVF indicates the proximity of cardiac axis to that lead.
- The axis lies at 90° to the isoelectric complex, i.e., positive and negative deflections are equal in any of the lead L_I, L_{II}, L_{III}, aVL, aVR, and aVF.

Normal axis is between –30° and +90°.

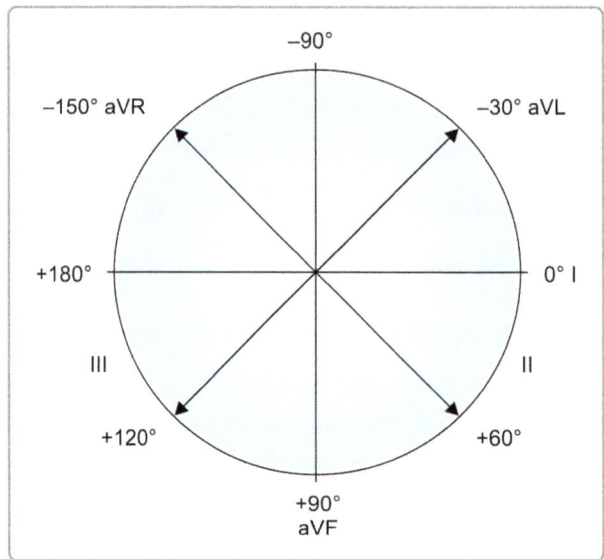

Type of axis deviation:
1. Left axis deviation
2. Right axis deviation
3. Indeterminate axis deviation

Chapter 1: Basic Concepts of ECG

Quick and Simple Way of Determination of Cardiac Axis

- Positive QRS in both L_I and aVF means axis is normal.
- Positive QRS in L_I and negative in aVF (tall R in L_I and deep S in aVF) means LAD. However, in such case, look at L_{II}. If negative in L_{II}, it is more likely to be LAD. But, if positive in L_{II}, axis may be normal.
- Negative QRS in L_I and positive in aVF (deep S in L_I and tall R in aVF) means RAD.
- If negative QRS in L_I and also aVF, the axis is indeterminate.

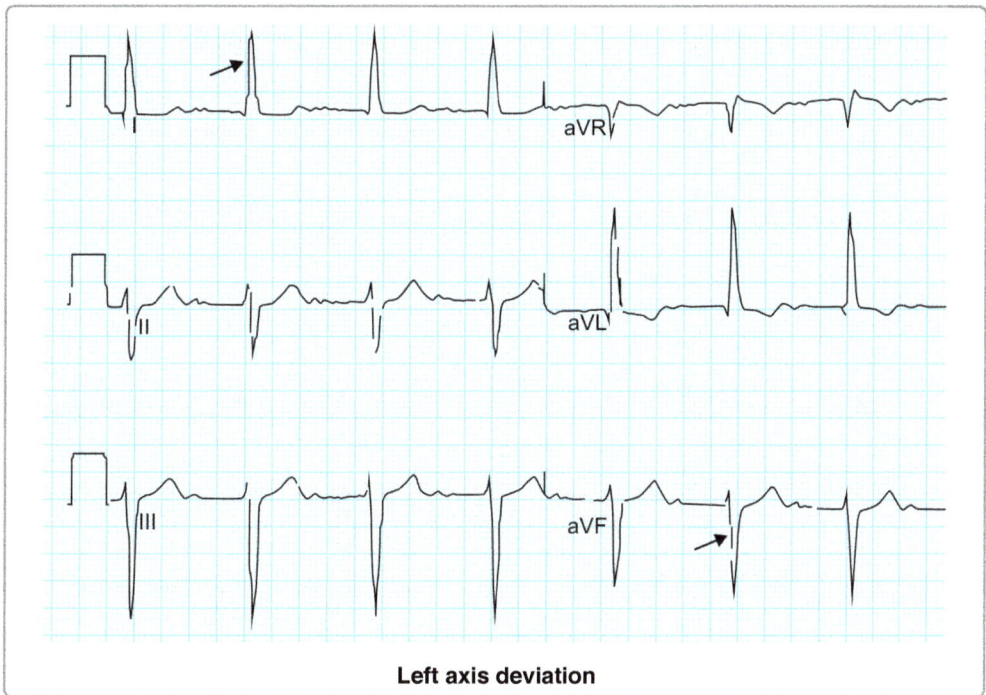

Left axis deviation

Left Axis Deviation

When the cardiac axis is between –30° and –90°. Causes are as follows:
- Normal variant (with increased age)
- Left ventricular hypertrophy
- Left anterior hemiblock
- Left bundle branch block
- Inferior myocardial infarction
- WPW syndrome (some)
- Ventricular ectopic
- Pacing from the apex of the right or left ventricle (endocardial pacing)

ECG in Medical Practice

Right Axis Deviation

When the cardiac axis is between +90° and +180°. Causes are as follows:
- Normal variant (common in children and young adult)
- RVH (due to any cause such as chronic cor pulmonale, pulmonary embolism, and congenital heart diseases, i.e., tetralogy of Fallot)
- Anterolateral myocardial infarction (high lateral myocardial infarction)
- Left posterior hemiblock
- Dextrocardia
- WPW syndrome (type A)
- Right bundle branch block
- Epicardial pacing
- Ventricular ectopic

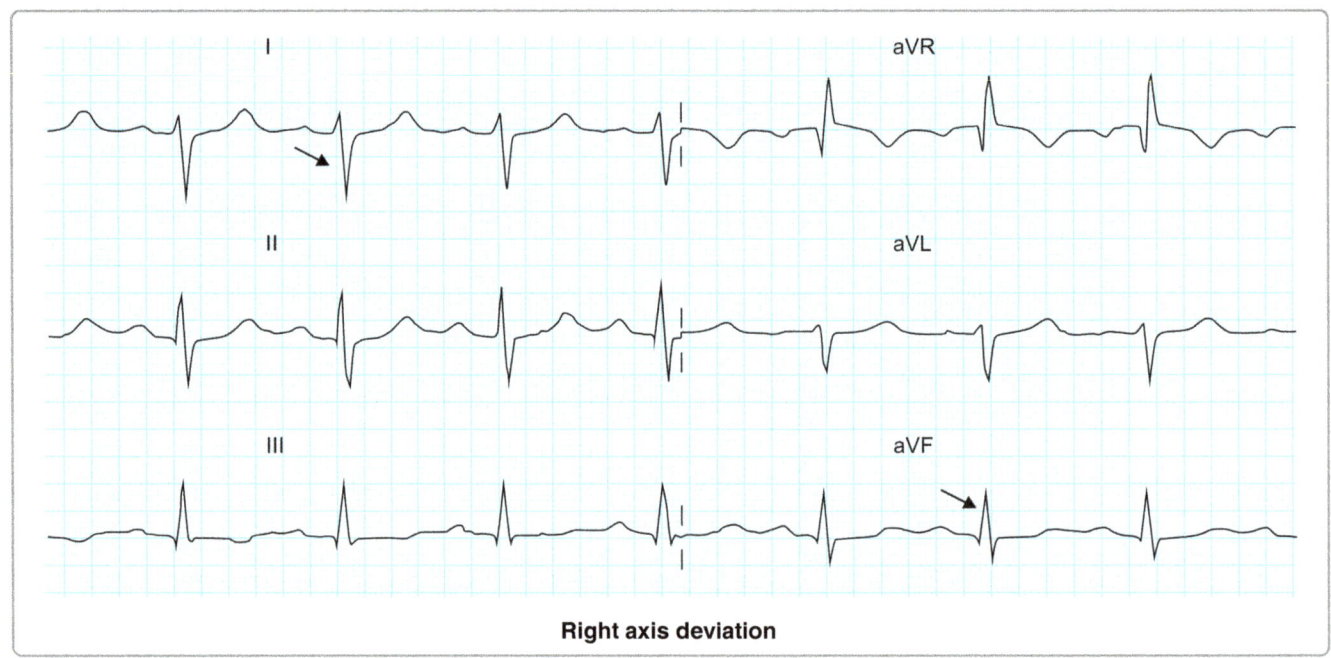

Right axis deviation

Indeterminate Axis

Occurs when QRS lies between +180° and −90°. This term is used when exact axis can not be determined (all six limb leads are biphasic). It may be found in:
- Severe right ventricular hypertrophy.
- Aneurysm of left ventricular apex.

NB: Remember the following points:
- Axis deviation may be used to diagnose fascicular block or hemiblock, as follows:
  - When there is left axis deviation, it is called left anterior hemiblock.
  - When there is right axis deviation, it is called left posterior hemiblock.
  - When associated with right bundle branch block, it is called bifascicular block.

Chapter 1: Basic Concepts of ECG

NORMAL VARIANTS IN ELECTROCARDIOGRAM

In an ECG, occasionally, there are certain findings detected, which are the normal variants, may be observed in healthy individuals. These are commonly found in young adults and children. Some examples are:
- Sinus arrhythmia
- Early repolarization syndrome (in young black males)
- Inverted P (in inferior leads)
- Short P-R interval
- QRS in V_1 (not >0.12 second) and RBBB pattern
- Q wave in L_{III} (disappears with deep inspiration)
- Tall R in V_1 (R/S ratio ≥1)
- T inversion in L_{III}, aVR, and V_1
- Left ventricular hypertrophy (in children and young adults)
- RAD (in children and young adults)
- Mild LAD or left anterior hemiblock, in the absence of cardiac disease
- Wandering pacemaker
- Low voltage in obese people
- First-degree heart block
- Wenckebach phenomenon
- Juvenile T wave pattern in children and young adults.

Careful interpretation is essential for the diagnosis. This should not be confused with underlying pathology. Detailed history and physical findings should be correlated with the ECG findings.

Ques. What are the possible ECG features of healthy athletes?

Ans. There may be change in normal rhythm and ECG pattern in healthy athletes, which are usually normal findings. The following may be the variations in rhythm and variations in ECG pattern.

1. *Variations in rhythm*:
   - Sinus bradycardia
   - Marked sinus arrhythmia
   - Junctional rhythm
   - Wandering atrial pacemaker
   - First-degree heart block
   - Second-degree heart block (Wenckebach phenomenon)
2. *Variations in ECG pattern*:
   - Tall P waves
   - Prominent septal Q waves
   - Tall R and deep S waves
   - Counterclockwise rotation
   - Slight ST segment elevation
   - Tall symmetrical T waves
   - T wave inversion, especially in lateral leads
   - Biphasic T waves
   - Prominent U waves

EXERCISE ELECTROCARDIOGRAM (EXERCISE TOLERANCE TEST OR ETT)

Exercise ECG is a technique used to assess the cardiac response during exercise. The 12-lead ECG is recorded, while the patient walks or runs on a motorized treadmill. The traditional Bruce protocol is followed. The limb leads are placed on the shoulders and hips, rather than on the wrists and ankles. Blood pressure is recorded, symptoms such as anginal pain are assessed, and ST depression or elevation is noted.

The test is positive, if there is:
- Anginal pain
- Blood pressure falls or fails to rise
- ST depression >1 mm (planar or downsloping depression is more important rather than upsloping ST depression which is nonspecific)
- ST elevation may occur, which indicates transmural ischemia due to coronary spasm or critical stenosis.

The patient who can perform exercise <6 minutes, generally have poor prognosis. Sustained fall of blood pressure indicates severe coronary artery disease.

Exercise tolerance test (ETT) may be false positive (20%), or false negative. It has a specificity of 80% and sensitivity of 70%.

Indications of Exercise Testing

- To confirm the diagnosis of ischemic heart disease
- To evaluate stable angina
- Selecting patient for coronary artery bypass grafting (CABG), percutaneous transluminal coronary angioplasty (PTCA), and cardiac catheterization
- To assess prognosis following myocardial infarction
- To assess outcome after coronary revascularization (coronary angioplasty)
- To diagnose and evaluate the treatment of exercise-induced arrhythmias

Contraindications of Exercise Testing

- Acute myocardial infarction within preceding 4–6 days
- In presence of unstable angina
- Decompensated heart failure
- Severe hypertension (systolic >220 mm Hg and diastolic >120 mm Hg)
- Acute myocarditis or pericarditis.
- Severe aortic stenosis
- Severe hypertrophic obstructive cardiomyopathy
- Untreated life-threatening arrhythmia
- Deep vein thrombosis
- Dissecting aortic aneurysm
- Any acute systemic illness

Causes of false positive exercise test:
- Digoxin toxicity
- Hypokalemia
- Ventricular hypertrophy
- Bundle branch block
- WPW syndrome
- Mitral valve prolapse
- Significant aortic or mitral valve insufficiency
- Significant aortic valve stenosis
- Female sex

False negative ETT may occur if the patient is on: β-blocker, verapamil, diltiazem, and nitrate group of drugs.

Reasons for stopping of ETT: During ETT, if any of the following is detected, the procedure should be stopped.
1. *Sign and symptoms*:
    - If the patient request stopping, because of severe fatigue
    - Severe chest pain, dyspnea, or dizziness or syncope
    - Fall in systolic blood pressure (>20 mm Hg).
    - Hypertensive response (SBP >260 mm Hg and DBP >130 mm Hg)
    - Ataxia
2. *ECG criteria*:
    - Severe ST-segment depression (>3 mm)
    - ST-segment elevation >1 mm in non-Q wave lead
    - Frequent ventricular extrasystoles (unless the test is to assess ventricular arrhythmia)
    - Onset of ventricular tachycardia
    - New atrial fibrillation or supraventricular tachycardia
    - Development of new bundle branch block
    - New second- or third-degree heart block
    - Cardiac arrest

HOLTER MONITORING (AMBULATORY ELECTROCARDIOGRAM)

Holter monitor is a battery-operated portable ECG. It records the electrical activity of the heart continuously over 24–48 hours or longer depending on the type of monitoring used. The patient is provided with a pocket-sized device, which can record and store a short segment of ECG. Electrodes, which are small, plastic patches that stick to the skin, are placed at certain points on the chest and abdomen. The electrodes are connected to an ECG machine by wires, which is kept at the belt of waist. It does not interfere with patient's physical activity. The electrical activity of the heart can be measured, recorded, and printed. No electricity is sent into the body.

Indications:
- To detect suspected arrhythmia in patient with symptoms such as palpitation, dizziness, or syncope.
- To determine the risk or type of arrhythmia or conduction defect.
- To assess the rate control in patient with atrial fibrillation.
- To detect transient myocardial ischemia using ST segment analysis.
- To monitor the efficacy of antiarrhythmic drug therapy.

Patients with the following disease that may require documentation of an arrhythmia:
- Structural heart diseases such as postmyocardial infarction, dilated or hypertrophic cardiomyopathy, and valvular heart disease.
- Primary electrical heart disease such as sick sinus syndrome, WPW syndrome, and high grade AV block.
- Family history of sudden death or arrhythmia.

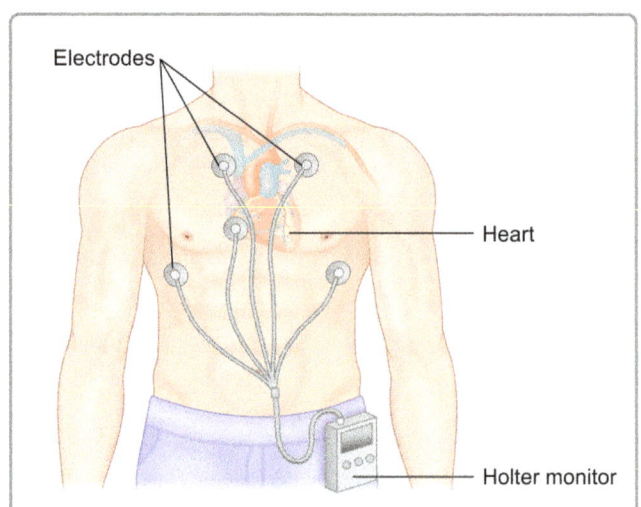

CHAPTER 2

ECG Changes in Different Diseases

*"ECG by itself is not to be all and end of the diagnosis.
Correlation of clinical diagnosis is essential and very vital"*

LEFT VENTRICULAR HYPERTROPHY

Electrocardiogram (ECG) Criteria of Left Ventricular Hypertrophy (LVH) (Voltage Criteria): Commonly used any one of the following:
- S in V_1 + R in V_6 or V_5 >35 mm (S V_1 + R V_6 >35 mm). These criteria are applicable only >25 years of age.
- R in V_5 (or V_6) >26 mm

Other Criteria of LVH
- R in aVL >11 mm (or 13 mm)
- R in aVF >20 mm (also in L_{II} and L_{III})
- R in V_6 is ≥R in V_5 (normally R in V_5 is taller than R in V_6)
- R in L_I + S in L_{III} >25 mm
- R in L_I >15 mm
- S in V_1 or V_2 >25 mm
- Sum of all QRS in all 12 leads >175 mm
- Left axis deviation (LAD) (QRS between –30° and –90°)

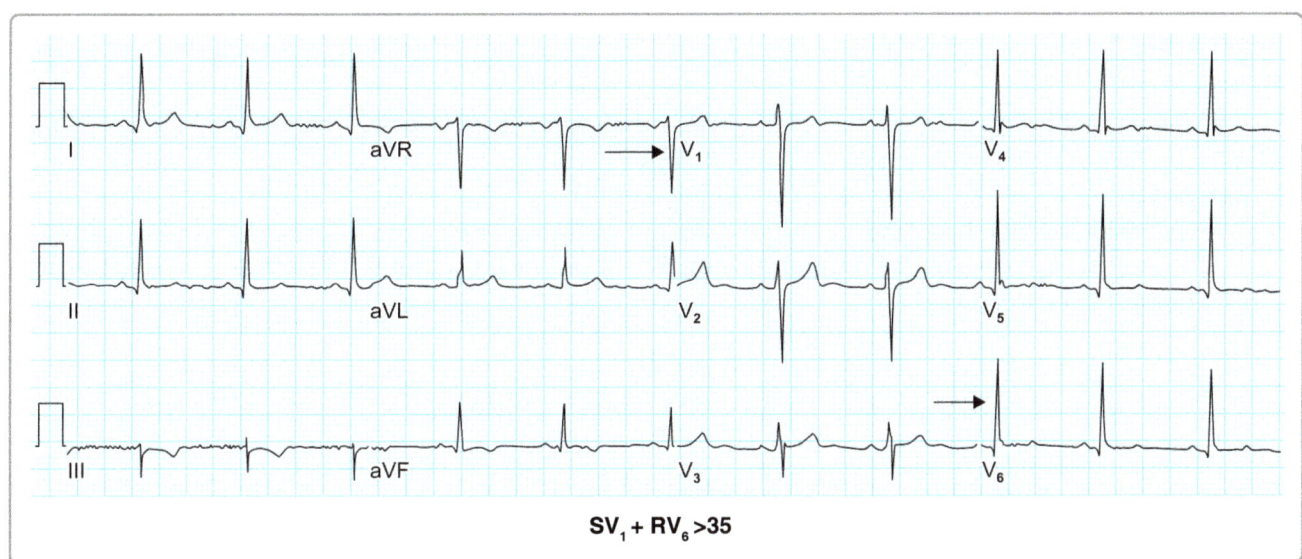

$SV_1 + RV_6 >35$

NB: In a young and thin person, these voltage criteria are not diagnostic (in a younger person, S in V_1 + R in V_5 or V_6 should be >40 mm).

Ques. How to confirm the diagnosis of LVH?
Ans. By echocardiography (M-mode).

Ques. How to diagnose LVH clinically or what is the character of apex beat in LVH?
Ans. Apex beat is heaving in nature.

Ques. Does apex beat shift in LVH?
Ans. Apex beat is not shifted, as the hypertrophy is of concentric type (at the expense of the cavity).

ECG in Medical Practice

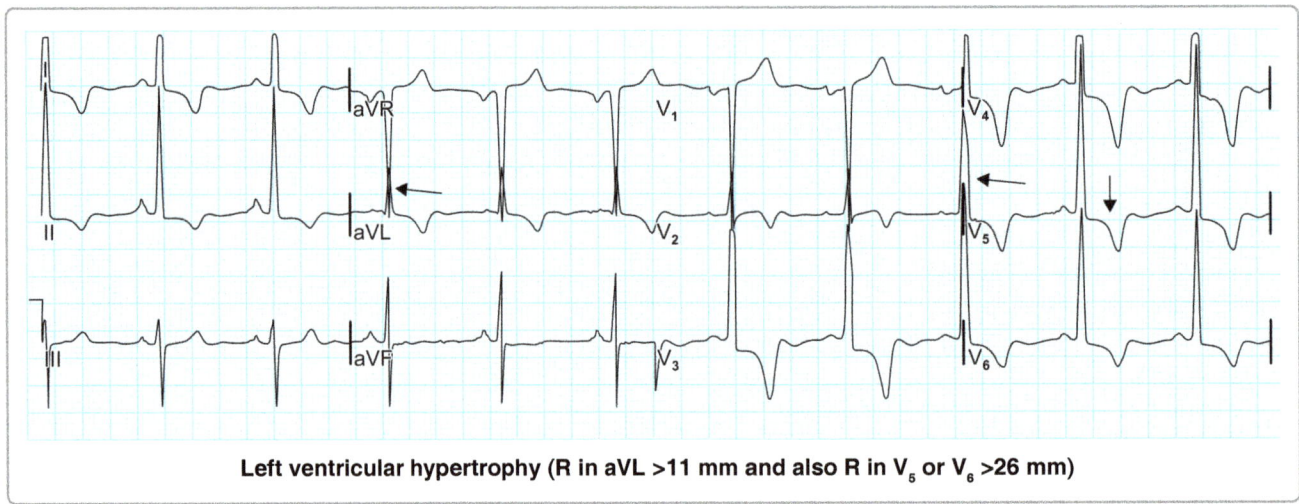

Left ventricular hypertrophy (R in aVL >11 mm and also R in V_5 or V_6 >26 mm)

ECG Criteria of LVH with Strain

- Findings of LVH
- ST depression and T inversion (in L_1, aVL, and V_4 to V_6), which is 1 mm or more in these leads.

Ques. What are the differential diagnoses of LVH with strain?

Ans. As follows:
- Hypertrophic cardiomyopathy
- Subendocardial myocardial infarction non-ST-elevation myocardial infarction (NSTEMI) or non-q myocardial infarction.

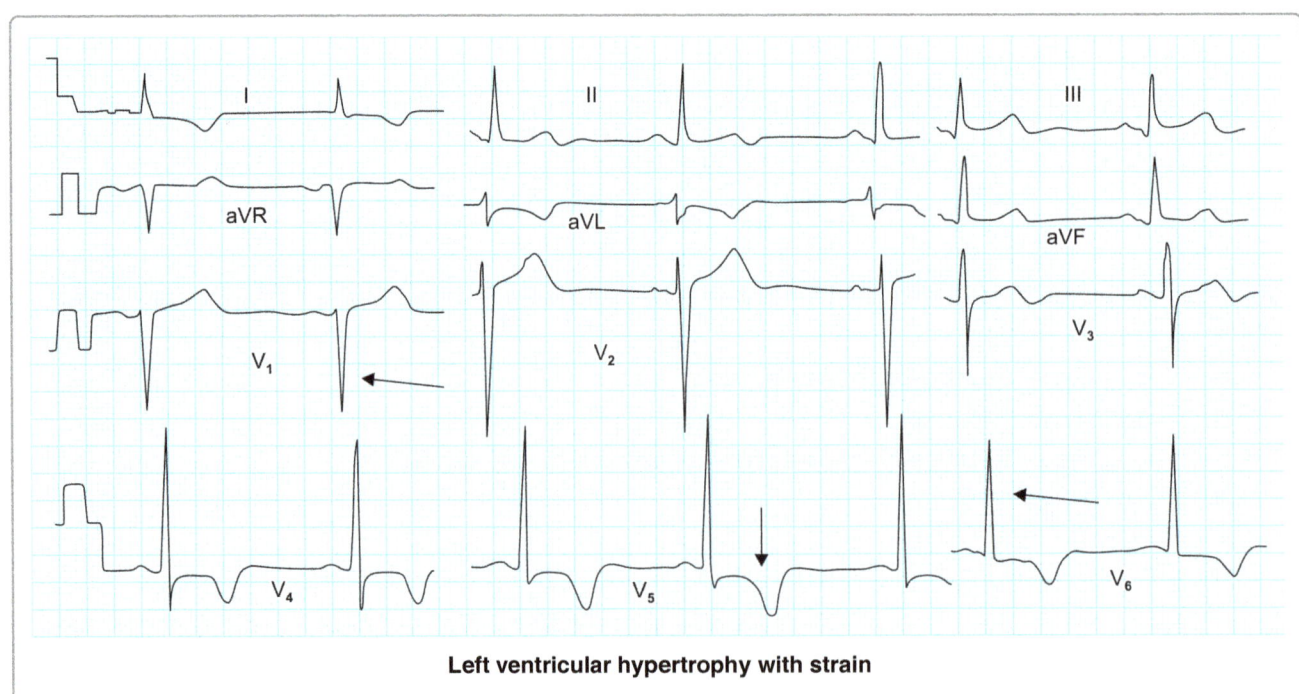

Left ventricular hypertrophy with strain

Ques. **How to differentiate LVH with strain from subendocardial myocardial infarction?**
Ans. As follows:
- If in ECG, there is LVH with T inversion, it is likely to be LVH with strain.
- But if in ECG, there is symmetrical T inversion in all chest leads, it is likely to be subendocardial myocardial infarction (NSTEMI).

Ques. **How to confirm the diagnosis?**
Ans. By echocardiography (2D or M-mode).

Ques. **What are the causes of LVH?**
Ans. As follows:
- Systemic hypertension
- Aortic stenosis
- Coarctation of aorta
- Hypertrophic cardiomyopathy
- Ventricular septal defect (VSD)
- Mitral regurgitation (MR)
- Aortic regurgitation
- Patent ductus arteriosus (PDA)
- Coronary artery disease (long-standing)

Ques. What are the types of electrocardiographic pattern of LVH?
Ans. There are two types of electrocardiographic pattern:
- Pressure overload (systolic overload): It is associated with concentric hypertrophy of ventricular muscles (at the expense of cavity, which is small). Causes are hypertension, aortic stenosis, coarctation of aorta, and hypertrophic cardiomyopathy. ECG shows tall R in V_5 and V_6. It may be also associated with ST depression and T inversion (strain pattern).
- Volume overload (diastolic overload): It is associated with eccentric and dilated left ventricular cavity. Cause are aortic regurgitation, MR, VSD, PDA, severe anemia, and thyrotoxicosis. ECG shows tall R V_5, V_6 with narrow Q waves in V_4 to V_6. ST and T are often normal. Also, negative U wave in V_4 to V_6 is common.

Ques. How to diagnose LVH clinically?
Ans. As follows:
- On palpation: Apex beat is heaving in nature. (However, apex beat is usually not shifted, as the hypertrophy is due to concentric left ventricular hypertrophy. It is at the expense of left ventricular cavity, not due to dilatation).
- To be confirmed, 2D or M-mode echocardiography should be done.

RIGHT VENTRICULAR HYPERTROPHY

ECG Criteria of Right Ventricular Hypertrophy (RVH)

- Tall R wave in V_1 >7 mm (also deep S in V_5 or V_6).

Other Criteria (less used for the diagnosis)
- R/S ratio in V_1 >1 (R is >S in V_1)
- R in V_1 + S in V_5 or V_6 is ≥10.5 mm
- S in V_1 <2 mm
- R in V_5 and V_6 <5 mm
- Negative T wave in V_1 in the presence of R >5 mm
- R in aVR >5 mm
- S in V_1 <2 mm
- S in V_6 >7 mm
- Incomplete right bundle branch block (RBBB) (rSR in V_1)
- QRS is wide (>0.12)
- Small q in V_1
- Right axis deviation (RAD) (between +90° and +180°)

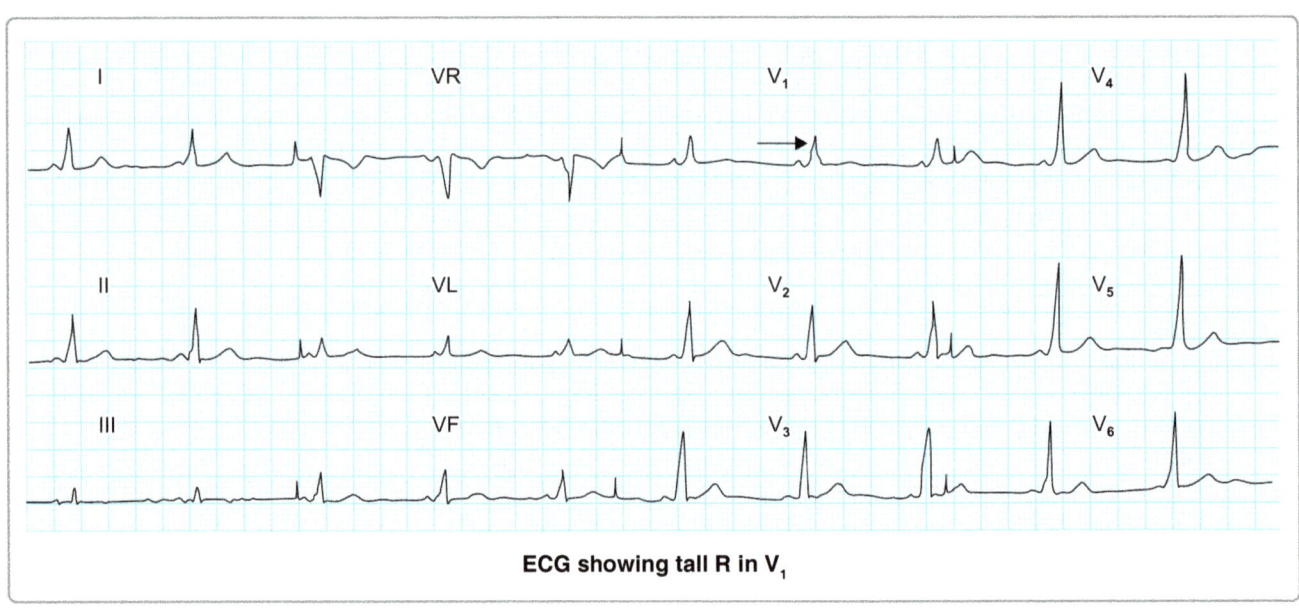

ECG showing tall R in V_1

Ques. What are the causes of tall R in V_1?
Ans. As follows:
- Normal variant
- RVH
- True posterior myocardial infarction
- Wolff–Parkinson–White (WPW) syndrome type A
- Dextrocardia

Ques. What are the causes of RVH?

Ans. As follows:
- Chronic cor pulmonale
- Mitral stenosis (MS) with pulmonary hypertension
- Pulmonary hypertension (due to any cause)
- Pulmonary stenosis
- Eisenmenger's syndrome
- Tetralogy of Fallot
- Atrial septal defect (ASD)
- VSD
- Tricuspid regurgitation

Ques. How to diagnose RVH clinically?

Ans. By palpation of precordium:
- Left parasternal heave
- Epigastric pulsation
- Features of pulmonary hypertension

Ques. What are the signs or features of pulmonary hypertension?

Ans. As follows:
- Low volume pulse
- Prominent "*a*" wave in jugular venous pressure (JVP)
- Palpable P_2
- Left parasternal heave
- Epigastric pulsation
- Loud P_2 on auscultation
- Early diastolic murmur due to pulmonary regurgitation

Ques. How to confirm RVH?

Ans. Echocardiography (M-mode or 2D)

Right Ventricular Hypertrophy with Strain

ECG Criteria

- Features of RVH
- ST depression and T inversion (in V_1 and V_2)

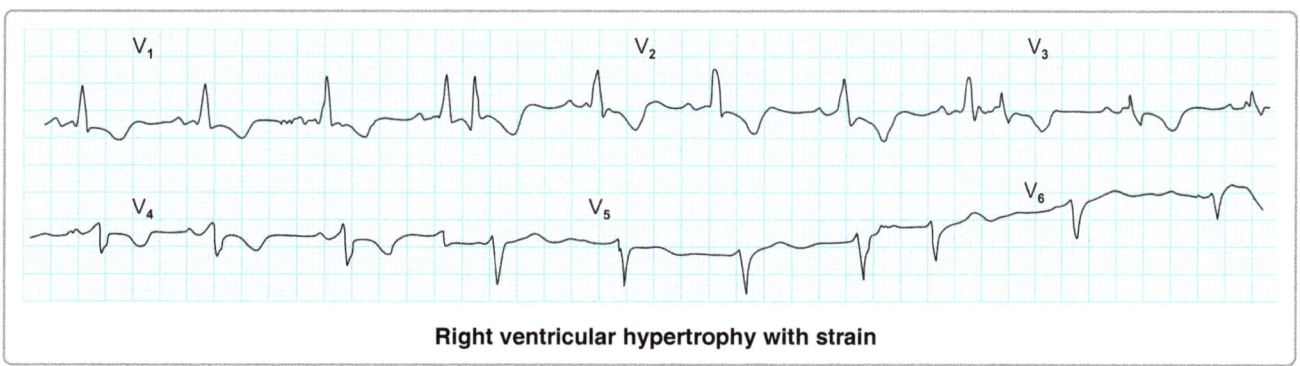

Right ventricular hypertrophy with strain

Ques. How to confirm RVH with strain?

Ans. Echocardiography (M-mode or 2D).

Ques. What are the electrocardiographic patterns of RVH?

Ans. Two types of electrocardiographic patterns of RVH are:
- Volume overload pattern: It is similar to incomplete or partial RBBB. Usual causes are MS with pulmonary hypertension and also, ASD.
- Pressure overload pattern: It manifests as tall R in V_1. It is common in pulmonary stenosis, and also, in pulmonary hypertension, due to any cause, and in cor pulmonale.

Both patterns are associated with RAD. Also, there may be ST depression and T inversion in the chest leads.

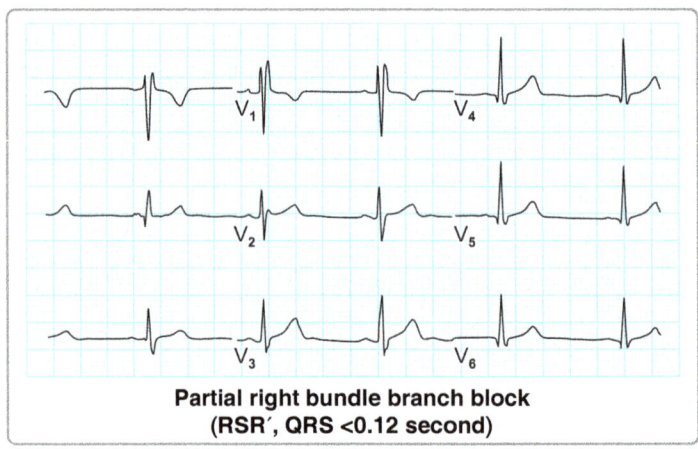

Partial right bundle branch block (RSR′, QRS <0.12 second)

Ques. How to diagnose RVH clinically?

Ans. As follows:
- Left parasternal heave or lift
- Palpable P_2 (indicates pulmonary hypertension also)
- Epigastric pulsation

BIVENTRICULAR HYPERTROPHY (COMBINED LEFT VENTRICULAR HYPERTROPHY AND RIGHT VENTRICULAR HYPERTROPHY)

ECG Criteria of Combined LVH and RVH

- Findings of LVH and RVH as described above (such as tall R V_1 and also V_5 and V_6).

Other findings:
In the presence of LVH, the following findings are suggestive of RVH:
- RAD
- R > S in V_1
- Presence of prominent S wave in V_5 and V_6
- ECG signs of right atrial abnormality
- Unusually tall biphasic R/S complexes in chest leads (commonly V_2, V_3, and V_4)

Ques. How to confirm the diagnosis?
Ans. Echocardiography (M-mode or 2D).

Ques. What are the causes of biventricular hypertrophy?
Ans. As follows:
- Eisenmenger's syndrome (VSD or ASD or PDA with reversal of shunt)
- Hypertrophic cardiomyopathy
- Multiple valvular heart diseases (e.g., aortic stenosis + pulmonary stenosis)

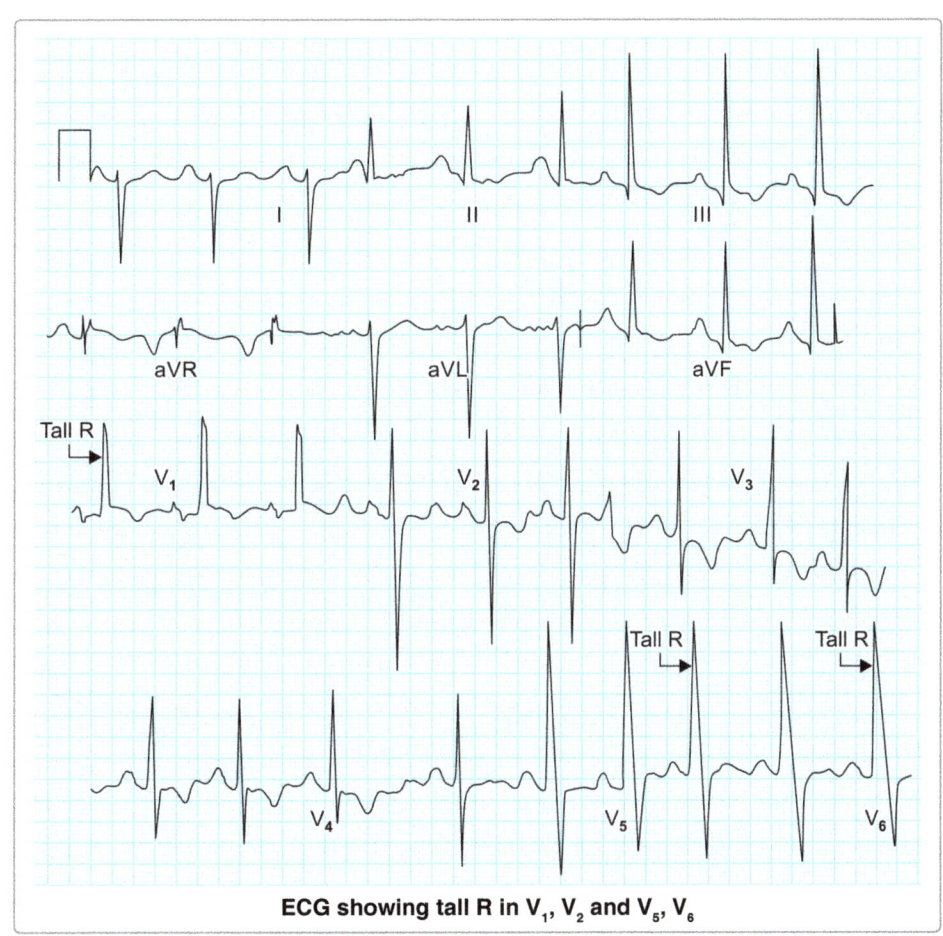

ECG showing tall R in V_1, V_2 and V_5, V_6

LEFT ATRIAL HYPERTROPHY

ECG Criteria of Left Atrial Hypertrophy (LAH)

- P is wide >0.12 second (>2.5 small squares), P may be notched or bifid (like M), called P mitrale (it is better seen in L_{II}, also in L_I and aVL).
- P in V_1-biphasic with small initial positive deflection and prominent, and deep negative deflection (>1 mm depth).

Ques. What does P mitrale indicate?

Ans. It indicates LAH or enlargement.

Ques. How to confirm?

Ans. Echocardiography (M-mode or 2D).

Ques. What are the causes of P mitrale?

Ans. As follows:
- MS (the most common)
- MR

Ques. What are the causes of LAH?

Ans. As follows:
- Mitral valvular disease (MS or MR)
- Secondary to LVH due to any cause
- ASD

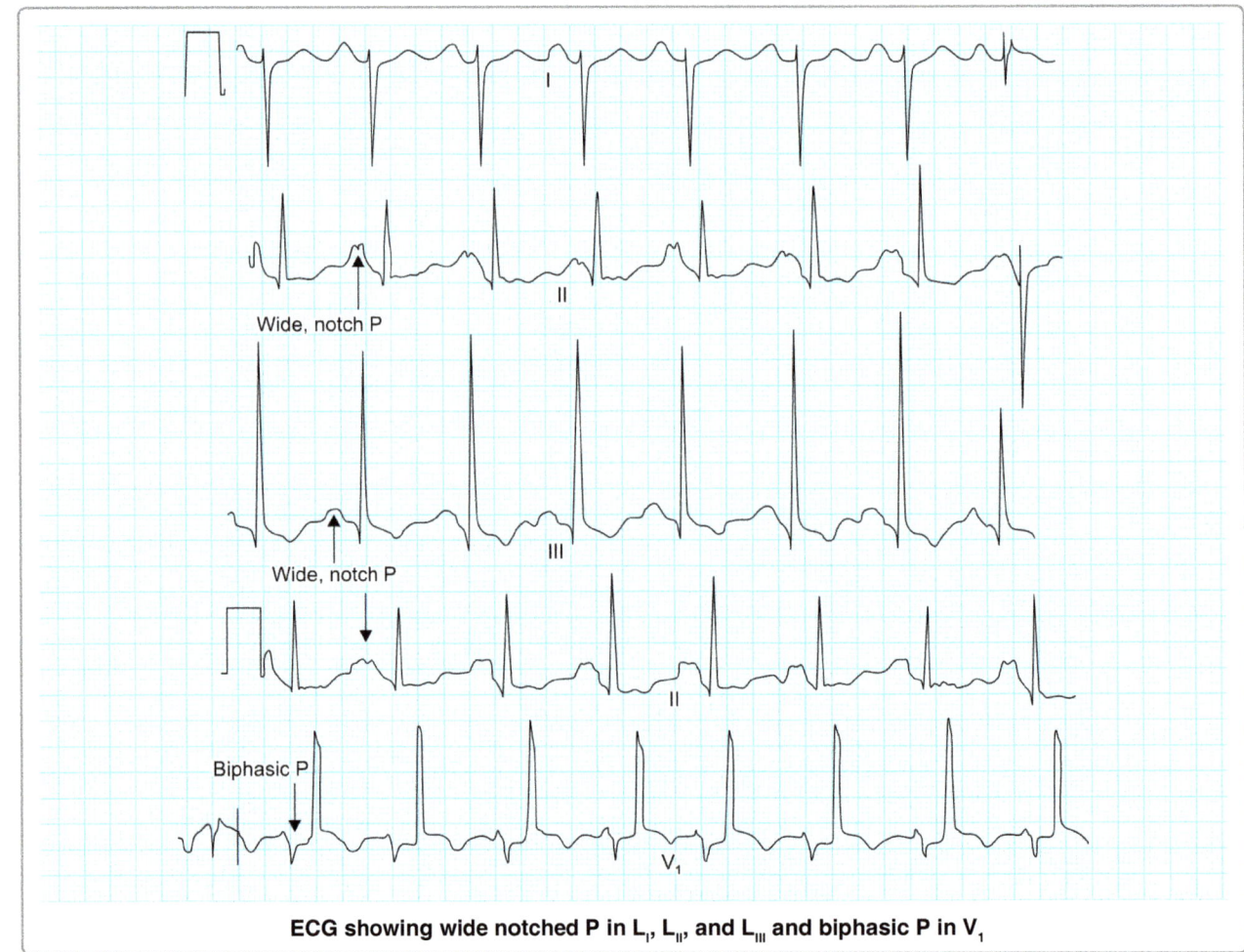

ECG showing wide notched P in L_I, L_{II}, and L_{III} and biphasic P in V_1

RIGHT ATRIAL HYPERTROPHY

ECG Criteria of Right Atrial Hypertrophy (RAH)

- P is tall, >2.5 mm (>2.5 small squares), better seen in L_{II}, L_{III}, and aVF and sometimes in V_1 (Tall P is called *P pulmonale*).
- P in V_1: Biphasic, tall initial positive deflection (>1.5 mm) with a small negative deflection (only positive deflection may be present).

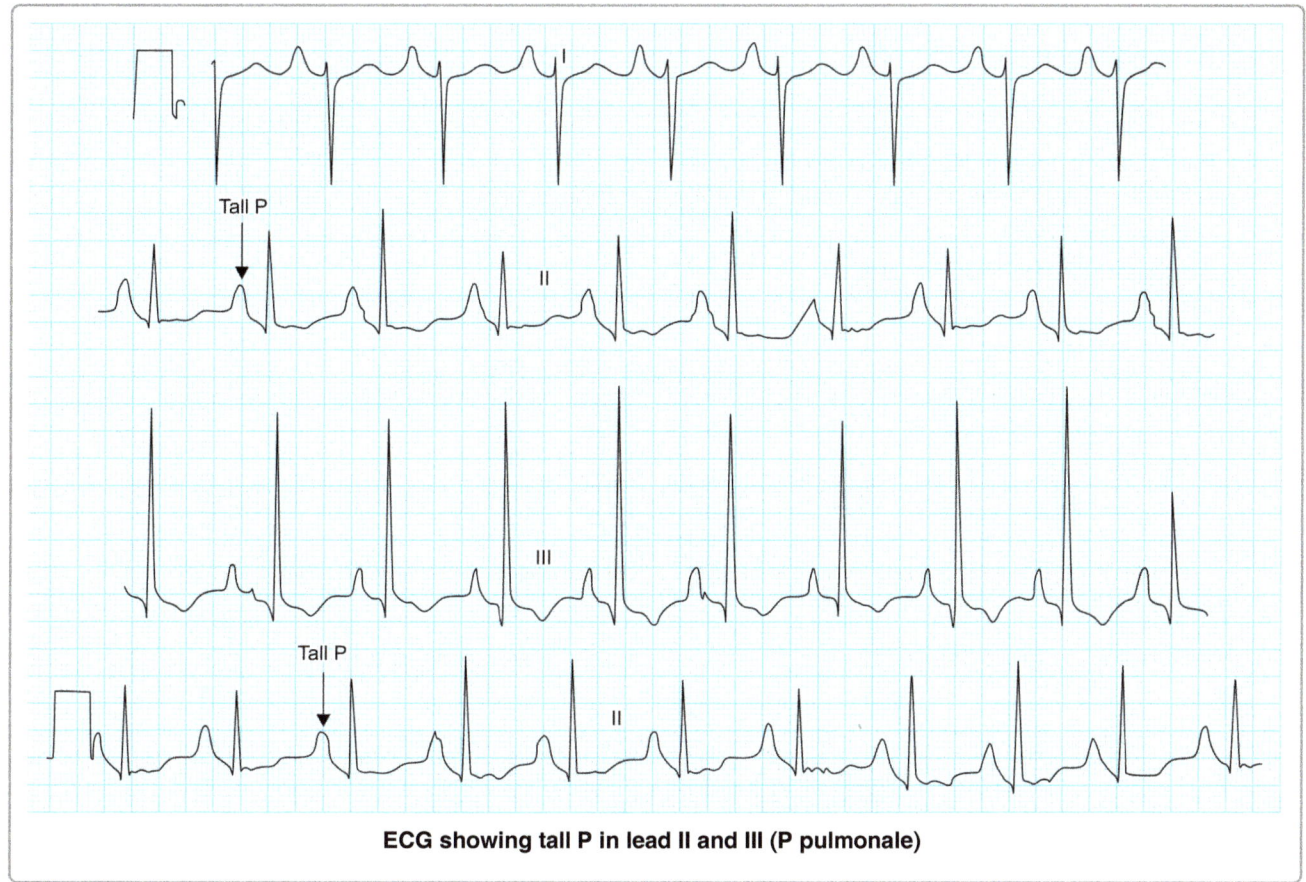

ECG showing tall P in lead II and III (P pulmonale)

Ques. What are the causes of right atrial hypertrophy (RAH)?

Ans. As follows:
- Tricuspid stenosis
- Tricuspid regurgitation
- Atrial septal defect
- Pulmonary hypertension due to any cause

Ques. What does P pulmonale indicate?

Ans. It indicates RAH or enlargement (it is called P pulmonale, because it is commonly seen in severe pulmonary disease).

Ques. How to confirm?

Ans. Echocardiography (M-mode or 2D).

Ques. What are the causes of P pulmonale?

Ans. As follows:
- Chronic obstructive pulmonary disease (COPD) with chronic cor pulmonale (the most common)
- Chronic lung diseases
- ASD
- Tricuspid regurgitation
- Tricuspid stenosis
- Pulmonary stenosis
- Pulmonary hypertension (due to any cause)
- Transient P pulmonale occurs in acute pulmonary embolism and acute severe asthma

Ques. How to confirm RAH?

Ans. Echocardiography (M-mode or 2D).

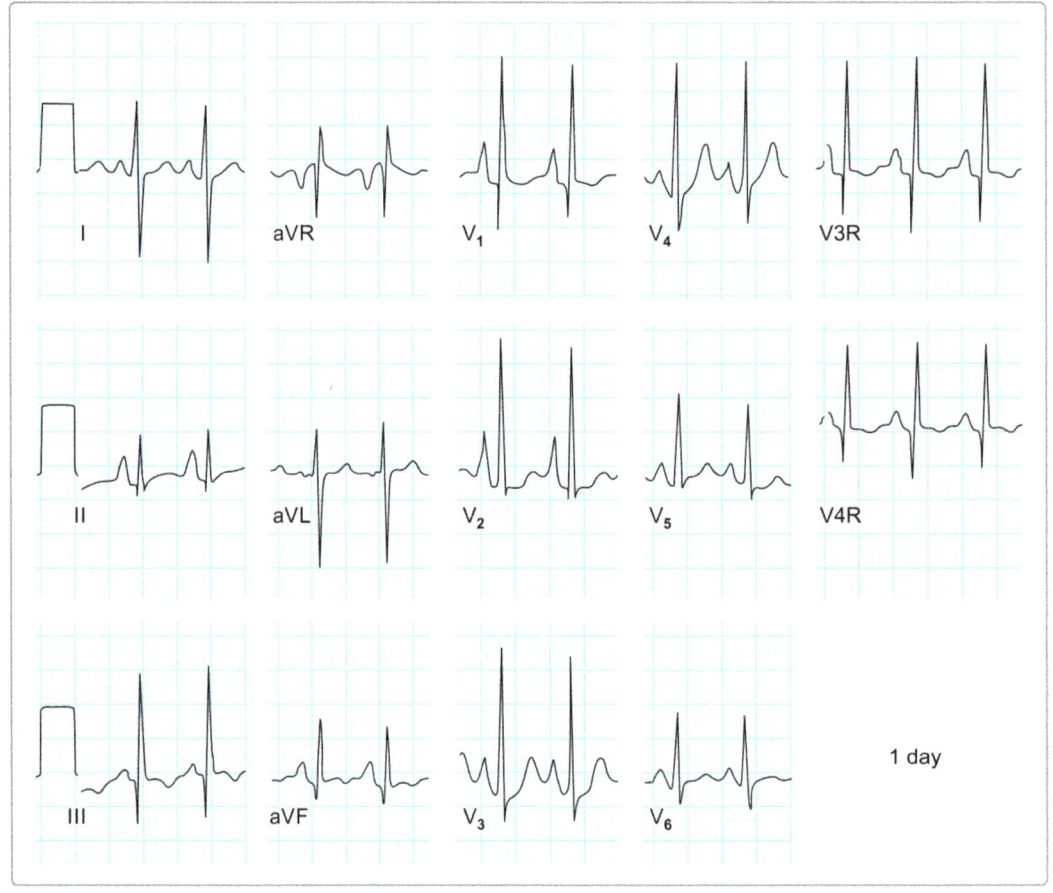

1 day

COMBINED LEFT AND RIGHT ATRIAL HYPERTROPHY (BIATRIAL HYPERTROPHY)

ECG Criteria of Combined LAH and RAH

- Wide and notched P wave in all limb leads, also in V_4 to V_6
- Tall P in all limb leads, also in V_2 and V_3

Ques. What are the causes of biatrial enlargement?

Ans. As follows:
- MS with pulmonary hypertension
- ASD
- Lutembacher's syndrome (ASD with acquired MS)
- MS with tricuspid regurgitation or tricuspid stenosis

Ques. How to confirm biatrial enlargement?

Ans. As follows:
- Echocardiography (M-mode or 2D)
- Also, color Doppler echocardiography to find out the cause

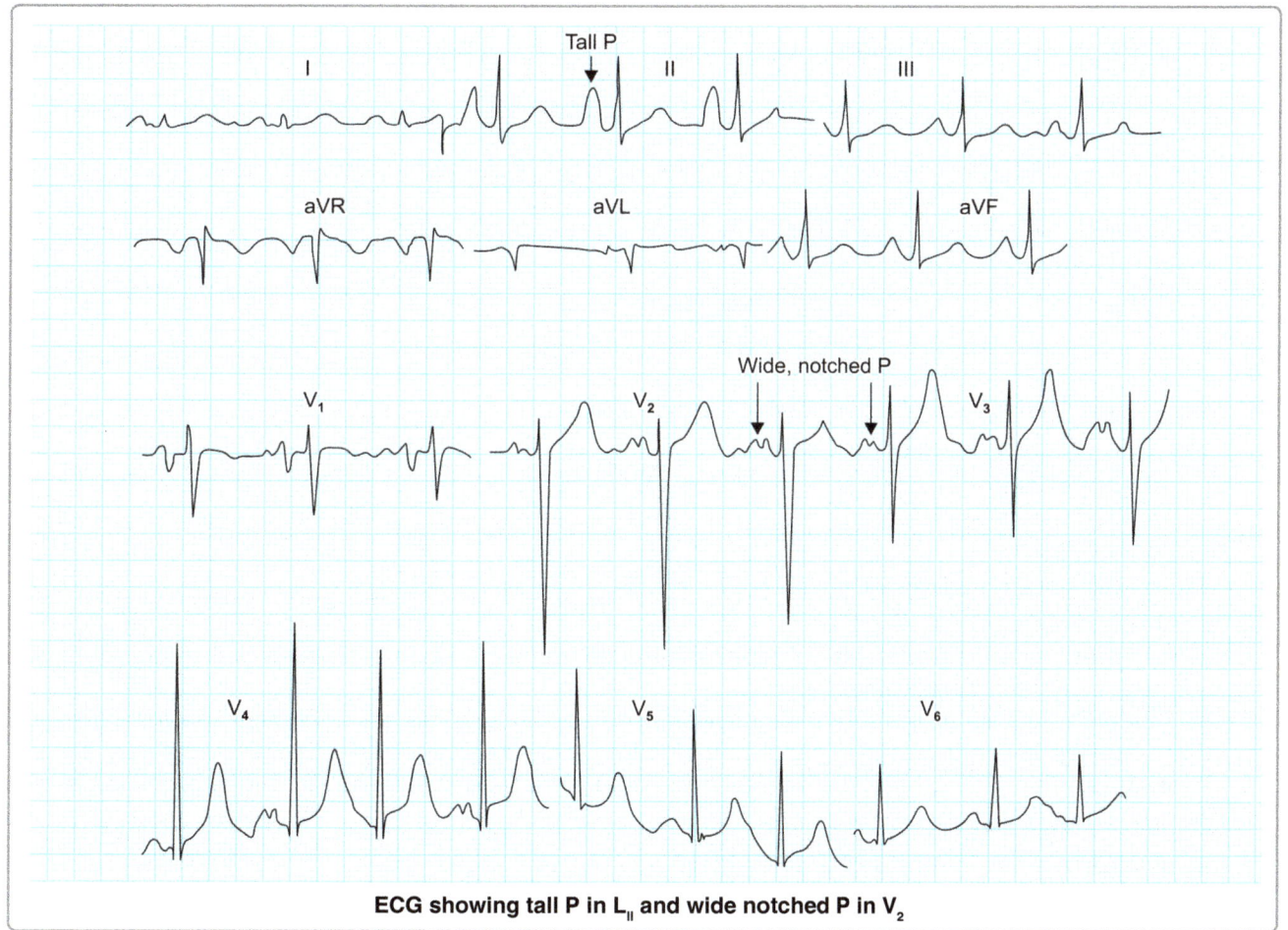

ECG showing tall P in L_{II} and wide notched P in V_2

SINUS ARRHYTHMIA

ECG Criteria of Sinus Arrhythmia

- *PP or RR interval:* Short in inspiration and long in expiration
- *Rhythm:* Irregular (PP or RR interval is irregular)
- *PQRST:* Normal

Ques. What is sinus arrhythmia?

Ans. It refers to a changing sinus node rate with respiratory cycle. In this arrhythmia, heart rate increases in inspiration and decreases in expiration. Sinus arrhythmia is well seen, if the sinus rate is slow.

Ques. What is the mechanism?

Ans. It is the normal manifestation of autonomic activity which varies with respiration.
- In inspiration, parasympathetic activity diminishes, so the heart rate increases. It reverses during expiration.
- Sinus arrhythmia is a benign condition, common in children and young adults. It is sometimes seen in healthy old people.
- It has no clinical significance
- It is absent in autonomic neuropathy
- Since it is affected by vagal tone, sinus arrhythmia cannot be seen in a patient who has received atropine or who has undergone vagotomy.

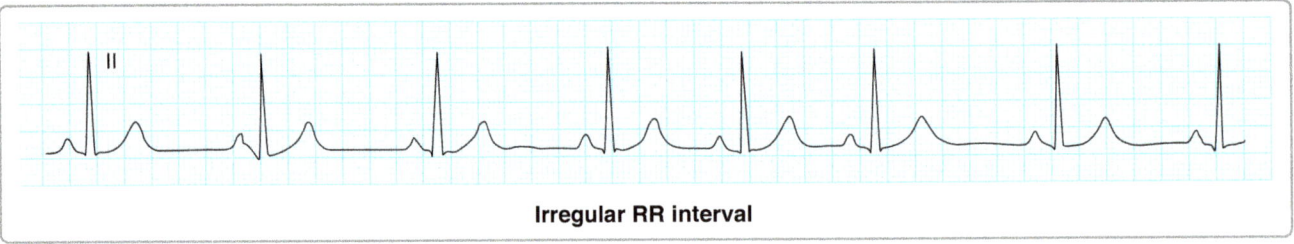

Irregular RR interval

Ques. What are the diseases associated with sinus arrhythmia?

Ans. Sinus arrhythmia may be associated with:
- Sinus bradycardia
- Wandering pacemaker
- Sinus tachycardia

Ques. What are the types of sinus arrhythmia?

Ans. Sinus arrhythmia may be of two types:
- *Respiratory sinus arrhythmia:* It is related to respiration. It is common in children and young adults. It is a benign condition, usually physiological.
- *Nonrespiratory sinus arrhythmia:* It has no relation to respiration. It may be associated with any cardiac disease (myocardial infarction and heart failure), sinus bradycardia, digoxin therapy, enhanced vagal tone, etc. It may be idiopathic in many cases. It is common in the elderly. Full evaluation of cardiac function should be done.

Ques. How to treat such case?

Ans. It is benign condition. No treatment is necessary.

SINUS TACHYCARDIA

ECG Criteria of Sinus Tachycardia

- Heart rate—>100 beats/min
- P, QRS, and T—normal
- Rhythm—regular

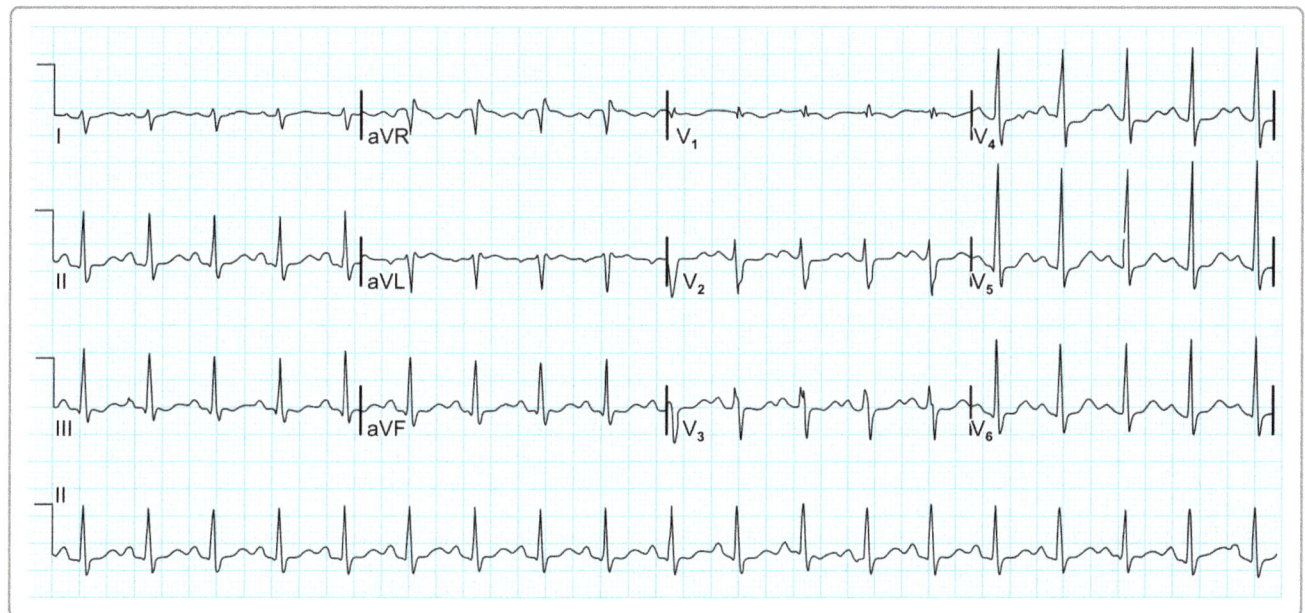

Ques. What is sinus tachycardia?

Ans. Sinus tachycardia means heart rate is >100/min with sinus rhythm.

Ques. What are the causes of sinus tachycardia?

Ans. As follows:
- Physiological—anxiety, emotion, exercise, pain, and pregnancy
- *Pathological*:
    - Anemia
    - Fever
    - Thyrotoxicosis
    - Shock (except vasovagal attack in which bradycardia is present)
    - Heart failure
    - Sick sinus syndrome
    - Bleeding
    - Hypovolemia due to any cause (such as vomiting and diarrhea)
    - Hypoglycemia
    - Hypoxia
    - Myocarditis
    - Massive pulmonary embolism
    - Chronic constrictive pericarditis
    - Acute anterior myocardial infarction (bradycardia is common in acute inferior myocardial infarction)
    - Drugs (salbutamol, atropine, adrenaline, isoprenaline, ephedrine, propantheline, and thyroxine)

Ques. What are the differences between sinus tachycardia and supraventricular tachycardia (SVT)?

Ans. See in topic SVT (later).

Ques. What is inappropriate sinus tachycardia?

Ans. Persistent increase in resting heart rate unrelated to or out of proportion with the level of physical activity or emotional stress. It is common in women and also in health professionals.

Ques. What is tachycardia?

Ans. When the heart rate is >100/min, it is called tachycardia.

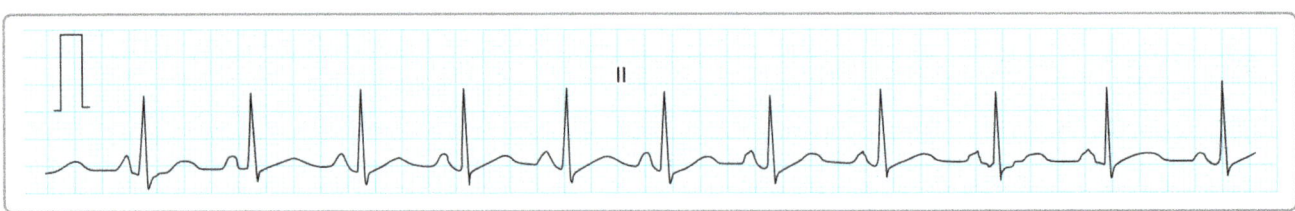

Ques. What are the types of tachycardia?

Ans. Depending on the width of QRS, tachycardia is divided into two types:
- Narrow-complex tachycardia
- Broad-complex tachycardia

Ques. What are the ECG criteria of narrow-complex tachycardia?

Ans. As follows:
- Rate >100/min
- QRS <0.12 second (<3 small squares)

Ques. What are the ECG criteria of broad-complex tachycardia?

Ans. As follows:
- Rate >100/min
- QRS >0.12 second (>3 small squares)

Ques. What are the causes of narrow-complex tachycardia?

Ans. As follows:
- Sinus tachycardia
- Atrial tachycardia
- Atrial flutter
- Atrial fibrillation
- Atrioventricular reentry tachycardia (AVRT)
- Atrioventricular nodal reentry tachycardia (AVNRT)

Ques. What are the causes of broad-complex tachycardia?

Ans. As follows:
- Ventricular tachycardia
- SVT with aberrant conduction
- WPW syndrome

Ques. How to treat sinus tachycardia?

Ans. Treatment should be given according to the cause.
- If the patient is on any offending drug, this should be withdrawn.
- To prevent anxiety, mild tranquilizer and β-blocker therapy may be given.
- Other treatment: According to the cause of tachycardia.
- Also, treatment should be given according to the type of tachycardia, such as supraventricular tachycardia (SVT), ventricular tachycardia (VT) or atrial tachycardia, etc.

NB: Remember the following points:
- For 1° increase in temperature, pulse rate increases by 8–10 beats/min. Sinus tachycardia at a rate less than expected in fever is called "relative bradycardia," which is found in enteric fever and brucellosis.
- Sinus tachycardia more than expected or predicted is found in myocarditis, rheumatic fever, and bacterial endocarditis.
- Failure to develop sinus tachycardia due to physiological or pathological stimulus in the absence of β-blocker or calcium channel blocker therapy indicates sinus node dysfunction. Also, autonomic neuropathy.

SINUS BRADYCARDIA

ECG Criteria of Sinus Bradycardia

- Heart rate—<60 beats/min
- P, QRS, and T—normal
- Rhythm—regular

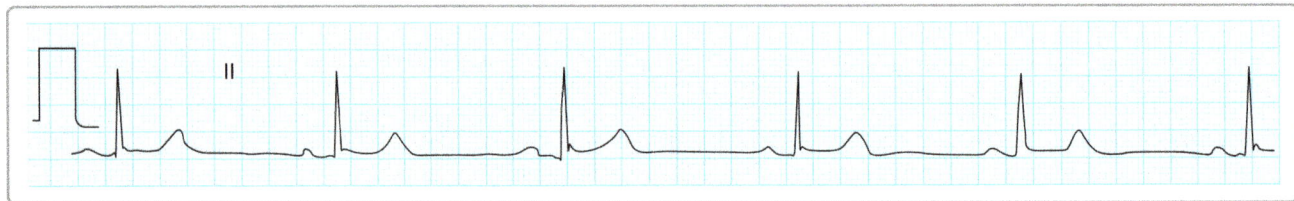

Ques. What is sinus bradycardia? What are the causes of sinus bradycardia?

Ans. Sinus bradycardia means heart rate is <60/min with sinus rhythm. Causes are:
- *Physiological (due to increased vagal tone)*:
  - Athlete
  - Sleep
  - Occasionally, healthy elderly
- *Pathological*:
  - Hypothyroidism
  - Hypothermia
  - Raised intracranial pressure (it is due to due to inhibitory effect on sympathetic outflow)
  - Drugs (digoxin, β-blockers, and verapamil)
  - Acute inferior myocardial infarction
  - Obstructive jaundice (it is due to the deposition of bilirubin in the conducting system)
  - Sick sinus syndrome
  - Electrolyte imbalance (e.g. hypokalemia)
  - Neurally mediated syndromes, due to a reflex (Bezold–Jarisch), which causes bradycardia and reflex peripheral vasodilatation. These are—carotid sinus syndrome and neurocardiogenic (or vasovagal) syncope, which present as syncope or presyncope.

NB: Remember the following points:
- If the heart rate is <40/min, it is less likely to be sinus bradycardia.
- Always think of complete heart block, if the pulse rate is very low.
- Sinus bradycardia may be associated with sinus arrhythmia.

Ques. What should be done, if the patient presents with sinus bradycardia?

Ans. As follows:
- In asymptomatic case or in athlete, no treatment is needed.
- If it is secondary to any disease, treatment of primary cause should be done.

Chapter 2: ECG Changes in Different Diseases

Ques. **What is bradycardia? What are the causes of bradycardia?**

Ans. When the pulse rate is <60/min, it is called bradycardia. It may occur due to any cause including the impulse originating from the sinus node. Causes are:
- Sinus bradycardia due to any cause
- Sick sinus syndrome
- Second-degree heart block (Mobitz type II)
- Complete heart block
- Nodal rhythm
- Idioventricular rhythm
- Drugs (β-blocker, digoxin, etc.)

Ques. **How to treat bradycardia?**

Ans. As follows:
- If it is sinus bradycardia:
  - In asymptomatic case, no specific drug is necessary.
  - If due to any drug, such as digoxin or beta-blocker, these should be stopped.
  - Also if any cause is found, such as myxedema, acute inferior myocardial infarction or obstructive jaundice, these should be treated accordingly.
- If the bradycardia is due to other cause, such as sick sinus syndrome, second-degree heart block (Mobitz type II), complete heart block or nodal rhythm, these should be treated accordingly.

SUPRAVENTRICULAR TACHYCARDIA

ECG Criteria of SVT

- P—absent
- QRS—narrow
- Rhythm—regular
- Heart rate—high (150–250/min)

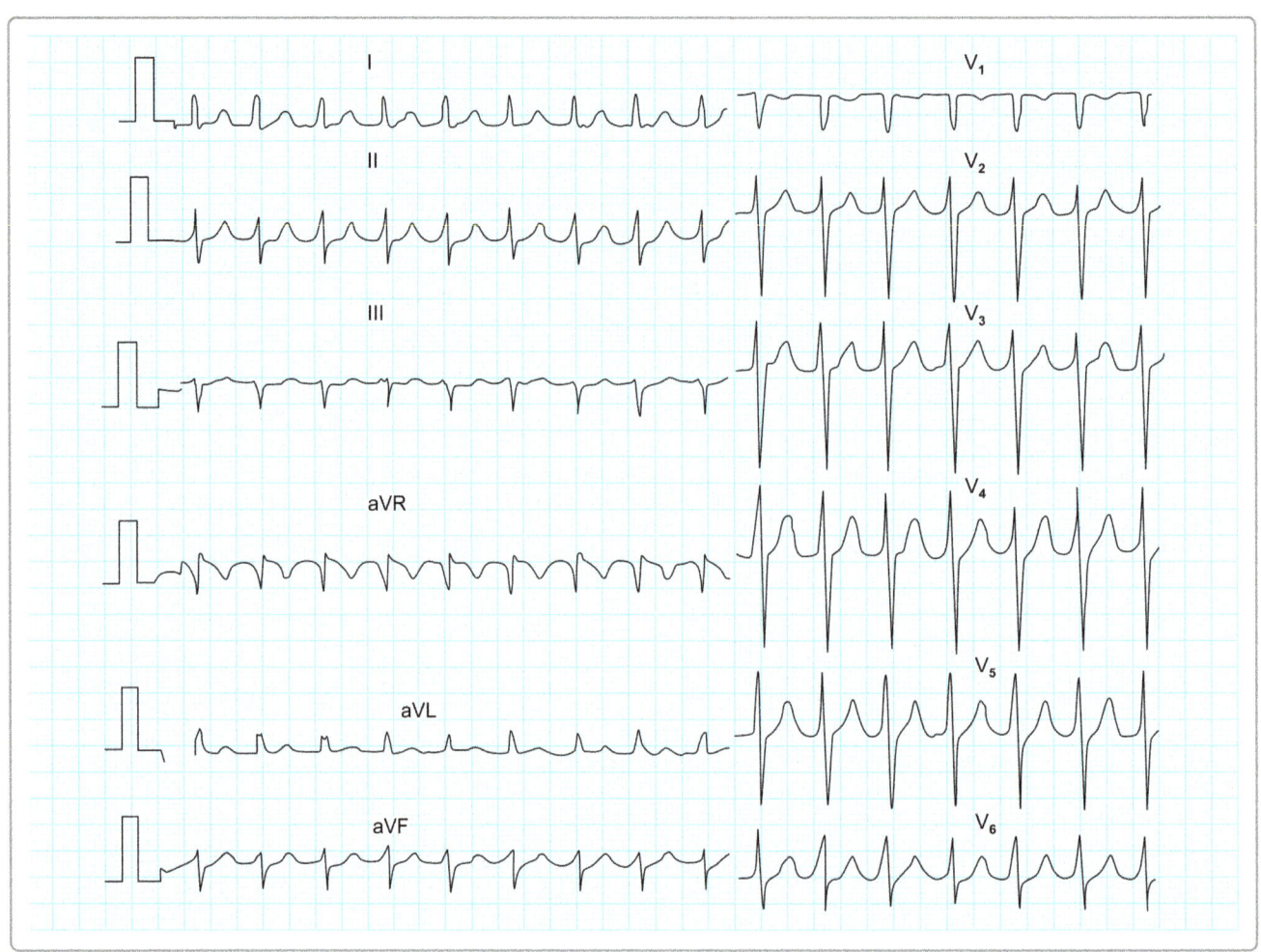

Ques. What are the causes of SVT?

Ans. As follows:
- *Physiological:* Anxiety, tension, tea, coffee, and alcohol
- *Pathological:*
  - Thyrotoxicosis
  - Ischemic heart disease
  - WPW syndrome
  - Digoxin toxicity

Chapter 2: ECG Changes in Different Diseases

Ques. What are the presentations of SVT?

Ans. As follows:
- Sudden onset of palpitation
- Dizziness or giddiness
- Dyspnea or breathlessness
- Anxiety and weakness
- Syncope may occur
- Polyuria may occur due to release of atrial natriuretic peptide (ANP), in response to increase in atrial pressure during tachycardia.
- Prominent jugular venous pulsation may be seen

Ques. What are the differences between sinus tachycardia and supraventricular tachycardia?

Ans. As follows:

Points	Sinus tachycardia	Supraventricular tachycardia
1. Onset	Gradual	Sudden
2. Pulse	<160/min	>160/min (140–220)
3. ECG	P, QRS, and T-normal	P absent (buried in QRS) and QRS is narrow
4. Carotid sinus massage or Valsalva maneuver	No or little response	May respond abruptly
5. Symptoms	Palpitation, usually present	Sudden palpitation, dizziness, syncope, and breathlessness. There may be polyuria after attack (due to release of ANP)
6. Prognosis	Not serious	Hemodynamic instability is common

Ques. What is the complication of SVT?

Ans. In SVT, because of rapid heart rate, there is short diastolic filling time. This results in reduction of stroke volume and may precipitate heart failure.

Ques. How to treat SVT?

Ans. As follows:

During acute attack:
- Rest and reassurance
- Mechanical or physiological method such as carotid sinus massage or Valsalva maneuver or splashing ice cold water on the face or supraorbital pressure. These procedures act by increasing vagal tone.
- *If no response*:
  - *Intravenous (IV) adenosine:* 3 mg over 2 seconds. If no response in 1-2 minutes, then 6 mg IV.
  - If still no response in 1-2 minutes, then 12 mg (maximum dose).
  - Or IV verapamil 10 mg slowly over 5-10 minutes may be given (verapamil should be avoided if QRS >0.12 second or history of WPW syndrome or if the patient is on β-blocker).

- *Other drugs*: β-blocker (propranolol, metoprolol, and esmolol), flecainide may be used.
- If the patient is hemodynamically unstable (hypotension and pulmonary edema), then direct current (DC) shock should be given.

Long-term management:
- *If the attack is frequent or disabling:* Prophylactic oral therapy with β-blocker, verapamil, diltiazem, and flecainide may be given.
- *If there is no response:* Catheter ablation may be done.
- *In WPW syndrome:* Transvenous radiofrequency catheter ablation is the treatment of choice.

Ques. What is the mode of action of adenosine? What are the side effects and contraindications of adenosine therapy?

Ans. As follows:
- *Mode of action of adenosine*: It causes transient atrioventricular (AV) block, lasting for few seconds (half-life is 8–10 seconds).
- *Side effects (all are transient)*:
  - Chest pain and dyspnea
  - Bronchospasm and choking sensation
  - Transient flushing
  - Hypotension
  - Heaviness in the limbs
  - Sense of impending doom
- *Contraindications*:
  - H/O bronchial asthma
  - Second- or third-degree heart block
  - Sick sinus syndrome

Ques. What are the types of SVT?

Ans. Usually, there are three types:
- *AVNRT:* There is abnormal circuit of impulse within the AV node by two pathways (a superior "fast," short effective refractory period and an inferior "slow" longer effective refractory period).
- *AVRT:* In this case, there is an abnormal accessory pathway or bypass tract that connects the atria and ventricles. In about 50% of cases, this pathway conducts impulse in a retrograde direction (from ventricles to atria) and in other case, it conducts in an antegrade direction (from atria to ventricles).
- *Atrial tachycardia:* The impulse arises from an ectopic atrial focus. There is rapid discharge of impulses from an ectopic atrial focus causing atrial tachycardia. It is rare.

NB: Remember the following points:
- SVT may be confused with sinus tachycardia. However, sinus tachycardia neither starts abruptly nor stops abruptly.
- If SVT is associated with WPW syndrome, verapamil should not be given intravenously. Adenosine is safe in such case.
- Look for carotid bruit before carotid sinus massage. Otherwise, thrombus may be dislodged and may cause cerebral embolism.

SVT with WPW Syndrome

ECG Criteria

- Heart rate—high (>200/min)
- QRS—wide (>0.12)
- Delta wave—in V_3 to V_6

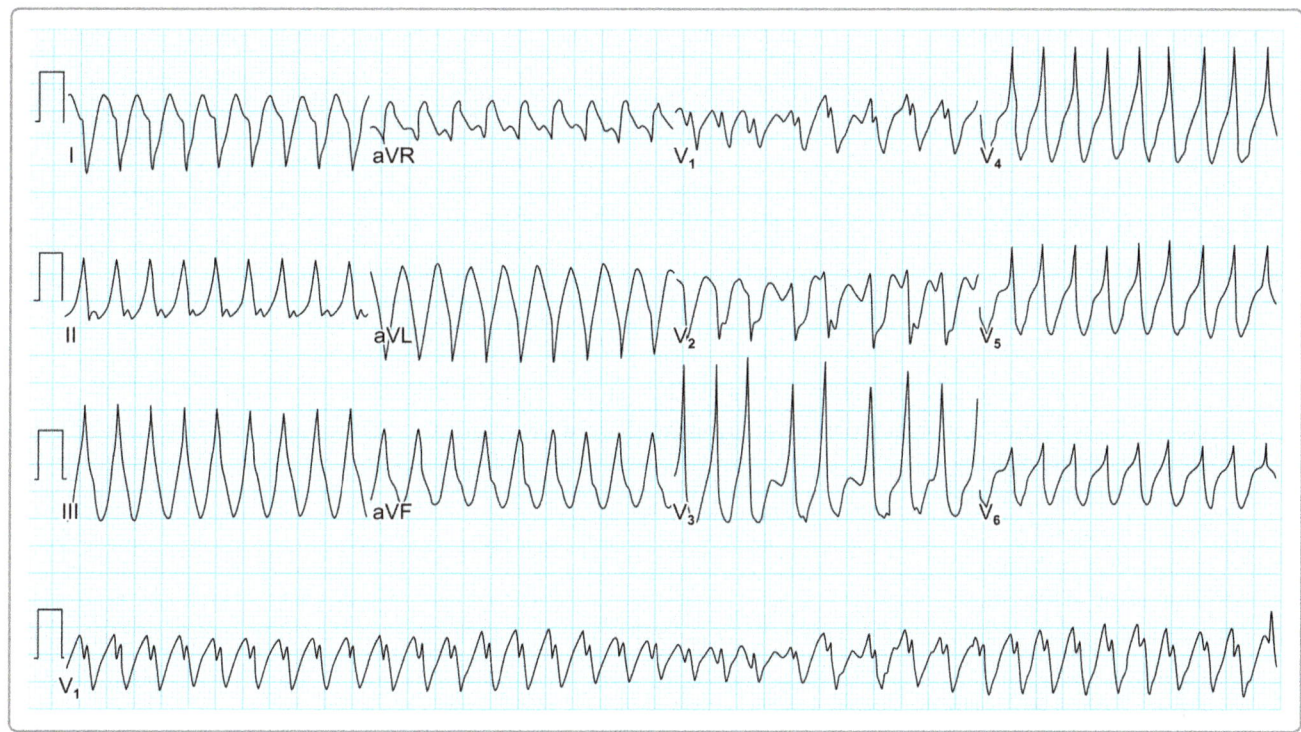

Ques. How to treat this case?

Ans. As follows:
- To reduce the rate: Mechanical measures and rate reducing drugs should be given. However, IV verapamil and digoxin should not be given.
- Transvenous radiofrequency catheter ablation is the treatment of choice (see above).

ATRIAL TACHYCARDIA

ECG Criteria of Atrial Tachycardia

- P—small and abnormal shape (may be upright or inverted)
- Atrial rate—140–220/min
- QRS—normal
- Rhythm—normal
  (There may be 2:1, 3:1, or variable AV block. Atrial tachycardia with AV block is common in digoxin toxicity).

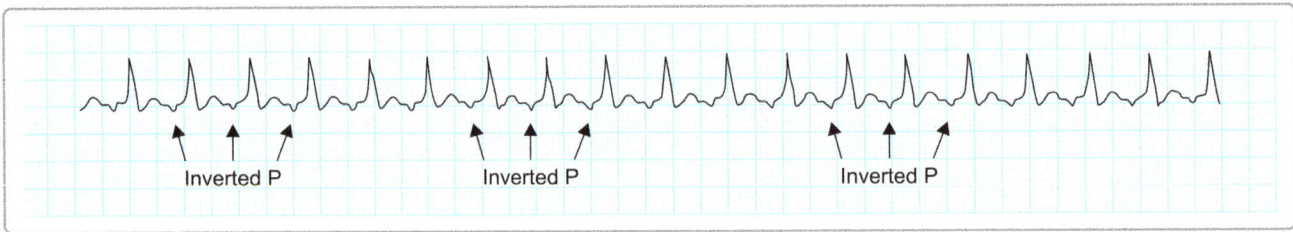

Ques. What is the mechanism of atrial tachycardia? What are the causes of atrial tachycardia?

Ans. It is due to the ectopic focus that arises from any part of atrial myocardium. Causes are:
- Ischemic heart disease
- Rheumatic heart disease
- Cardiomyopathy
- Sick sinus syndrome
- Digoxin toxicity

Ques. How to treat atrial tachycardia?

Ans. As follows:
- If due to digoxin—it should be stopped.
- *If not due to digoxin*:
  - To control the heart rate—digoxin, β-blocker, and verapamil may be used. Other drugs such as amiodarone and flecainide also may be used.
  - If no response—DC cardioversion may be done.
  - Atrial overdrive pacing may also be done in selected cases if other measures fail.
  - Occasionally, transvenous radiofrequency catheter ablation may be done (especially with persistent and troublesome symptoms).

NB: Remember the following points:
- Carotid sinus massage will not terminate atrial tachycardia. However, it increases the AV block, thereby facilitates the diagnosis.
- Atrial tachycardia is usually paroxysmal, so it is called paroxysmal atrial tachycardia (PAT).
- In atrial tachycardia, heart rate is usually >100/min, P wave morphology is abnormal with normal QRS.
- When atrial tachycardia occurs with 2:1 AV block, the more likely cause is digoxin toxicity.

Ques. What is multifocal atrial tachycardia (MAT)?

Ans. It is a rapid and irregular conduction rhythm originating from two or more sites of atrium. ECG shows at least three different ectopic P waves of different configurations and PR is variable, also rhythm is irregular. It is common in COPD (due to hypoxemia). It may also be found in pulmonary embolism, hypoxemia, hypokalemia, and theophylline toxicity.

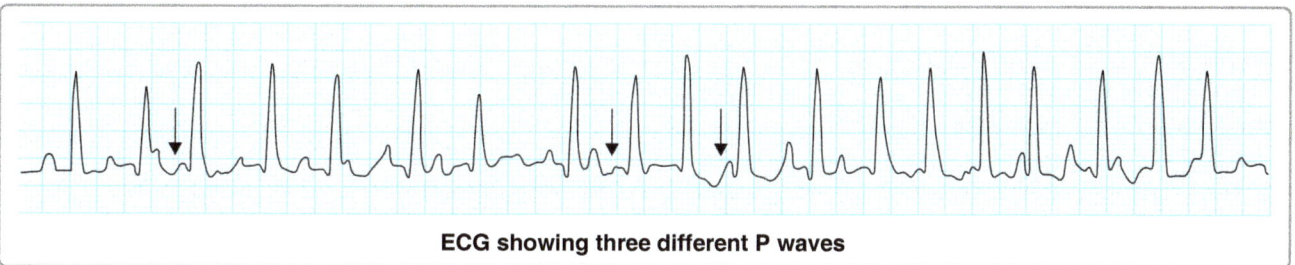

ECG showing three different P waves

Ques. How to treat multifocal atrial tachycardia?

Ans. As follows:
- Treatment of underlying cause such as COPD.
- To reduce the rate, antiarrhythmic drugs should be given.
- If no response or if there is haemodynamic instability, cardioversion may be done.
- In selected cases, transvenous radiofrequency catheter ablation may be needed.

NODAL RHYTHM (JUNCTIONAL RHYTHM)

ECG Criteria of Nodal Rhythm

- Heart rate—40-60 beats/min
- P—small and inverted (P may not be seen, buried in QRS or after QRS)
- PR interval—short

Nodal rhythm may be of three types:
- *High nodal*: Small inverted P before QRS (simulate low atrial ectopic)
- *Mid nodal*: P is not seen (buried in QRS)
- *Low nodal*: P is present after QRS

Ques. What is nodal rhythm?

Ans. When the impulse originates from the AV node, it is called nodal or junctional rhythm. If the rate is high, it is called junctional tachycardia. Usually, it occurs due to depressed activity of the sinoatrial (SA) node.

Nodal rhythm may be transient or permanent.
- Transient—may occur in normal people
- *Also transient or permanent nodal rhythm may occur in*:
    - Digoxin toxicity
    - Ischemic heart disease (commonly, inferior myocardial infarction)
    - Rheumatic myocarditis
    - Myocarditis due to any cause
    - Pericarditis
    - Thyrotoxicosis
    - Cardiac surgery

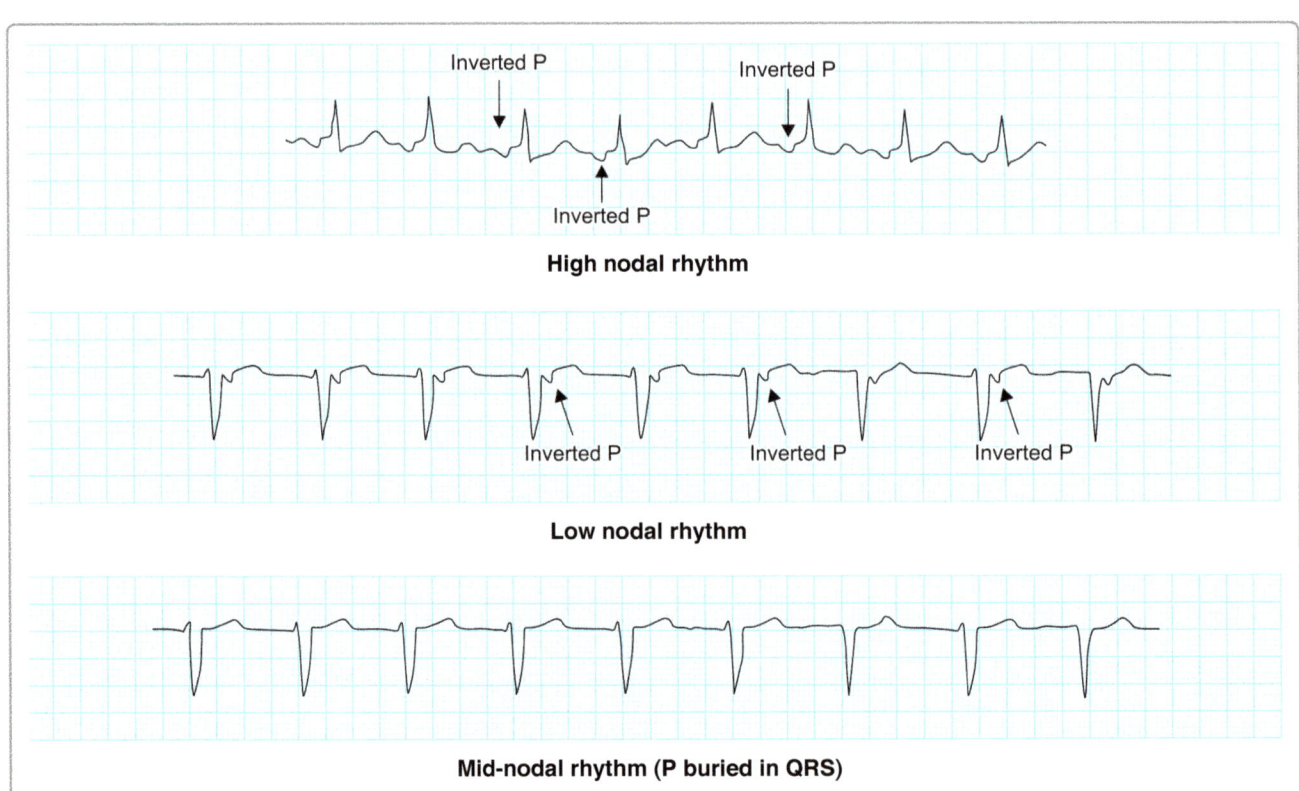

Ques. **What are the presentations of nodal rhythm?**

Ans. May be asymptomatic. There may be:
- Palpitation
- Missing of beat
- Neck pulsation

Ques. **How to treat nodal rhythm?**

Ans. As follows:
- If asymptomatic, no specific drug is necessary
- If it is due to drugs, such as digoxin, it should be stopped
- Treatment of primary cause

WANDERING PACEMAKER

ECG Criteria of Wandering Pacemaker

- P-variable configuration (some inverted, some small, and some upright)
- PR interval—variable
- QRS—normal

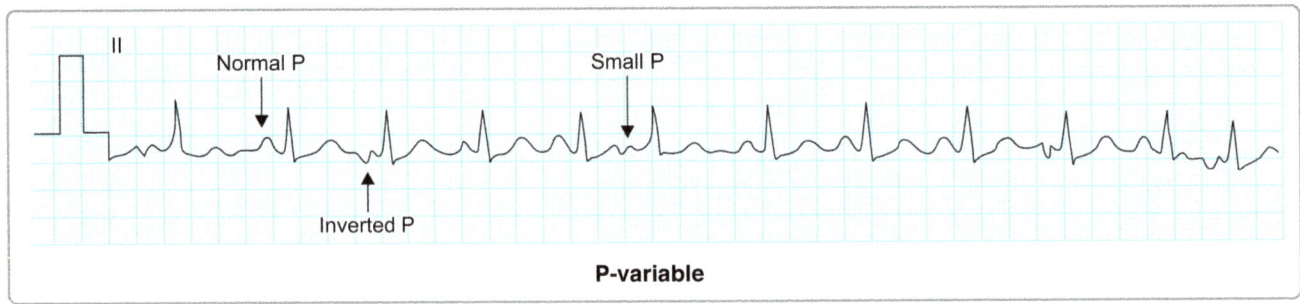

P-variable

Ques. What is wandering pacemaker?

Ans. It is an arrhythmia in which there are multiple pacemaker impulses originating from two or more sites in or around the SA node, the atrium, or the AV junction. The pacemaker wanders from one focus to other. So, P-wave configuration is variable from beat to beat and PR interval is also variable. Upright P wave occurs when the impulse arises from the SA node or high atrial and the P wave is inverted when impulse arises from low atrial or the AV node.

Ques. What are the causes of wandering pacemaker?

Ans. As follows:
- Normal individual (due to increase in vagal tone). It is found in athlete.
- Digoxin toxicity
- Rheumatic carditis
- Chronic lung disease
- Valvular disease (mitral and tricuspid valve disease)

NB: Wandering pacemaker may be associated with sinus arrhythmia.

Ques. What investigations should be done?

Ans. As follows:
- Chest X-ray (CXR)
- Echocardiography
- Serum digoxin level (if the history of taking digoxin)

Ques. How to treat?

Ans. No active treatment in an asymptomatic case.
- Digoxin should be stopped, if the patient is on digoxin.
- Treatment of cause, such as rheumatic carditis.
- *If symptomatic bradycardia*: Injection atropine may be given.

Ques. **What is the prognosis?**

Ans. It is usually benign, often found in a young healthy individual. So, prognosis is good. Actually it is completely harmless, it is insignificant variation of sinus rhythm. Its significant is: It is sometimes confused with significant arrhythmia.

NB: Remember the following points:

- In the presence of wandering pacemaker, rhythm may be irregularly irregular which is confused with atrial fibrillation. However, in wandering pacemaker, there is a distinct P wave which excludes atrial fibrillation, in which P is absent or replaced by fibrillary F wave.
- Sometimes, wandering pacemaker is confused with MAT. In MAT, there are multiple distinct P wave morphology, irregular PP interval, and rapid ventricular rate of 100–150/min. The heart rate is 60–100/min in wandering pacemaker (excludes MAT).

ATRIAL FIBRILLATION

ECG Criteria of Atrial Fibrillation

- *P wave*: Absent (P may be replaced by fibrillary F wave)
- *Rhythm*: Irregularly irregular (RR interval is irregular)
  (Atrial rate is very high and ventricular rate is less)

According to the rate, atrial fibrillation may be of two types:
- *Fast atrial fibrillation*: Heart rate >100 beats/min (also called atrial fibrillation with fast ventricular rate)
- *Slow atrial fibrillation*: Heart rate <100 beats/min (also called atrial fibrillation with slow ventricular rate)

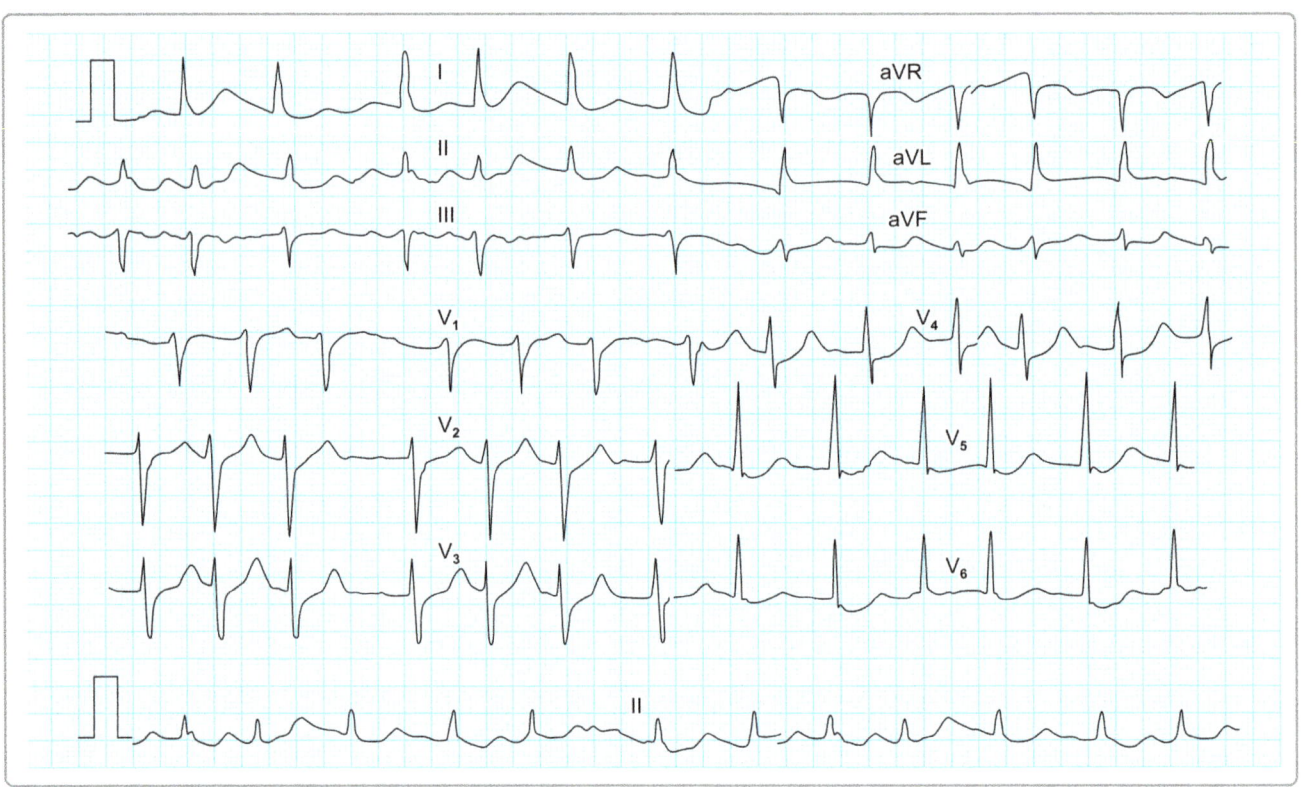

Ques. What is atrial fibrillation?

Ans. It is an arrhythmia where atria beat rapidly, chaotically, and ineffectively, while the ventricles respond at irregular intervals, producing irregularly irregular pulse. Any conditions causing raised atrial pressure, increased atrial muscle mass, atrial fibrosis, inflammation, and infiltration of the atrium can cause atrial fibrillation.

Atria usually fires impulse at the rate of 350–600/min and ventricles respond at irregular intervals usually at the rate of 100–140/min. Many of the atrial impulses reach the AV node in the refractory period. So, not all are conducted.

Ques. What are the types of atrial fibrillation?

Ans. There are three types:
- *Paroxysmal*: Intermittent self-limiting episodes, terminate within 7 days.
- *Persistent*: Fibrillation usually persists >7 days. It can be converted to sinus rhythm by cardioversion.
- *Permanent*: Fibrillation continues indefinitely and conversion to sinus rhythm is not possible by cardioversion.

Ques. **What are the causes of atrial fibrillation?**
Ans. As follows:
- Chronic rheumatic heart disease with valvular lesions, commonly MS
- Coronary artery disease (commonly, acute myocardial infarction)
- Thyrotoxicosis
- Hypertension
- Lone atrial fibrillation (idiopathic in 10% cases)
- Others—ASD, chronic constrictive pericarditis, acute pericarditis, cardiomyopathy, myocarditis, sick sinus syndrome, coronary bypass surgery, valvular surgery, acute chest infection (pneumonia), thoracic surgery, electrolyte imbalance (hypokalemia, hyponatremia), alcohol, and pulmonary embolism.

NB: Remember the following points:
- First five causes should always be mentioned sequentially at the top of the list.
- Mention the causes of atrial fibrillation according to the age of the patient (see below).

Ques. **If the patient is young, what are the causes of atrial fibrillation?**
Ans. As follows:
- Chronic rheumatic heart disease with valvular lesions, commonly MS
- Thyrotoxicosis
- Others: ASD, acute pericarditis, myocarditis, and pneumonia

Ques. **If the patient is middle aged or elderly, what are the causes of atrial fibrillation?**
Ans. As follows:
- Coronary artery disease (commonly acute myocardial infarction)
- Thyrotoxicosis
- Hypertension
- Lone atrial fibrillation (idiopathic in 10% cases)
- *Others*: See above (unusual or less in chronic rheumatic heart disease)

Ques. **What are the causes of temporary or paroxysmal atrial fibrillation?**
Ans. As follows:
- Acute myocardial infarction
- Myocarditis (due to any cause)
- Pneumonia
- Electrolyte imbalance

Ques. **What are the complications of atrial fibrillation?**
Ans. As follows:
- Systemic and pulmonary embolism (systemic from left atrium and pulmonary from right atrium). Annual risk is 5% (1–12%).
- Heart failure

Ques. **What is lone atrial fibrillation?**
Ans. Lone atrial fibrillation means atrial fibrillation without any cause. Genetic predisposition may be responsible. It is related to electrophysiological phenomenon (triggers) in a structurally normal atria.
- 50% patients with paroxysmal atrial fibrillation and 20% with persistent or permanent atrial fibrillation have no cause and heart is normal.
- Lone atrial fibrillation usually occurs below 60 years of age.
- It may be intermittent, later may become permanent.
- *Prognosis*: Usually life span is normal, low risk of CVD (0.5% per year).

ECG in Medical Practice

Ques. **What history would you like to take in atrial fibrillation?**

Ans. I would take the history of:
- Rheumatic fever
- Ischemic heart disease
- History of thyrotoxicosis
- Other history of any disease (according to cause)

Ques. **What are the clinical findings of atrial fibrillation?**

Ans. As follows:
- *Pulse*: Irregularly irregular (irregular in rate, rhythm and volume)
- *Blood pressure (BP)*: It may be hypertensive
- Examination of heart (heart rate to see pulse deficit, mitral valvular, or other cardiac disease)
- Thyroid status (warm sweaty hands, tremor, tachycardia, exophthalmos, and thyroid gland size)

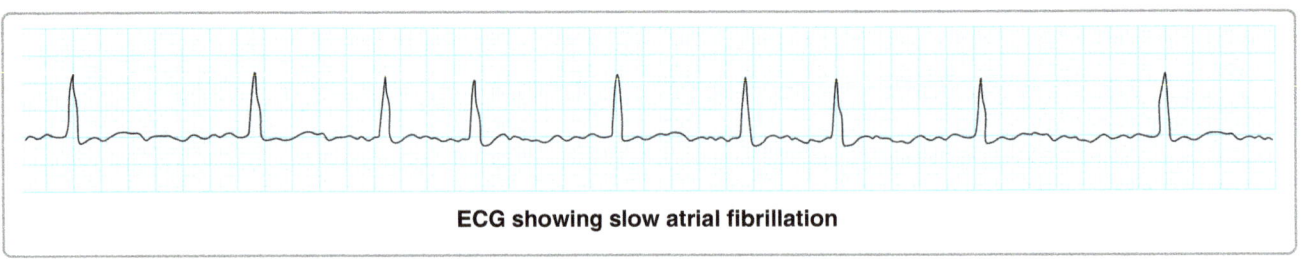

ECG showing slow atrial fibrillation

Ques. **If a patient with atrial fibrillation is unconscious, what is the likely cause?**

Ans. Cerebral embolism (usually with right-sided hemiplegia).

Ques. **How to treat atrial fibrillation?**

Ans. Aim of treatment is as follows:
- Control of heart rate
- Restoration of sinus rhythm and prevention of recurrence
- Treatment of primary cause

Acute management: If atrial fibrillation is due to an acute illness, such as alcohol toxicity, chest infection, or hyperthyroidism, this should be treated, which restores sinus rhythm. Otherwise, following treatment should be given:
- *To control rate*: Digoxin, β-blocker, or calcium channel blocker (verapamil or diltiazem) may be given.
- *If no response*:
    - Medical cardioversion by intravenous infusion of antiarrhythmic drug such as flecainide, propafenone, vernakalant, or amiodarone. Oral flecainide or propafenone may be given.
    - *If no response*: DC shock should be given. To prevent risk of thromboembolism, patient should be anticoagulated with warfarin or dabigatran 3 weeks before cardioversion (unless atrial fibrillation is less than 48 hours) and at least 4 weeks after the procedure.

Long-term treatment is given according to the type:
1. Paroxysmal atrial fibrillation:
    - *If asymptomatic*: Does not require any treatment, follow-up the case.
    - *If troublesome symptoms are present*: β-blocker. Other drugs, flecainide or propafenone, may be given.
    - Amiodarone is effective in prevention. Low-dose aspirin to prevent thromboembolism.
    - *If bradycardia is present (in SA disease)*: Permanent over drive atrial pacing (60% effective).
    - *In some intractable cases*: Radiofrequency ablation is required, if no structural heart disease (70% effective).

2. Persistent atrial fibrillation:
   - *Control of heart rate*: β-blocker, digoxin, or calcium channel blocker (verapamil and diltiazem). Combination of digoxin and atenolol may be used.
   - *To control rhythm*: DC cardioversion may be done safely. It may be repeated, if relapse occurs. Concomitant use of β-blocker or amiodarone may be used to prevent recurrence.
   - *If no response*: Transvenous radiofrequency ablation may be done (it induces complete heart block). So, permanent pacemaker should be given. This is known as *"patch and ablate strategy."*
3. Permanent atrial fibrillation: As in persistent atrial fibrillation.

Ques. **What is the role of anticoagulant in atrial fibrillation?**

Ans. Usually, warfarin is given to patients who are at risk of stroke. Target international normalized ratio (INR) is 2–3. It reduces stroke in two-thirds of cases. Aspirin reduces stroke in one-fifth of cases. Anticoagulation is indicated in atrial fibrillation related to rheumatic MS or in mechanical prosthetic heart valve. In patients with nonvalvular atrial fibrillation (in the absence of MS, artificial heart valves or mitral valve repair), a scoring system known as CHA_2DS_2-VASc is used to determine the need for anticoagulation. CHA_2DS_2-VASc risk score for assessing the risk of stroke and for selecting antithrombotic therapy for patients with atrial fibrillation.

\multicolumn{3}{c}{CHA_2DS_2-VASc risk score system}		
Risk factors		*Score/points*
C	Congestive heart failure	1
H	Hypertension	1
A_2	Age ≥75	2
D	Diabetes mellitus	1
S_2	Stroke/ transient ischemic attack (TIA)/thromboembolism	2
V	Vascular disease (aorta, coronary, or peripheral arteries)	1
A	Age 65–74 years	1
Sc	Sex category: Female	1

Annual risk of stroke:
- 0 points = 0% risk: No prophylaxis
- 1 point = 1.3% risk: Anticoagulant (oral) or aspirin
- 2+ points = 2.2% risk: Oral anticoagulant

ASHMAN PHENOMENON (ASHMAN BEATS)

Definition

It is a type of aberrant ventricular conduction that occurs during atrial fibrillation when a long RR interval is followed by a short RR interval.

ECG in Ashman phenomenon shows:
- Atrial fibrillation
- Followed by supraventricular impulse which are aberrantly conducted in ventricles, resulting wide QRS
- Confuses with ventricular ectopics, i.e., wide QRS in between atrial fibrillation
- Ashman beats are aberrantly conducted complex, not premature ventricular complex (PVC)
- Wide QRS has a RBBB pattern
- Ashman phenomenon is typically seen with atrial fibrillation but can also occur with other supraventricular arrhythmias.

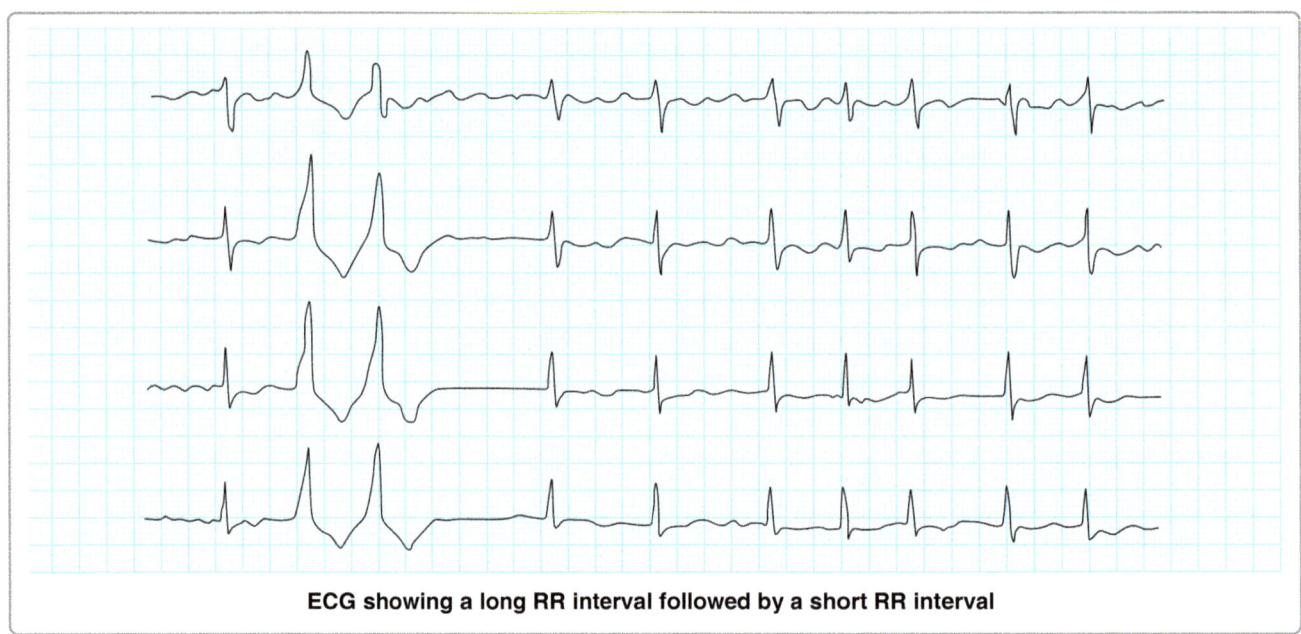

ECG showing a long RR interval followed by a short RR interval

Ques. What are the presentations?
Ans. It is usually asymptomatic.
Ques. How to treat?
Ans. As follows:
- No specific therapy
- Any underlying cardiac problem, if present, should be treated
- Correction of electrolyte abnormality

ATRIAL FLUTTER

ECG Criteria of Atrial Flutter

- P—saw-tooth appearance (normal P is replaced by flutter or F wave. It is better seen in lead II, III, aVF, and V_1).
- RR—regular (may be irregular, when there is variable block)
  (Atrial rate—250–350 beats/min, ventricular rate—variable, may be 2:1, 3:1, and 4:1, it is then called flutter with variable block).

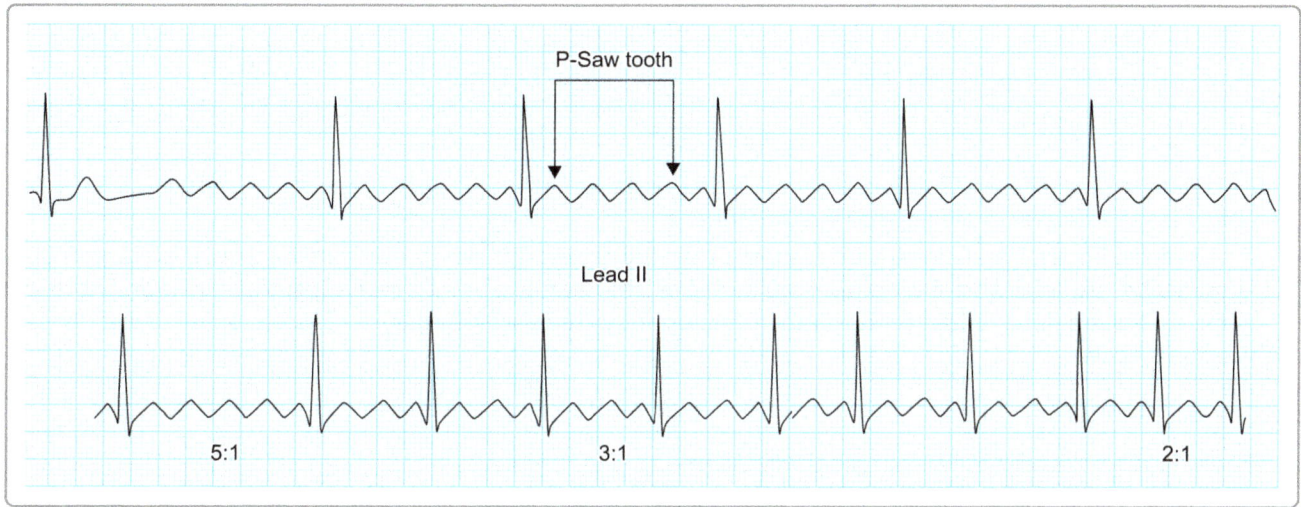

Ques. What is atrial flutter? What are the causes of atrial flutter?

Ans. Atrial flutter is characterized by large reentry circuit within the right atrium, usually encircling the tricuspid annulus. For causes, see in atrial fibrillation (same causes).

Ques. What is the mechanism of atrial flutter?

Ans. As follows:
- It is commonly due to macro-re-entrant circuit with in the right atrium and shares many etiological factors which are found in atrial fibrillation.

Ques. How to treat atrial flutter?

Ans. As follows:
- To control the heart rate: Digoxin, β-blocker, or verapamil may be used. Amiodarone, propafenone, or flecainide may be used and these can be used to prevent recurrence.
- If no response and the patient has troublesome symptoms: DC cardioversion or atrial overdrive pacing.
- In persistent or troublesome symptoms: Radiofrequency catheter ablation.
- Digoxin sometimes converts flutter to atrial fibrillation, due to shortening of atrial refractory period. This may be followed by conversion to normal rhythm, when digoxin is stopped.

Ques. What are appearance of wave of atrial flutter?

Ans. As follows:
- Individual flutter wave may be symmetrical resembling P waves
- Flutter waves may be asymmetrical resembling 'saw-tooth shaped'

NB: Occasionally, atrial fibrillation and flutter may be present together, it is called flutter fibrillation.

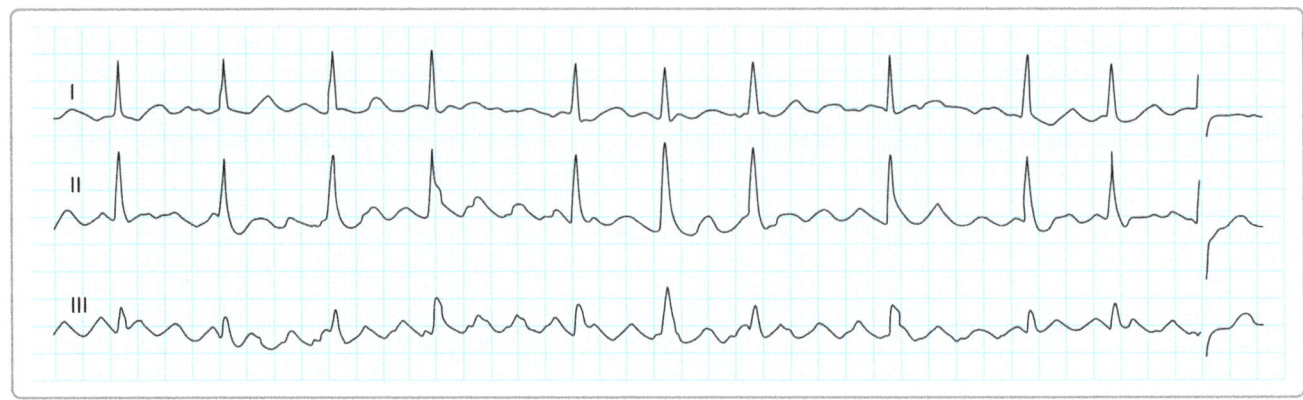

Ques. What is the differential diagnosis of atrial flutter?

Ans. When atrial flutter is associated with regular 2:1 AV block, it is difficult to differentiate from supraventricular or sinus tachycardia, because flutter waves are buried in QRS complex. In such case, diagnosis can be done by carotid sinus massage or intravenous adenosine which temporarily increases the degree of AV block and reveals the flutter waves (F wave).

NB: Remember the following points:
- Atrial flutter is always associated with organic heart disease.
- Drugs which can restore and maintain sinus rhythm are—sotalol, flecainide, disopyramide, and propafenone.
- DC cardioversion is the easiest way to convert sinus rhythm.

Chapter 2: ECG Changes in Different Diseases

ECTOPIC BEAT

ECG Criteria of Ectopic Beat

In ECG, sequence is as follows:
- *Normal* beat - *Short* pause - *Ectopic* beat - *Long* pause - *Strong* beat.

Ques. What is ectopic beat?

Ans. Ectopic beat or extrasystole is a premature extra beat that comes earlier than the normal beat. It arises from abnormal focus from the atria, the AV node, or the ventricle. By definition, ectopic beats are premature. Thus interval between the ectopic beat and the preceding normal beat is shorter, which is followed by long pause and strong beats.

Ques. What are the types of ectopic beat?

Ans. *There are three types according to their site of origin*:
- Atrial
- Nodal
- Ventricular

Atrial ectopics may be:
- *High atrial*: P is upright in L_I and aVF.
- *Low atrial*: P is inverted in L_{II}, L_{III}, and aVF (confuses with high nodal ectopic).

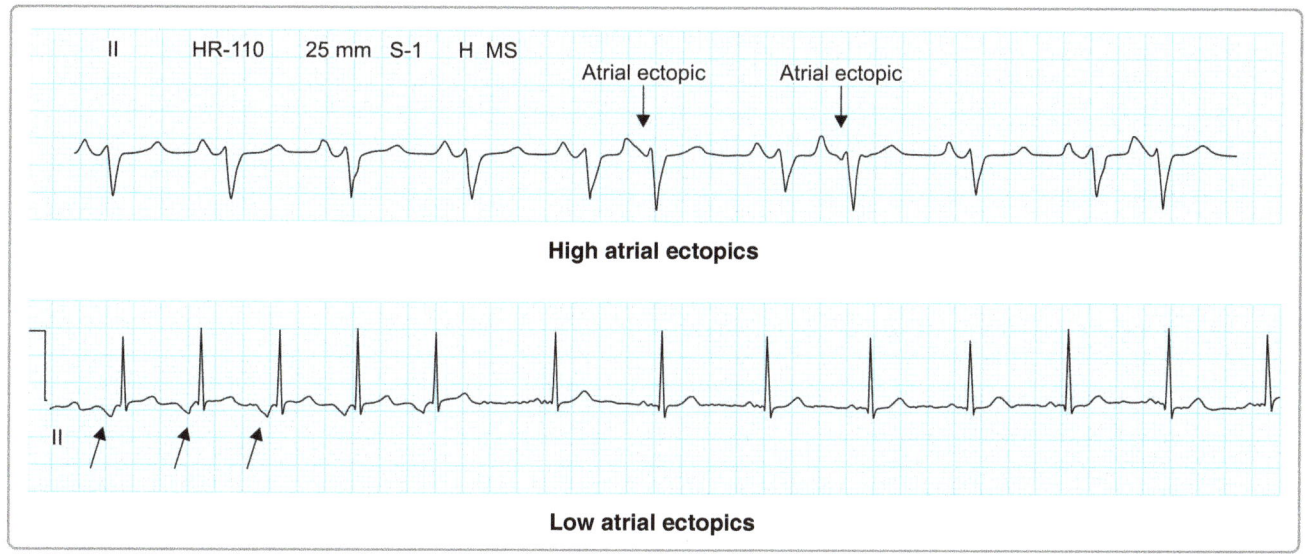

Nodal ectopics may be of three types:
- High nodal (P is inverted, confuses with low atrial)
- Mid nodal (P is not seen, buried in QRS)
- Low nodal (P is seen after QRS)

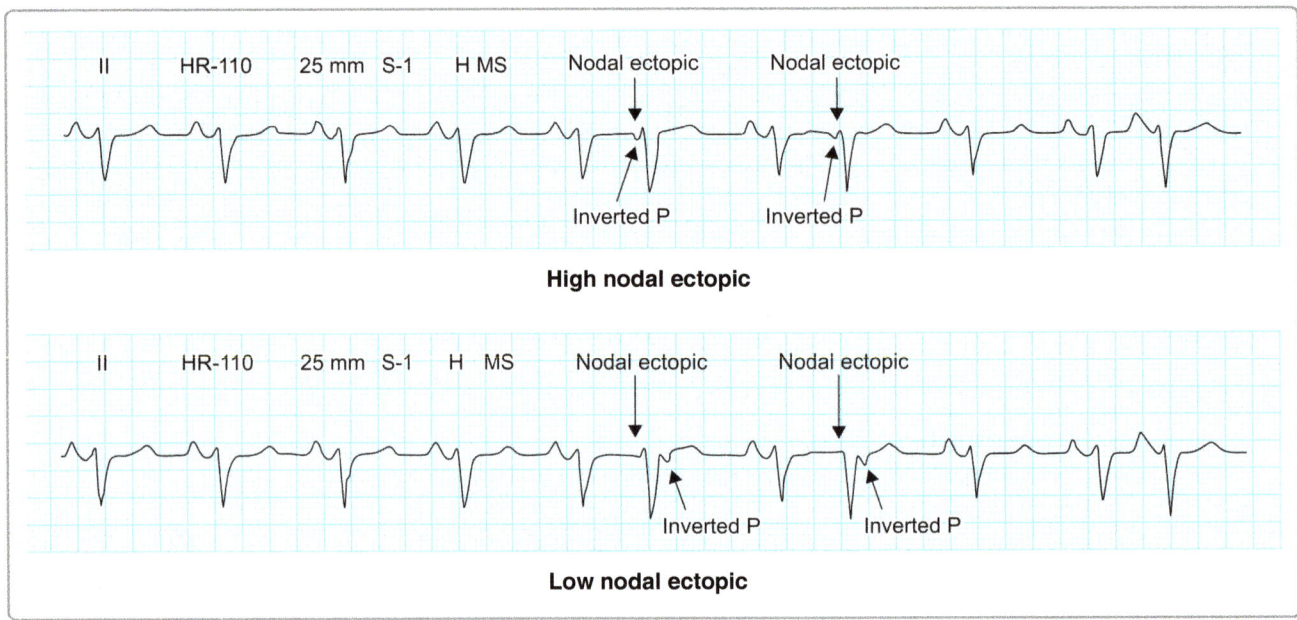

Ques. What are the causes of ectopic beat?

Ans. It may be cardiac and noncardiac.
- *Cardiac cause:*
  - Normally found in young adults, due to anxiety, excess caffeine, and alcohol
  - Acute myocardial infection
  - Myocarditis
  - Cardiomyopathy
  - Valvular heart disease
  - Mitral valve prolapse
  - Hypertensive heart disease
- *Noncardiac cause:*
  - Electrolyte imbalance (especially hypokalemia)
  - Hypocalcemia
  - Hypomagnesemia
  - Digoxin toxicity
  - Hypoxemia
  - Surgery

Ques. How to treat ectopic beat?

Ans. As follows:
- If it is asymptomatic, no treatment is needed
- If it is due to any drugs such as digoxin it should be stopped
- Electrolyte imbalance, if any, should be corrected
- Treatment of primary cause should be done

ATRIAL ECTOPIC

ECG Criteria of Atrial Ectopic

- P—small or inverted (abnormal shape)
- PR interval—short (followed by wide pause)
- PP interval—irregular
  (When atrial ectopic is associated with tachycardia, it is called chaotic or MAT. Atrial ectopic may not be followed by QRS. It is called blocked or nonconducted atrial ectopic).

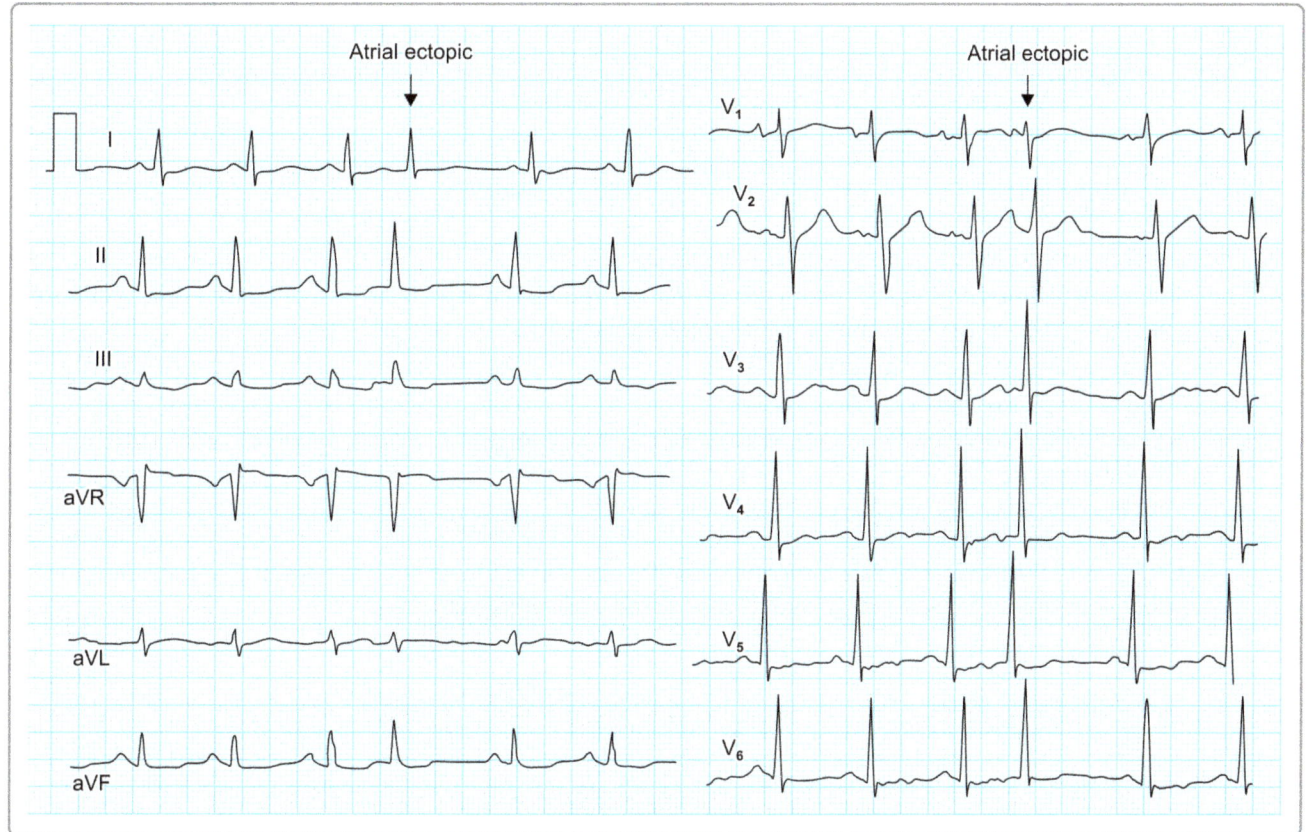

Ques. What are the causes of atrial ectopics?

Ans. As follows:
- Normal people found with anxiety, stress, excess intake of tea, coffee, and smoking
- Any organic heart disease (myocarditis and cardiomyopathy)
- Coronary artery disease
- Digoxin toxicity
- Electrolyte imbalance (e.g., hypokalemia)
- Hypomagnesemia
- *Drug*: Salbutamol and salmeterol
- COPD (usually MAT, due to hypoxemia)

Ques. What is the prognosis and how to treat?

Ans. It is usually benign. Avoidance of tea, coffee, alcohol, anxiety, and stress. Treatment of primary cause, if any.

VENTRICULAR ECTOPIC

ECG Criteria of Ventricular Ectopic

- P—absent
- QRS—wide >0.12 second (3 small squares)
- T—opposite to major deflection

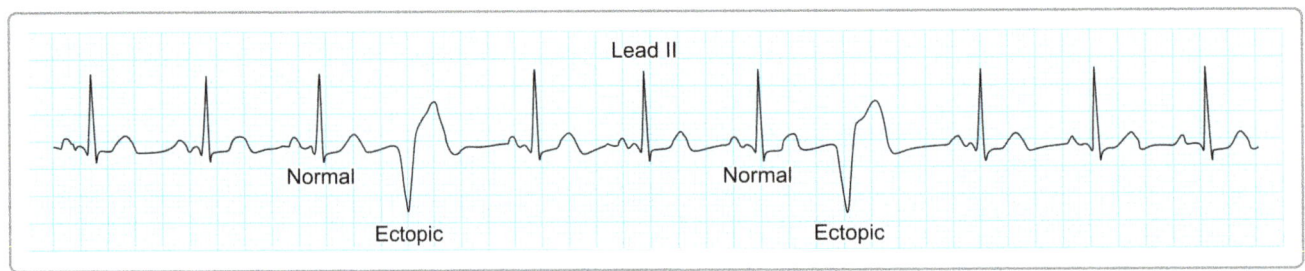

Ques. What are the presentations of ventricular ectopics?

Ans. The patient is usually asymptomatic, but may complain of irregular or extra heartbeat or missed beat or abnormally strong beat (due to increase in output of postectopic sinus beat).

Ques. What are the types of ventricular ectopics?

Ans. Ventricular ectopics may be of different types:
- *Unifocal*: Similar configuration of ectopics in all leads and originates from a single ectopic ventricular focus (QRS is similar).
- *Multifocal*: Variable configuration of ectopics in same lead, because ectopics originate from different focus of ventricle (QRS is variable).
- *Interpolated ventricular ectopics*: It means when ventricular ectopics occur between two normal sinus beats without compensatory pause (it is usually associated with sinus bradycardia).

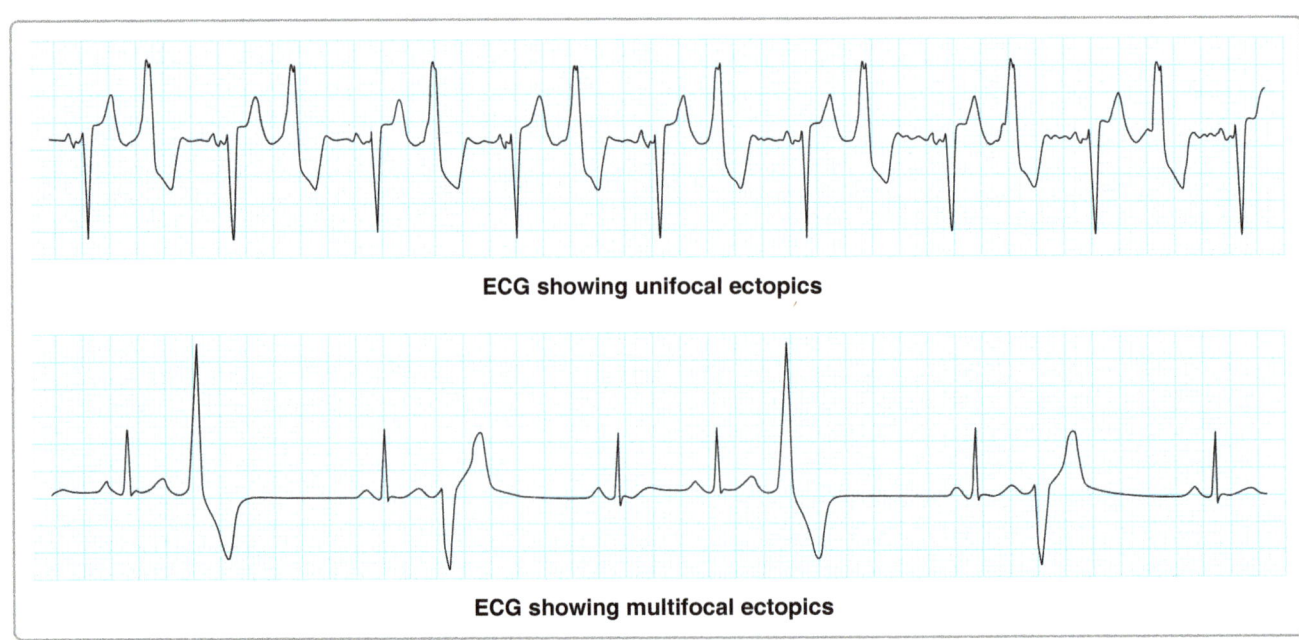

ECG showing unifocal ectopics

ECG showing multifocal ectopics

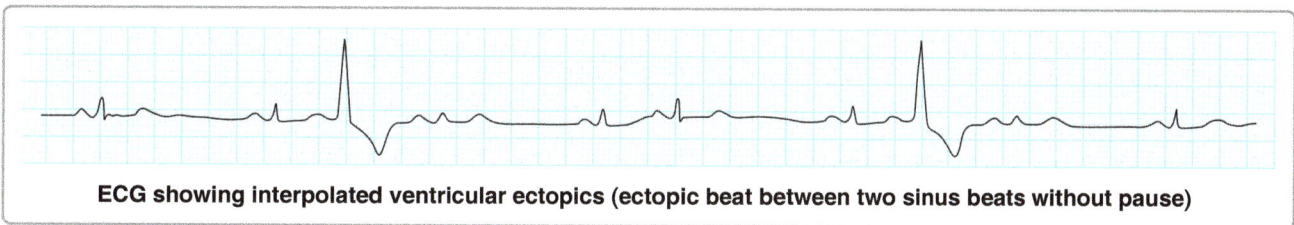
ECG showing interpolated ventricular ectopics (ectopic beat between two sinus beats without pause)

Other Types

- *Couplet*: Two ventricular ectopics in a row, multifocal.
- *Triplet*: Three ventricular ectopics in a row (runs of ectopic, three or more ventricular ectopics in a row, may be taken as ventricular tachycardia).
- *Runs of ectopics*: Consecutive multiple (>3) ventricular ectopics, also called Salvos.
- *Ventricular bigeminy*: Every one normal beat followed by ventricular ectopic (See later page).
- *Ventricular trigeminy*: Every two normal beats followed by ventricular ectopic (See later page).
- *Ventricular quadrigeminy*: Every three normal beats followed by ventricular ectopic (See later page).

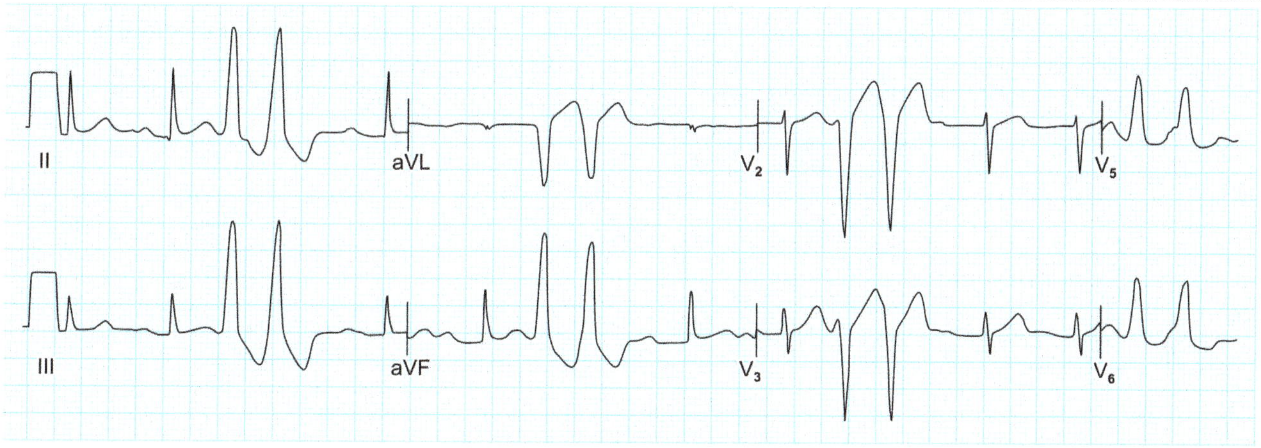

ECG showing couplet ectopics

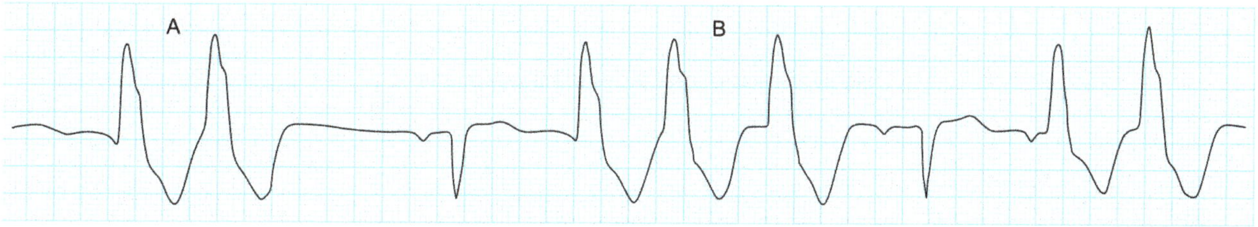

ECG showing couplet (A) and triplet (B) ectopics

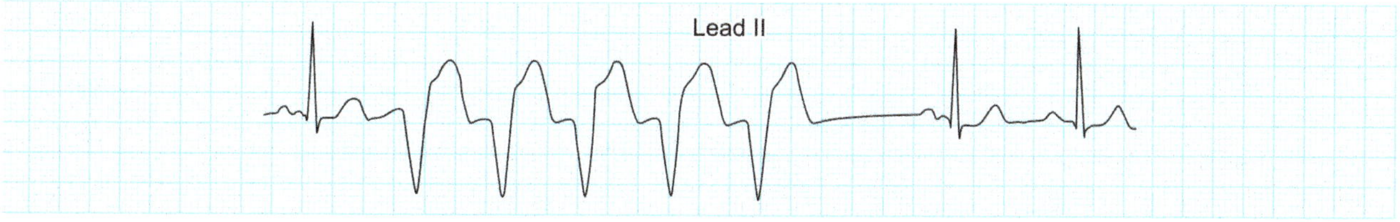

ECG showing runs of ventricular ectopics

NB: Remember the following points:

- Ventricular ectopics originating in left ventricle resembles RBBB pattern.
- Ventricular ectopics originating in right ventricle resembles left bundle branch block (LBBB) pattern.

Ques. What are the causes of ventricular ectopic?

Ans. As follows:
- Normally in young adults, also in anxiety, excess caffeine, and alcohol
- Acute myocardial infarction
- Myocarditis
- Cardiomyopathy
- Valvular heart disease
- Mitral valve prolapse
- Hypertensive heart disease
- Electrolyte imbalance (especially hypokalemia)
- Digoxin toxicity
- Hypoxemia

Ques. What is R on T phenomenon?

Ans. It means R wave of ventricular ectopic occurs on or near the peak of previous T wave. It is common in acute myocardial infarction (rare in other case). This is also called malignant ectopic, as it may induce ventricular fibrillation or ventricular tachycardia and sudden death. R on T phenomenon may be found in:
- Ventricular premature complex (VPC) after acute myocardial infarction
- VPC with underlying QT interval prolongation
- Electrical cardioversion during digoxin therapy
- Very premature stimuli during artificial pacing

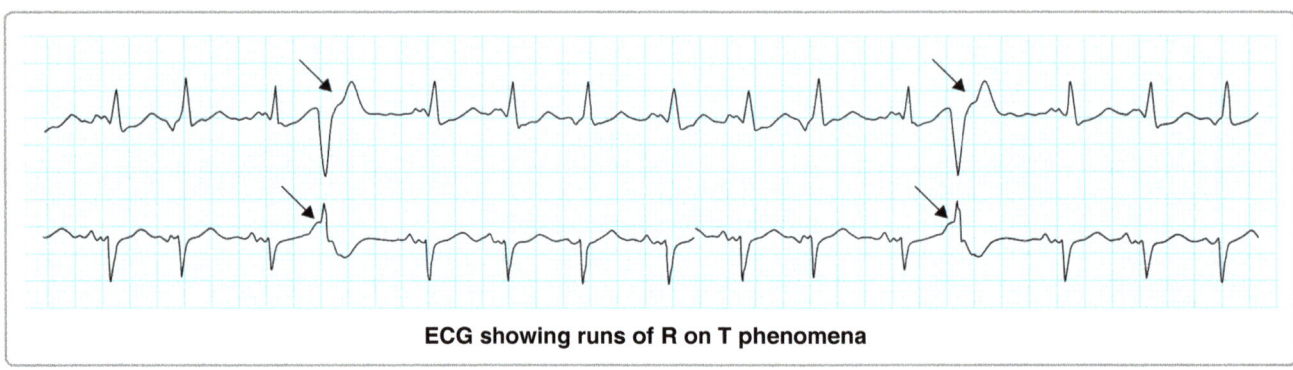

ECG showing runs of R on T phenomena

Ques. When ventricular ectopics are considered as dangerous or malignant?

Ans. VPCs are considered to be "dangerous" or "malignant" in the followings cases:
- Occurring frequently (six or more beats/minute)
- In showers with runs of ventricular tachycardia
- In couplets or VPCs in bigeminal rhythm
- With short coupling interval (R-on-T phenomenon)
- >0.14 second wide, bizarre, or multifocal
- Associated with serious organic heart disease and left ventricular dysfunction

Ques. How to assess the severity for ventricular ectopic?

Ans. Severity of ectopic is classified on the basis of *Lown classification*, as follows:

Category	Degree of ectopic
Class 0	No ectopic
Class 1	<30/hour
Class 2	>30/hour
Class 3	Multiform VPCs
Class 4A	Couplets
Class 4B	Runs of three or more
Class 5	R-on-T phenomenon

Ques. How to treat ventricular ectopics?

Ans. As follows:
- *In a normal person, if no organic heart disease and in an asymptomatic case*: No treatment.
- *If the patient is symptomatic*: Reassurance and β-blocker may be used.
- *If ectopics are very frequent*: Left ventricular dysfunction may develop and if ectopic stem from single focus, especially from right ventricle: catheter ablation can be very effective.
- *With organic heart disease*: Treatment of primary cause should be done.
- If VPCs occur after myocardial infarction, lidocaine or amiodarone may be used. Also, these are effective after cardiac surgery or catheterization.
- *If due to digoxin toxicity*: It should be stopped. Correction of electrolytes. If persistence, phenytoin sodium may be used.

NB: Remember the following points:
- Ventricular ectopics may be found in normal people, incidence increases with age.
- Ventricular ectopic in normal heart is prominent at rest and disappears with exercise. No treatment is necessary, occasionally β-blocker may be given for palpitation. Prognosis is good.
- Multifocal ventricular ectopics and also in pairs are always abnormal. It indicates serious myocardial disease.

VENTRICULAR BIGEMINY

ECG Criteria of Ventricular Bigeminy

- Every normal beat is followed by an ectopic beat.

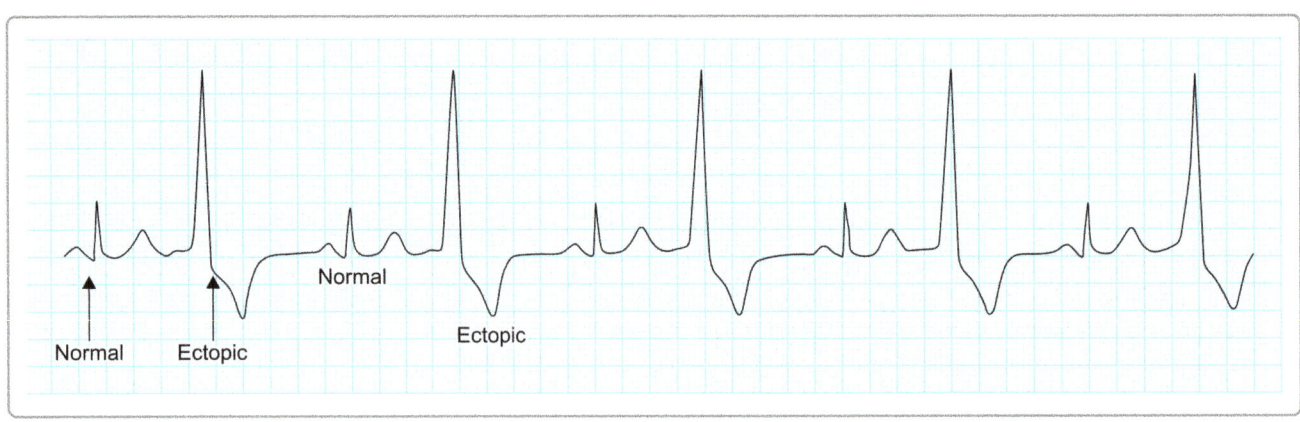

Ques. What are the causes of bigeminy?

Ans. As follows:
- Digoxin toxicity
- Myocarditis
- Cardiomyopathy
- After acute myocardial infarction
- Electrolyte imbalance (e.g., hypokalemia)
- Hypoxemia

Ques. What are the presentations of ventricular bigeminy?

Ans. Usually asymptomatic. Other features are:
- Palpitation
- Missing of beat
- *Pulse*: Drop beat present
- Features of primary disease

Ques. What investigation should be done?

Ans. As follows:
- ECG
- CXR posteroanterior (PA) view
- S. electrolytes
- S. calcium
- S. magnesium
- Echocardiogram
- S. digoxin level (if the patient was getting it)
- Other investigations according to suspicion of causes

Ques. How to treat ventricular bigeminy?

Ans. As follows:
- If due to any offending drug, it should be stopped.
- Correction of electrolytes, especially hypokalemia (also hyperkalemia and hypomagnesemia).
- Treatment of primary cause or any organic heart disease.
- If asymptomatic, no other treatment.
- If symptomatic, β-blocker should be given. Antiarrhythmic drugs should be avoided as they may worsen the prognosis.
- Reassurance should be given.

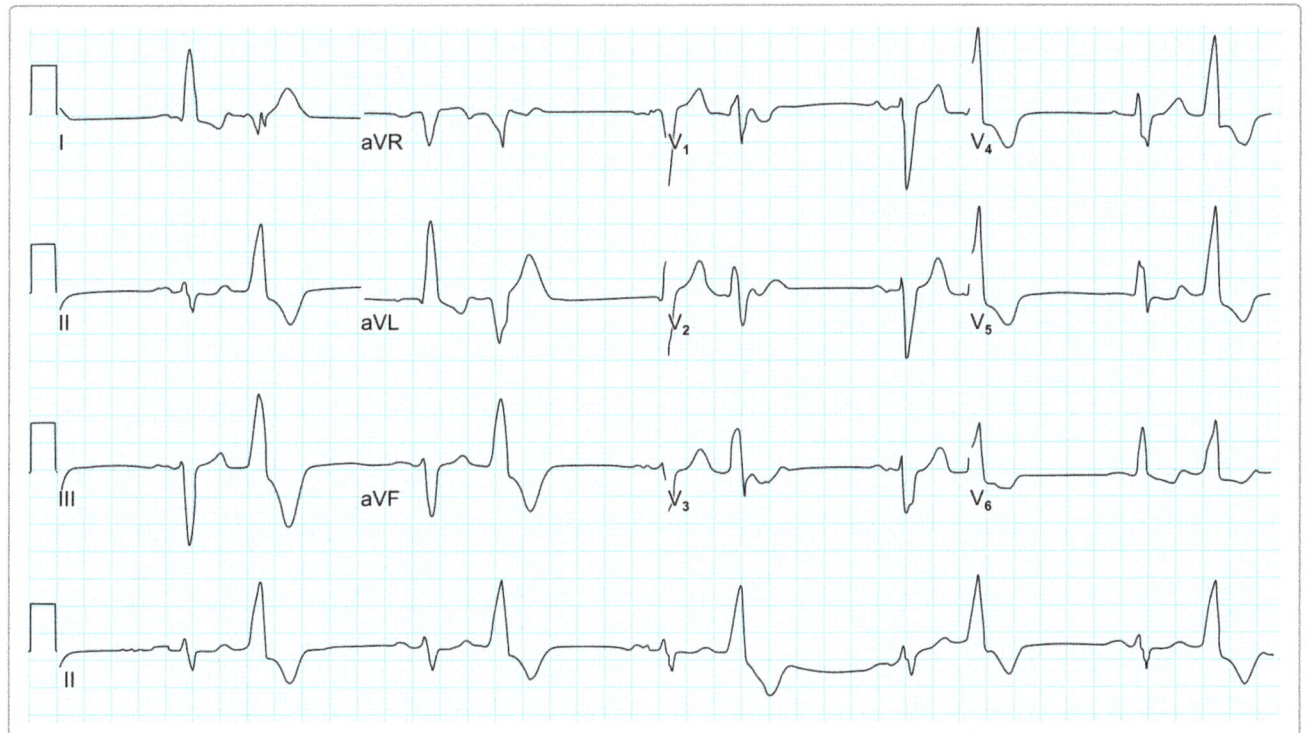

VENTRICULAR TRIGEMINY

ECG Criteria of Ventricular Trigeminy

- Every two normal beats are followed by an ectopic beat.

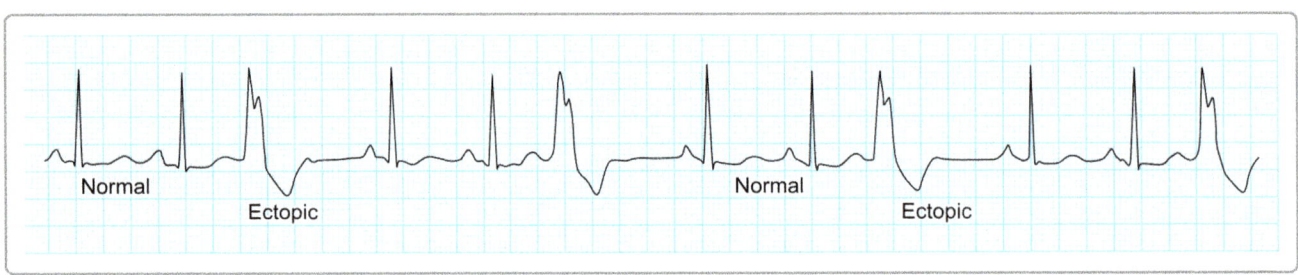

NB: Causes, investigations, and treatment as in bigeminy.

VENTRICULAR QUADRIGEMINY

ECG Criteria of Ventricular Quadrigeminy

Every three normal beats are followed by an ectopic beat.

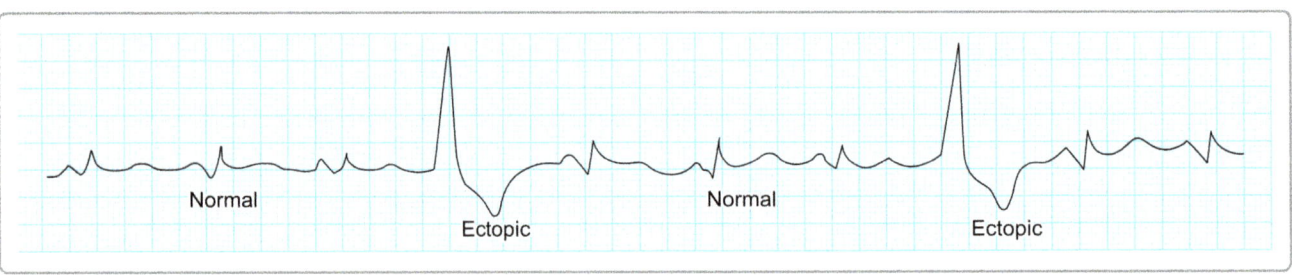

NB: Causes, investigations, and treatment as in bigeminy.

VENTRICULAR PENTAGEMINY

ECG Criteria of Ventricular Pentageminy

- Every four normal beats are followed by an ectopic beat.

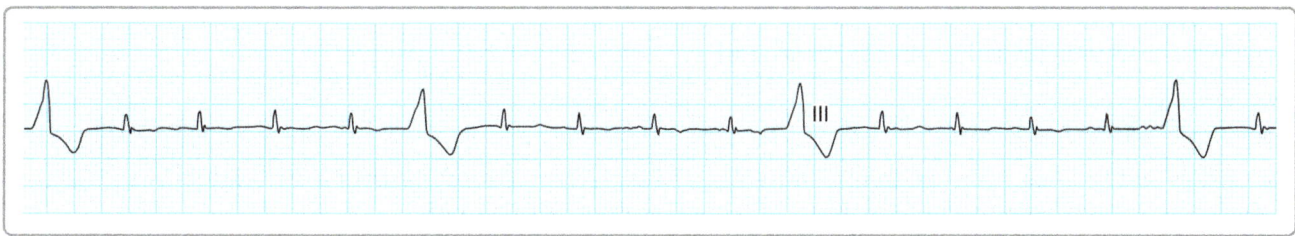

NB: Causes, investigations, and treatment as in bigeminy.

VENTRICULAR HEXAGEMINY

ECG Criteria of Ventricular Hexageminy

- Every five normal beats are followed by an ectopic beat.

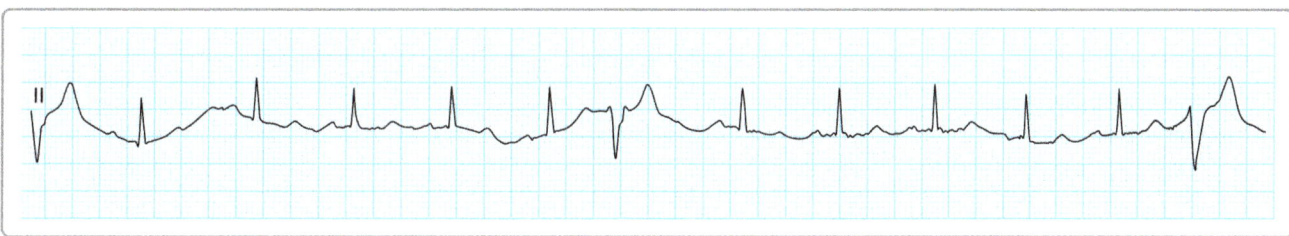

NB: Causes, investigations, and treatment as in bigeminy.

VENTRICULAR TACHYCARDIA

ECG Criteria of Ventricular Tachycardia

- P wave—absent (dissociated P wave may be seen)
- Three or more successive extra systoles in succession
- QRS—broad >0.14 second, abnormal, or bizarre pattern
- Rate >100 beats/min (usually, 140–220 beats/min)

Other Findings

- Occasional *capture beat* is present (normal sinus P, QRS, and T in between ventricular tachycardia).
- *Fusion beat* (conducted sinus impulse fuses with impulse from tachycardia).
- QRS: In chest leads (V_1 to V_6), either all positive or all negative (called ventricular *concordance*).

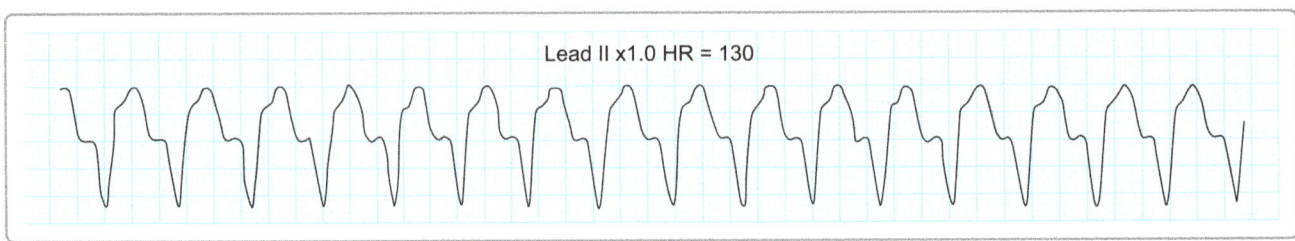

Ques. What is ventricular tachycardia?

Ans. It is defined as three or more successive extra systoles in succession with a rate >100/min.

Ques. What are the causes of ventricular tachycardia?

Ans. As follows:
- Acute myocardial infarction
- Myocarditis
- Cardiomyopathy
- Chronic ischemic heart disease (especially with poor left ventricular function)
- Ventricular aneurysm
- Mitral valve prolapse
- Electrolyte imbalance (mainly hypokalemia and hypomagnesemia)
- Postcardiac surgery
- Drugs (digoxin, quinidine, and theophylline)
- Idiopathic

Ques. What is the differential diagnosis of ventricular tachycardia?

Ans. Ventricular tachycardia is confused with SVT with bundle branch block or WPW syndrome (aberrant conduction). Ventricular tachycardia is more common.

Ques. How to differentiate between ventricular tachycardia and supraventricular tachycardia with bundle branch block?

Ans. In ECG, points suggesting ventricular tachycardia are as follows:
- History of myocardial infarction
- QRS >0.14 second
- Extreme LAD
- AV dissociation (dissociated P wave may be seen)
- Narrow QRS capture complex beat (normal sinus beat in the middle of ventricular tachycardia)

- Fusion beat (conducted sinus impulse fuses with impulse from ventricular tachycardia)
- Ventricular concordance (either all positive or all negative in chest leads)
- Bifid R in V_1 with a tall first peak in V_1 and deep S in V_6
- RR interval is regular
- No response to carotid sinus massage or IV adenosine (but it terminates SVT)

NB: When there is doubt, it is safe to manage as ventricular tachycardia.

Ques. What are the types of ventricular tachycardia?
Ans. *Usually, there are two types*:
- Sustained ventricular tachycardia (lasts >30 seconds). Heart rate is 150–250/min.
- Nonsustained ventricular tachycardia (NSVT) (lasts <30 seconds), consists of short salvos (3 or more).

Ventricular tachycardia may also be:
- *Monomorphic*: All ventricular beats have same configuration in same lead, the most common form of sustained ventricular tachycardia.
- *Polymorphic*: Ventricular beats have changing configuration. It may be of irregular rhythm, with beat-to-beat variation in QRS complex.

Ques. What is NSVT?
Ans. It is defined as ventricular tachycardia >3 or more consecutive beats, but lasts <30 seconds, at a rate >100/min.
- NSVT that occurs in normal heart (6%)—no treatment is necessary.
- NSVT with heart disease—treated with β-blocker. In some cases, especially with myocardial infarction and ejection fraction 30% or less, implantable cardioverter defibrillator (ICD) may be helpful.

Ques. How to treat sustained ventricular tachycardia?
Ans. As follows:
- If the patient is hemodynamically unstable (such as hypotension, systolic <90 or heart failure)—cardioversion (DC shock) is the treatment of choice.
- If the patient is hemodynamically stable—bolus IV amiodarone (5 mg/kg body weight over 1 hour) should be given, followed by continuous IV infusion 1,200 mg over 24 hours (about 15–20 mg/kg/day). *Or alternately IV lignocaine 100 mg bolus (1–2 mg/kg) can be used. It is followed by lignocaine infusion 2–4 mg/min for 24–36 hours. It depresses left ventricular function, may cause hypotension or acute heart failure.*
- If all fails—cardioversion should be done.
- To prevent recurrence—β-blocker and oral amiodarone may be used.
- Correction of hypokalemia, hypomagnesemia, hypoxemia, and acidosis should be done.
- If all fail—automatic ICD device or radiofrequency ablation of focus of ventricular tachycardia should be done.

Ques. What is accelerated idioventricular rhythm (AIVR)?
Ans. Monomorphic ventricular tachycardia with a rate <100/min (usually 40–100/min), also called slow ventricular tachycardia. Commonly, it is found in acute myocardial infarction.
- AIVR is most commonly seen within the first 48–72 hours of acute myocardial infarction and frequently after successful reperfusion during acute myocardial infarction (following thrombolysis or angioplasty). Also, after cardiac surgery.
- It is a benign arrhythmia, usually asymptomatic, transient, and self-limiting and does not require any treatment.
- It is differentiated from ventricular tachycardia by the ventricular rate only.

Ques. What are the causes of wide-complex tachycardia?
Ans. As follows:
- Ventricular tachycardia
- SVT with aberrant conduction
- WPW syndrome

ECG in Medical Practice

Ques. What is bidirectional ventricular tachycardia?

Ans. When ventricular tachycardia is associated with two different QRS complexes alternating with every other beat, it is called bidirectional ventricular tachycardia. It may occur in severe digoxin toxicity, prognosis is grave in that case.

Ques. What is the mechanism of ventricular tachycardia?

Ans. It is caused by abnormal automaticity or triggered activity in ischemic tissue or by reentry within scarred ventricular tissue.

Ques. Can ventricular tachycardia occur in a normal heart?

Ans. Ventricular tachycardia can occur in a healthy heart, called *normal heart ventricular tachycardia*. It is usually due to abnormal automaticity in the right ventricular outflow tract or one of fascicles of the left bundle branch. In these cases, prognosis is good and catheter ablation can be curative.

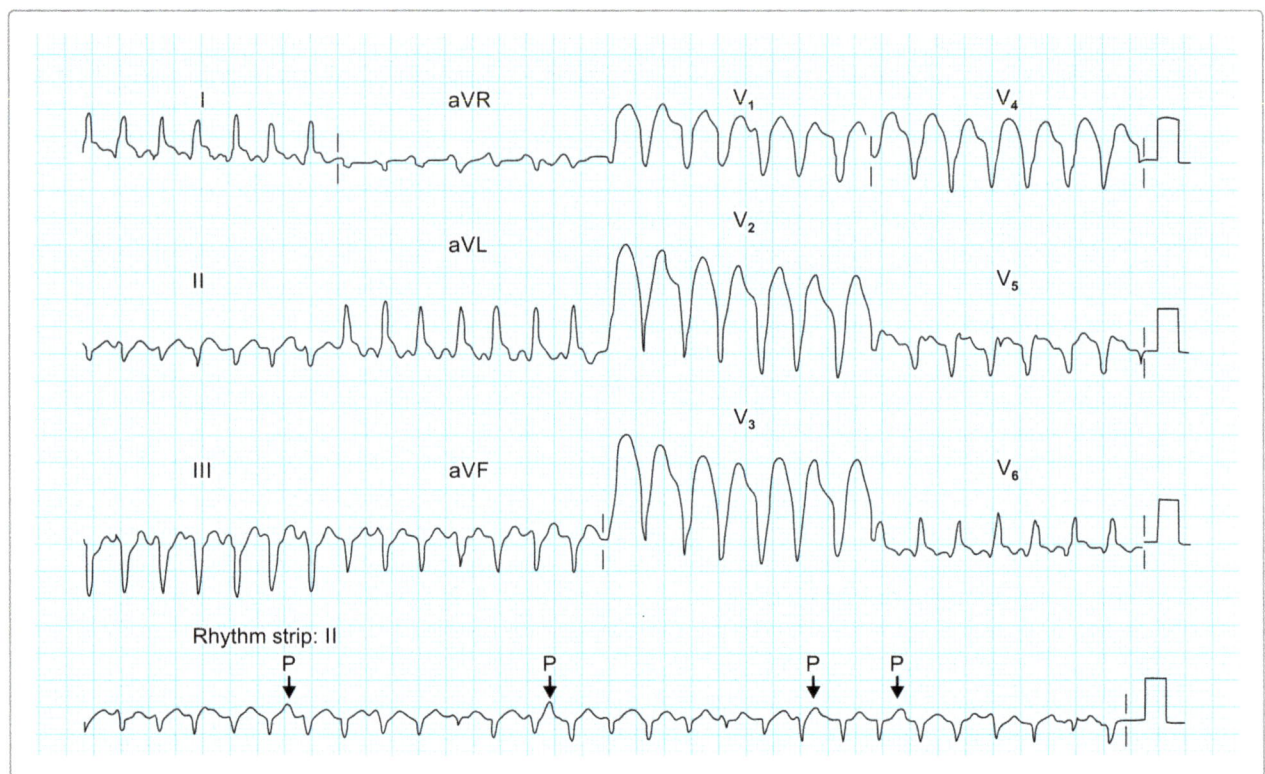

TORSADES DE POINTES

ECG Criteria of Torsades de Pointes

- *QRS*: Wide, bizarre, irregular or different or changing amplitude from upright to inverted position (different configuration of QRS)
- *QT*: Prolonged
  (ECG looks like ventricular tachycardia with different configuration of QRS).

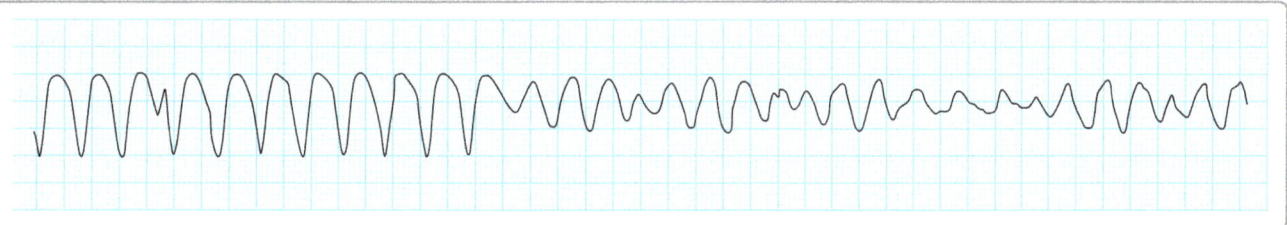

Ques. What is torsades de pointes?

Ans. It is a type of polymorphic ventricular tachycardia characterized by "twisting of the points" of QRS in ECG, which shows rapid irregular complex from upright to inverted position. During the period of sinus rhythm, ECG shows prolonged QT interval (> 0.42 second) at a rate of 60 beats/min.
- It is usually nonsustained, occurs in repetitive burst, lasting for few seconds. It may recur unless the underlying cause is corrected.
- It may progress to ventricular fibrillation and sudden death.
- Torsades de pointes is usually initiated by a ventricular ectopic with prolonged QT interval and broad T wave (may be R on T phenomenon).
- It is more common in women, triggered by multiple drugs and hypokalemia.

Ques. What are the causes of torsades de pointes?

Ans. As follows:
- Acute STEMI (ST-elevation myocardial infarction), NSTEMI, and also in unstable angina.
- Electrolyte imbalance—hypokalemia, hypomagnesemia, and hypocalcemia.
- Drugs—antiarrhythmic drugs (e.g., quinidine, procainamide, amiodarone, disopyramide, and sotalol), tricyclic antidepressant, erythromycin, cisapride, chlorpromazine, and other phenothiazines.
- Acute myocarditis
- Bradycardia (as in sinus node disease and complete heart block)
- Congenital syndrome such as Jervell and Lange-Nielsen syndrome (autosomal recessive) and Romano–Ward syndrome (autosomal dominant).

Ques. How to treat torsades de pointes?

Ans. Treatment should be directed at the underlying cause.
- Electrolyte imbalance should be corrected.
- Causative drugs should be stopped.
- *IV magnesium*: 8 mmol for 15 minutes, then 72 mmol over 24 hours should be given in all cases.
- The problem is best treated by cardiac pacing (atrial or in AV block—ventricular or dual chamber).
- If no pacing is available—isoprenaline infusion is a suitable alternative (it is avoided in congenital long QT syndrome).

- If all fail and there is history of sudden death in family—ICD.
- In congenital long QT syndrome—β-blocker is helpful. Other treatment—left stellate ganglion block, or ICD may help.

Ques. What is Brugada syndrome?

Ans. Brugada syndrome is a genetic disorder that may present with polymorphic ventricular tachycardia or sudden death. It is due to defect in sodium channel. ECG shows RBBB with ST elevation in V_1 and V_2, QT interval is normal.

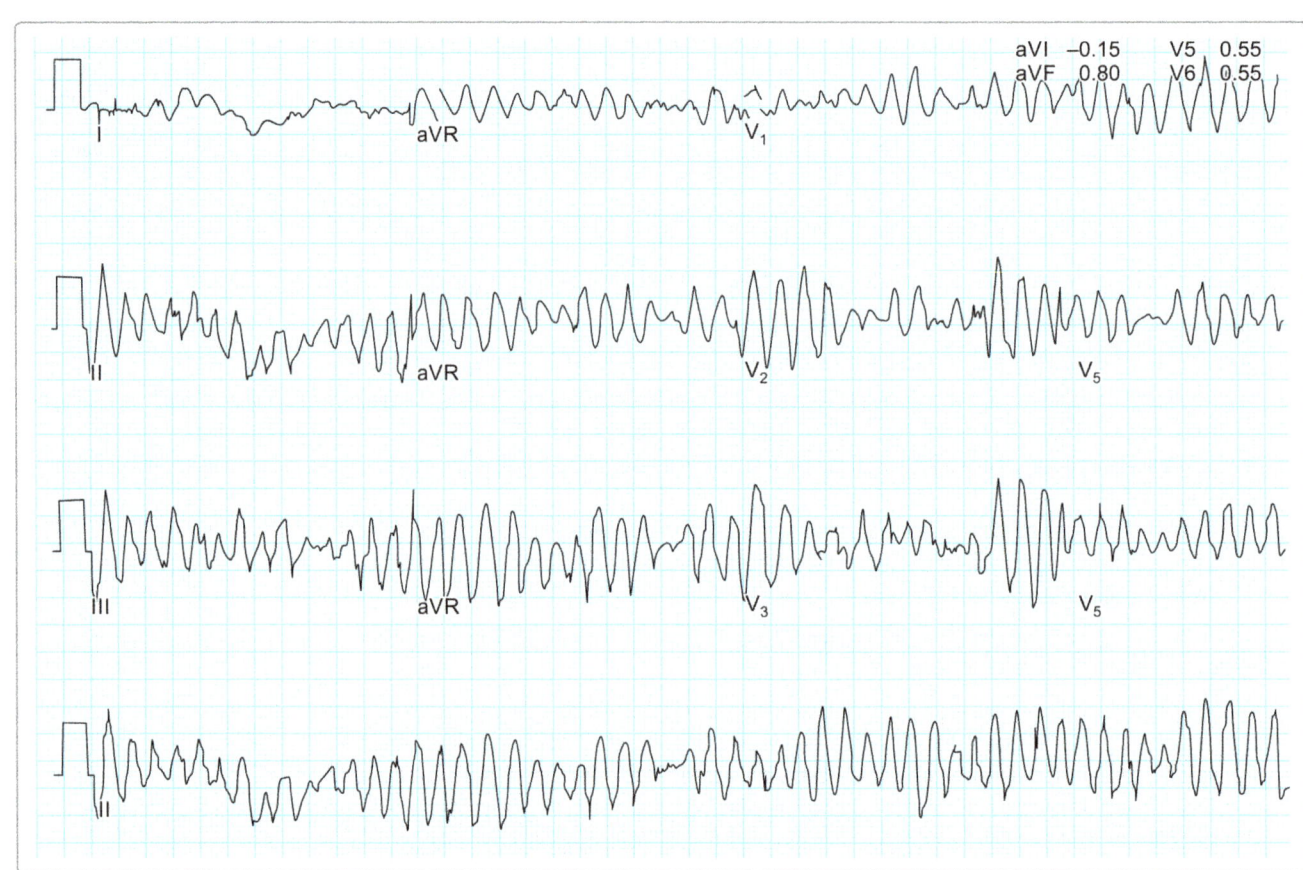

VENTRICULAR FIBRILLATION

ECG Criteria of Ventricular Fibrillation

- QRS—chaotic, wide, bizarre, and irregular pattern
- No identifiable P, QRS, or T wave
- Rapid rate. 150-500/min (difficult to count)

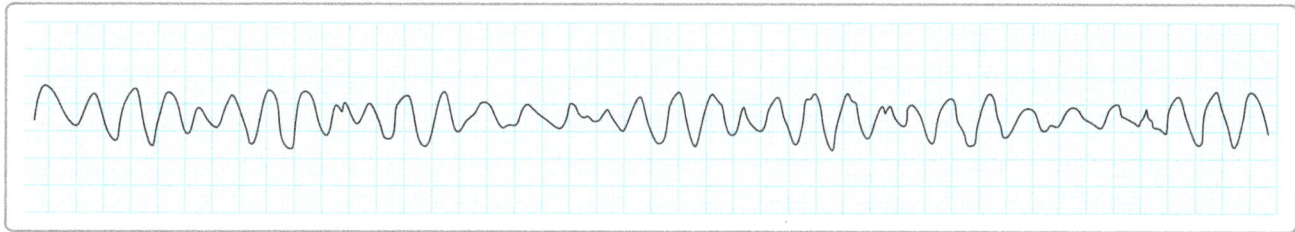

Ques. What is ventricular fibrillation?

Ans. This is a type of ventricular arrhythmia characterized by rapid, irregular, ineffective, and uncoordinated ventricular activation with no mechanical effect. There is chaotic electrical disturbance of ventricles, with impulse occurring irregularly at the rate of 300-500/min. Ventricular contraction is uncoordinated; ventricular filling and emptying cease. Cardiac output falls to zero. Ventricular fibrillation is the common cause of sudden death.

Ques. What are the findings, if you examine the patient clinically?

Ans. As follows:
- Pulse—absent
- BP—not recordable
- Respiration—ceases or absent
- Patient—unconscious
- Pupil—dilated, less, or no reaction to light
- Heart sounds—absent

Ques. What are the causes of ventricular fibrillation?

Ans. It may occur as a primary arrhythmia. Other causes are:
- As a complication in acute myocardial infarction
- Electrolyte imbalance (hypokalemia and hypomagnesemia)
- Electrocution
- Others—drowning and drug overdose (digoxin, adrenaline, and isoprenaline)

Ques. How to treat ventricular fibrillation?

Ans. As follows:
- Immediate defibrillation—200 J. If no response, another shock with 200 J is given. If still no response, another shock with 360 J is given.
- If three shocks unsuccessful—adrenaline is given IV, followed by cardiopulmonary resuscitation. IV amiodarone may be given.
- If one attempt of defibrillation fails, it may be repeated after IV bicarbonate to correct acidosis.
- If defibrillator is not available—cardiopulmonary resuscitation should be given.
- If recurrent ventricular fibrillation occurs, it can be prevented by antiarrhythmic drugs such as flecainide, phenytoin, sotalol, and propafenone.
- The patient who survives from ventricular fibrillation in the absence of identifiable cause is at a high risk of sudden death. This case is treated with ICD.

NB: Remember the following points:

- Ventricular fibrillation is invariably fatal, immediate treatment is necessary if death is to be prevented.
- Effective circulation and ventilation must be obtained within 4 minutes to prevent irreversible brain damage.
- Sinus rhythm can usually be restored by defibrillation.

VENTRICULAR FLUTTER

ECG Criteria of Ventricular Flutter

- QRS complex are wide and bizarre,
- P and T wave are not well seen, which gives rise a sine wave form

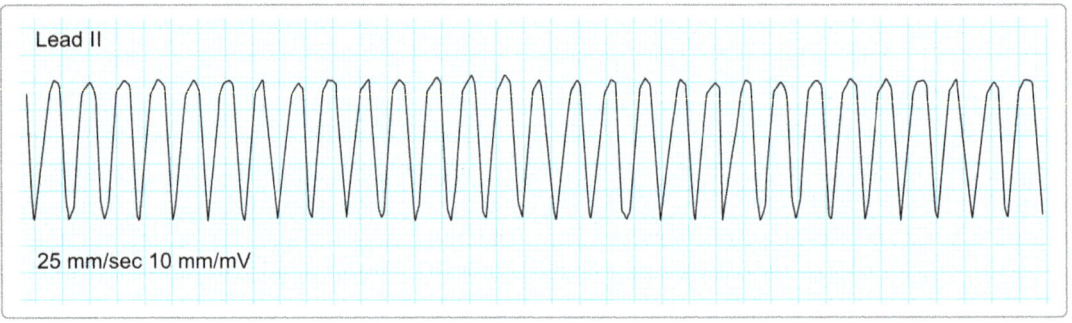

Ques. What is ventricular flutter ?

Ans. Ventricular flutter is an arrhythmia in which there is fast ventricular rhythm produced due to either rapid discharge of impulse from a ventricular pacemaker or repetitive circus movement of an impulse in a re-entrant circuit with a rate 250 to 350 beats/min. It looks like ventricular tachycardia.

Ques. What is the prognosis of ventricular flutter ?

Ans. It is considered as a possible transition stage between VT and fibrillation. It is a critically unstable arrhythmia, may result in VF and sudden cardiac death (SCD).

Ques. What is the treatment ventricular flutter ?

Ans. As it may turn to ventricular fibrillation so treatment is like ventricular fibrillation.

HEART BLOCK

Heart block or conduction block may occur at any level in the conductive system of the heart. Block in the AV node or His bundle results in the AV block and block lower in the conducting system produces bundle branch block.

Ques. What is heart block?

Ans. Heart block is defined as a "defect in either initiation or conduction of cardiac impulse."

Ques. What are the sites of heart block?

Ans. Sites may be:
- SA node
- AV node
- Bundle of His
- Branches of bundle of His

Ques. What are the types of heart block?

Ans. Heart block is of different types, depending on the sites, such as:
- SA block
- *AV block: It is of three types—*
  - First-degree AV block
  - *Second-degree AV block. It is of two types:*
    - Mobitz type 1 (Wenckebach phenomenon)
    - Mobitz type 2
- Complete heart block or third-degree heart block
- *Bundle branch block: It is of two types—*
  - RBBB
  - LBBB

Ques. What is hemiblock?

Ans. It means when there is a block involving one of the fascicles of left bundle branch. It is diagnosed by seeing the axis deviation in ECG.
- When there is LAD—it is called left anterior hemiblock.
- When there is RAD—it is called left posterior hemiblock.

NB: Remember the following points:
- There may be more block, one or more sites.
- If the block is on two sides, it is called bifascicular.
- If the block is on three sides, it is called trifascicular block.

ECG Criteria of Bifascicular

It may be of two types—RBBB with LAD and RBBB with RAD.
Right bundle branch block with LAD:
- QRS—wide >0.14 (RSR´ indicates RBBB)
- LAD (indicates left anterior hemiblock)

ECG in Medical Practice

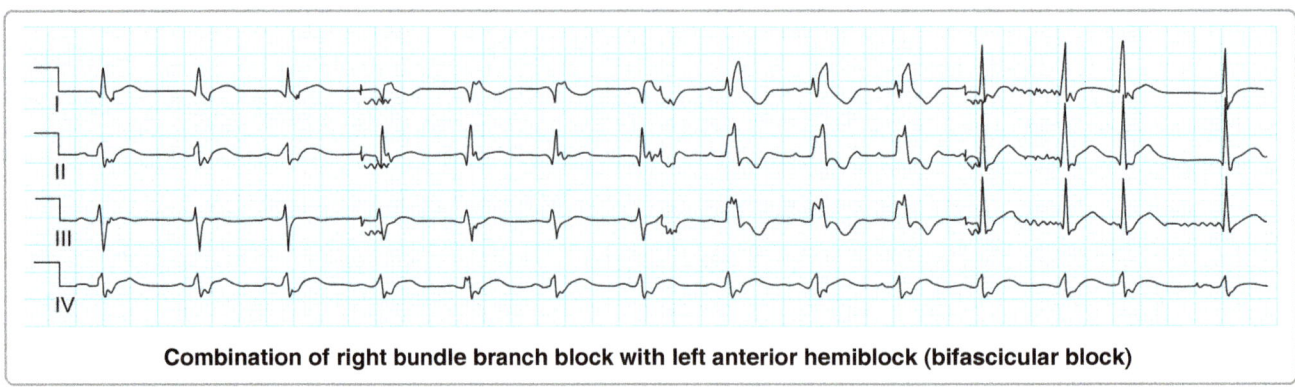

Combination of right bundle branch block with left anterior hemiblock (bifascicular block)

Right bundle branch block with RAD:
- QRS—wide >0.14 (RSR' indicates RBBB)
- RAD (indicates left posterior hemiblock)

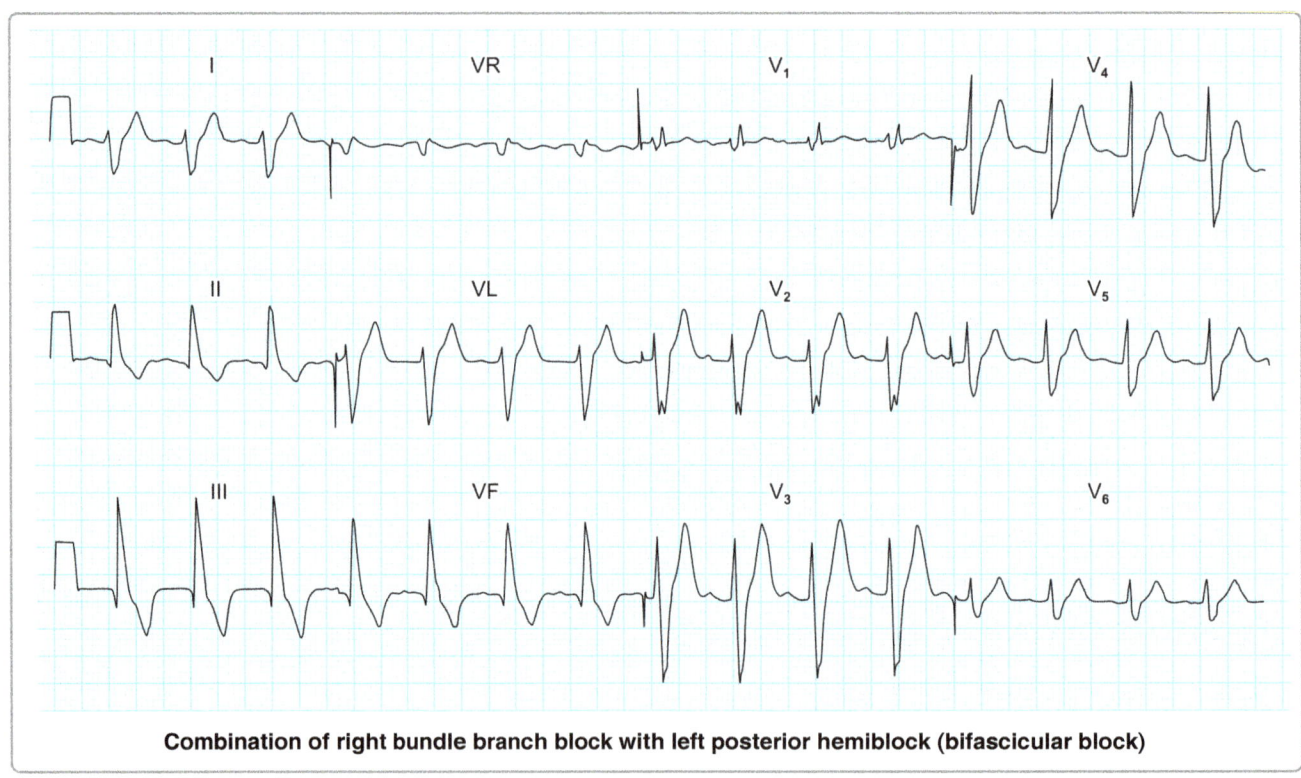

Combination of right bundle branch block with left posterior hemiblock (bifascicular block)

Ques. What is prognosis or complication of bifascicular block?
Ans. May develop complete heart block.
Trifascicular block: Two types are shown below.

ECG Criteria of Trifascicular

- QRS—wide >0.14 (RSR´ indicates RBBB)
- LAD (indicates left anterior hemiblock)
- PR prolonged >0.2 second (indicates first-degree heart block)

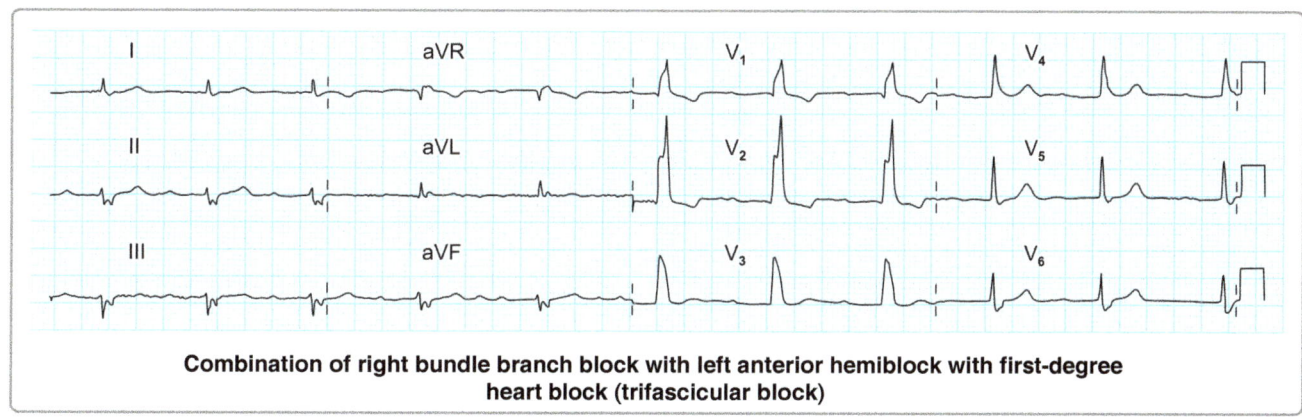

Combination of right bundle branch block with left anterior hemiblock with first-degree heart block (trifascicular block)

ECG Criteria of Trifascicular

- QRS—wide >0.14 (RSR´ indicates RBBB)
- LAD (indicates left anterior hemiblock)
- PR prolonged >0.2 second (indicates second-degree heart block, 2:1)

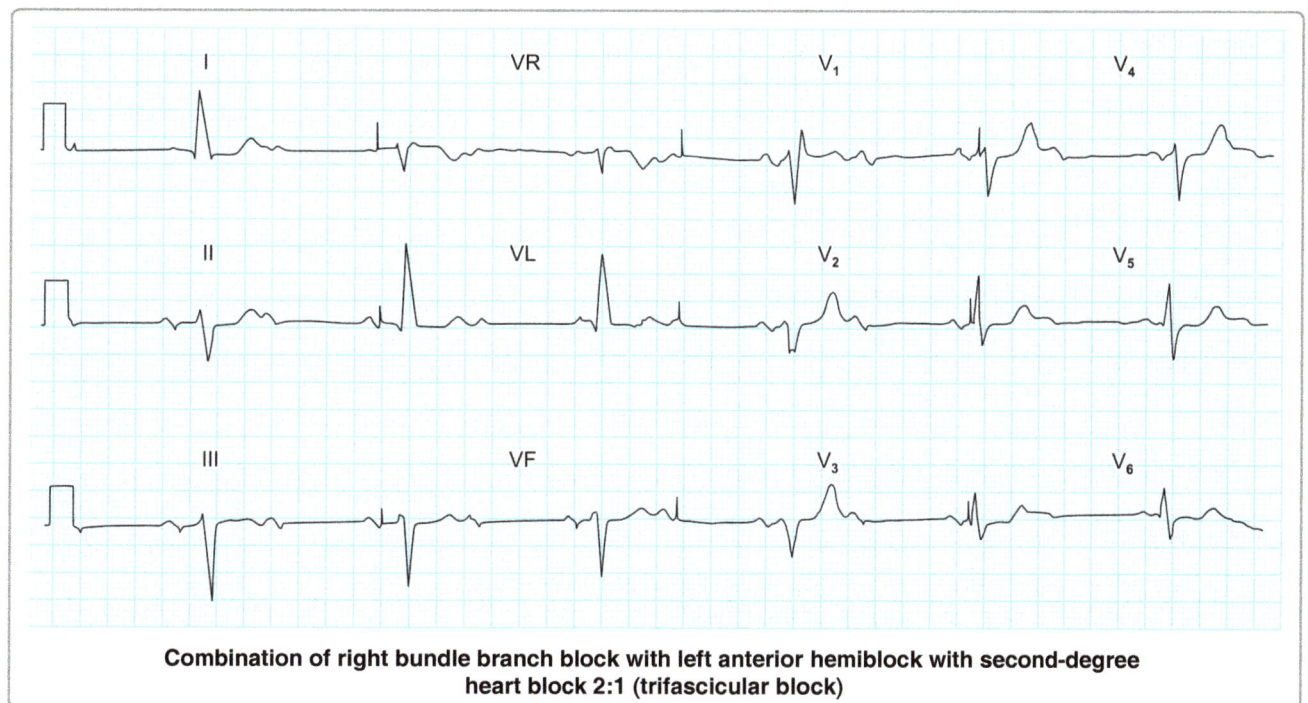

Combination of right bundle branch block with left anterior hemiblock with second-degree heart block 2:1 (trifascicular block)

SA BLOCK

ECG Criteria of SA Block

- Absence of one P-QRS-T complex
- P-P (or R-R) is double than the next P-P (or R-R)

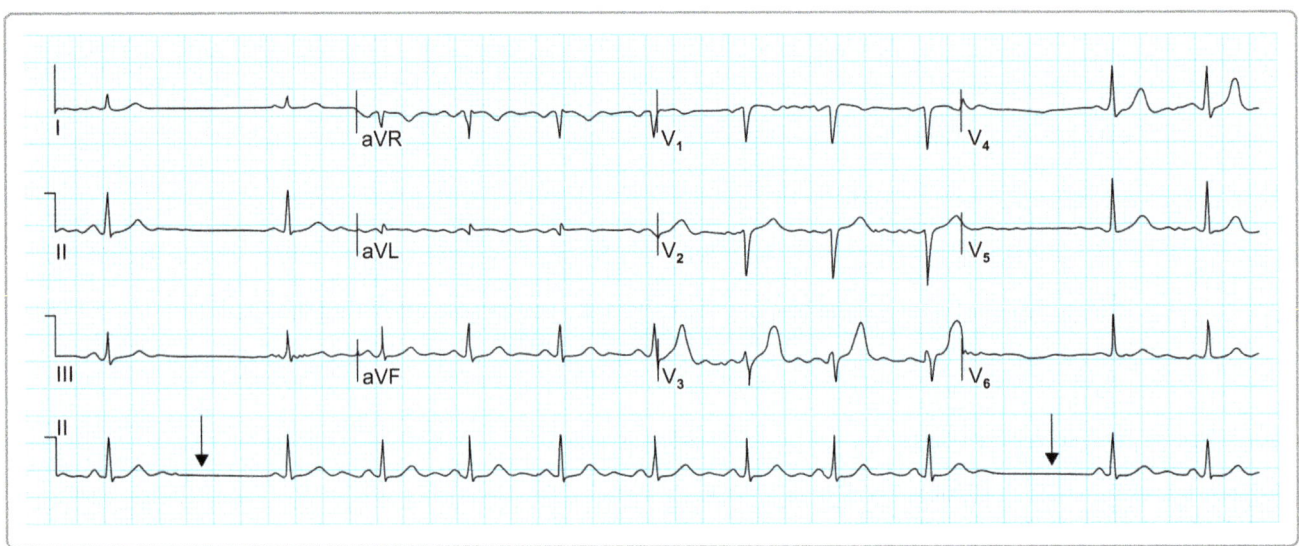

Ques. What are the differential diagnoses?

Ans. As follows:
- Sinus arrest
- Sinus standstill

Ques. How to differentiate between these two?

Ans. In sinus arrest, P-P (R-R) is not exactly the double of next normal beat.

Ques. What are the causes of SA block?

Ans. As follows:
- Degenerative changes in elderly
- Ischemic heart disease (involving SA node)
- Drugs (digoxin)
- Increased vagal tone

Ques. What are the presentations of SA block?

Ans. Usually asymptomatic. Sometimes, may present as sick sinus syndrome.

Ques. How to diagnose SA block?

Ans. As follows:
- Clinically—drop beat and no heart sound at the time of drop beat
- ECG—complete absence of one complex (P-QRS-T)
- Holter monitoring—may show the block

Ques. **How to treat SA block?**

Ans. As follows:
- No treatment, if asymptomatic
- Withdraw the offensive drug, if any
- Treatment of primary cause
- If any syncopal attack or sick sinus syndrome—permanent pacemaker should be given

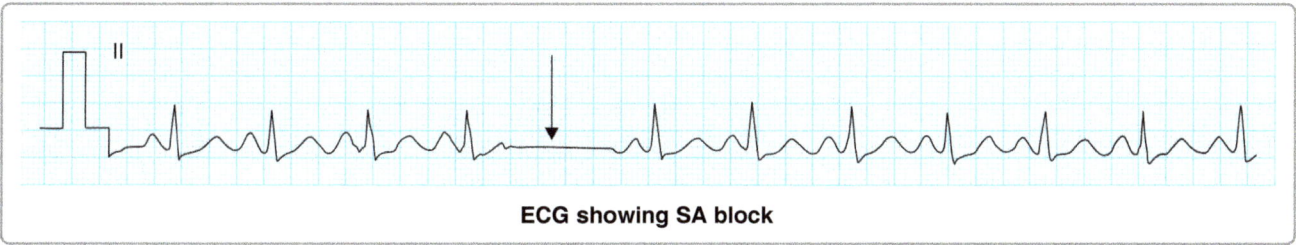

ECG showing SA block

Ques. **What is the prognosis of SA block?**

Ans. As follows:
- Prognosis depends on the cause
- In asymptomatic cases and without any cause, prognosis is good

SICK SINUS SYNDROME

ECG Criteria of Sick Sinus Syndrome

- Sinus arrest
- Sinus bradycardia and sinus tachycardia (or tachy-brady syndrome)
- Junctional rhythm

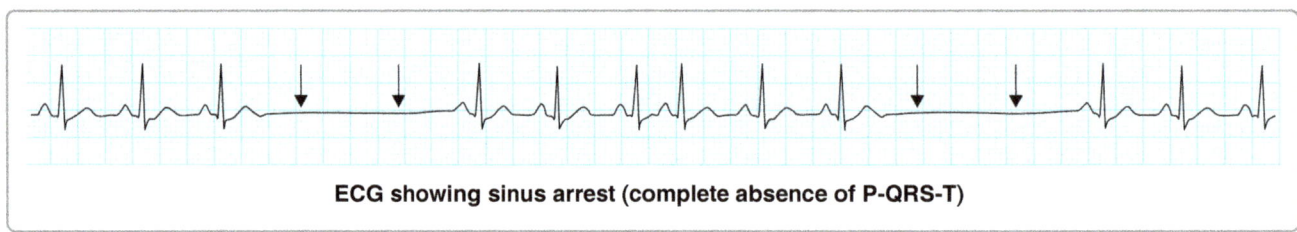

ECG showing sinus arrest (complete absence of P-QRS-T)

Ques. What is sick sinus syndrome?

Ans. It is the dysfunction of the SA node with impairment of its ability to generate and conduct impulses. It is characterized by attacks of sinus bradycardia, sinus arrest, or junctional rhythm, which may lead to palpitation, dizziness, or even syncope.

Ques. What is tachy-brady syndrome?

Ans. Tachy-brady syndrome is characterized by runs of tachycardia followed by episodes of bradycardia. It means tachycardia alternates with bradycardia. It is common in sick sinus syndrome.

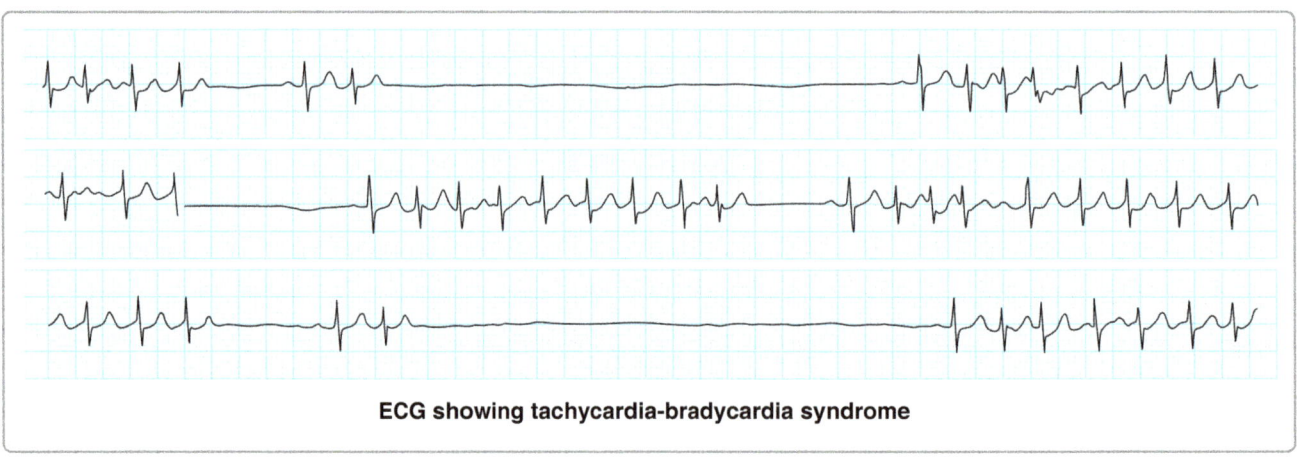

ECG showing tachycardia-bradycardia syndrome

Ques. What are the causes of sick sinus syndrome?

Ans. It is due to fibrosis, degenerative changes, or ischemia of the SA node or high vagal tone. Probable causes are:
- Elderly (due to degeneration) or idiopathic degenerative fibrosis (common cause)
- Ischemic heart disease
- Drug (digoxin, lithium, and ivabradine)
- Cardiomyopathy
- Myocarditis
- Rheumatic heart disease
- Infiltrative diseases (sarcoidosis, hemochromatosis, and amyloidosis)

Ques. What are the presentations of sick sinus syndrome?
Ans. As follows:
- Occasional palpitation even angina (due to coronary artery disease) may occure
- Frequent attack of dizziness
- Frequent fainting attack and syncope may occur
- Dyspnoea and fatigue (due to heart failure), may be postural hypotension
- Mental confusion even dementia

Ques. Why bradycardia or tachycardia occurs in sick sinus syndrome?
Ans. As follows:
- Bradycardia due to—sinus bradycardia, SA block or arrest, and junctional bradycardia.
- Tachycardia due to—atrial fibrillation, atrial flutter, or PAT.

Ques. How would you diagnose sick sinus syndrome?
Ans. By Holter monitoring (single ECG may sometimes be normal).

Ques. How to treat sick sinus syndrome?
Ans. As follows:
- If asymptomatic—no specific therapy. Follow-up the case
- If symptomatic — permanent pacemaker, usually dual chamber pacemaker is given
- Antiarrhythmic drug may be required in some case

Ques. What are the ECG criteria of sick sinus syndrome?
Ans. As follows:
- Sinus bradycardia
- Sinus arrest (pause >3 seconds)
- Escape rhythm
- Tachycardia-bradycardia syndrome (common)
- Atrial fibrillation with slow ventricular rate
- Sinoatrial block

ATRIOVENTRICULAR BLOCK (AV BLOCK)

Atrioventricular block occurs when atrial depolarization fails to reach the ventricle. It is of three types:
- *First degree*: In this block, there is only delay of AV conduction in all beats.
- *Second degree*: There is intermittent failure of conduction between the atria and the ventricles. So, there is drop of one or more beats.
- *Third degree (complete heart block)*: In this block, no sinus beat or impulse conducts to the ventricle as all of them get blocked in the AV node. Atria and ventricles work independently of each other and asynchronously leading to AV dissociation.

FIRST-DEGREE AV BLOCK

ECG Criteria of First-degree Block

- PR interval—prolonged >0.22 second (normal 0.12–0.20 second)
- QRS—normal
- Rhythm—normal

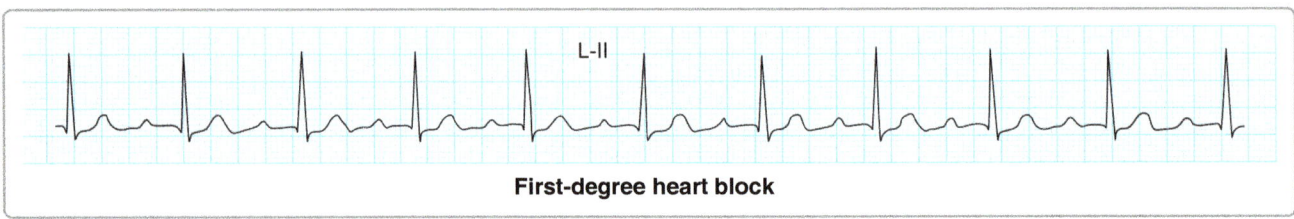

First-degree heart block

Ques. What are the causes of first-degree AV block?

Ans. As follows:
- Normally in athlete (due to increased vagal tone)
- Drugs (e.g., digoxin toxicity. Other drugs are β-blocker, calcium channel blocker, amiodarone, disopyramide, quinidine, and procainamide)
- Acute myocardial infarction (common in inferior myocardial infarction)
- Acute rheumatic carditis
- Diphtheric myocarditis
- In elderly (due to atherosclerosis)
- Electrolytes imbalance (e.g., hypokalemia and hypomagnesemia)
- *Others*: Cardiac surgery, catheter ablation for tachyarrhythmia, collagen diseases, e.g., rheumatoid arthritis and systemic lupus erythematosus (SLE).

Ques. What is first-degree heart block?

Ans. It is the simple prolongation of PR >0.22 second. Every atrial depolarization is followed by conduction to the ventricles, but with delay.

Ques. What are the clinical features of first-degree AV block?

Ans. Usually asymptomatic.

Ques. What other investigation should be done?

Ans. Investigation should be done according to the cause.

Ques. How to treat first-degree AV block?

Ans. As follows:
- No specific treatment is necessary, usually it is benign.
- Treatment of the primary cause should be done.

NB: Markedly prolonged PR interval may progress to Wenckebach AV heart block.

SECOND-DEGREE AV BLOCK

Second-degree AV block may be of three types:
- Mobitz type I (Wenckebach phenomenon)
- Mobitz type II
- 2:1 or 3:1 heart block

Mobitz Type I (Wenckebach Phenomenon)

ECG Criteria of Mobitz Type I

- Progressive lengthening of PR interval, followed by absent QRS complex (it means one P is not followed by a QRS complex)
- PP—constant
- RR—irregular
  (Progressive shortening of RR interval until block occurs)

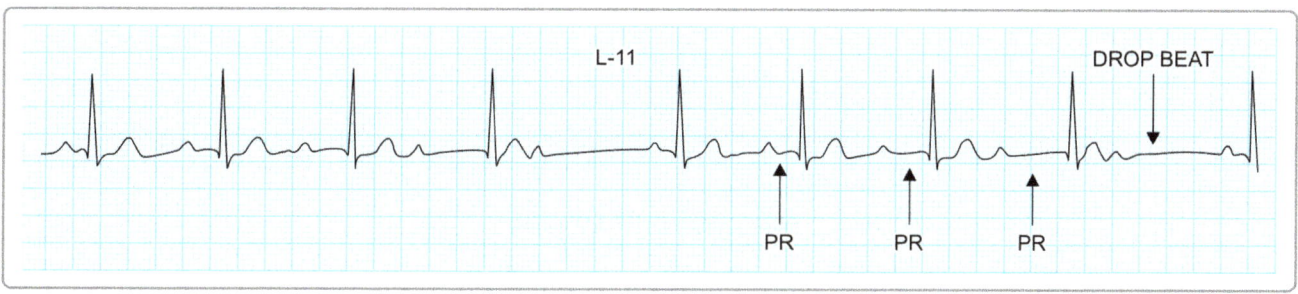

Ques. What is Mobitz I block?

Ans. Progressive prolongation of PR interval until a P wave fails to conduct. PR interval before the blocked P wave is much longer than the PR interval after the blocked P wave. PR interval is the shortest immediately after the drop beat. It is due to progressive fatigue of AV node followed by recovery.

Ques. What is the site of block in Mobitz type I AV block?

Ans. The block is in the higher area of AV node (proximal to the bundle of His).

Ques. What are the causes of Wenckebach phenomenon?

Ans. As follows:
- Physiological—in athlete, during rest, and sleep (due to increased vagal tone)
- Drugs—digoxin toxicity, also β-blocker, calcium channel blocker, and amiodarone
- Acute myocardial infarction (commonly inferior myocardial infarction)
- Myocarditis

Ques. What are the features of Mobitz type I AV block?

Ans. As follows:
- Usually asymptomatic
- Features of primary disease
- Pulse is irregular (drop beat occurs)

ECG in Medical Practice

Ques. How to treat Mobitz type I AV block?

Ans. As follows:
- No treatment is necessary
- Primary cause should be treated

Ques. What is the prognosis of Wenckebach phenomenon?

Ans. It is a benign condition. Prognosis is good.

Mobitz Type II AV block

ECG Criteria of Mobitz Type II Block

- Some P waves are not followed by QRS complex
- PR interval is constant (also PP interval constant)
- QRS—wide
  (In 2:1 AV block, alternate P wave is conducted. It may be 3:1 and 4:1)
  This type of AV block is rare and more severe. It is generally a sign of severe conduction system disease.

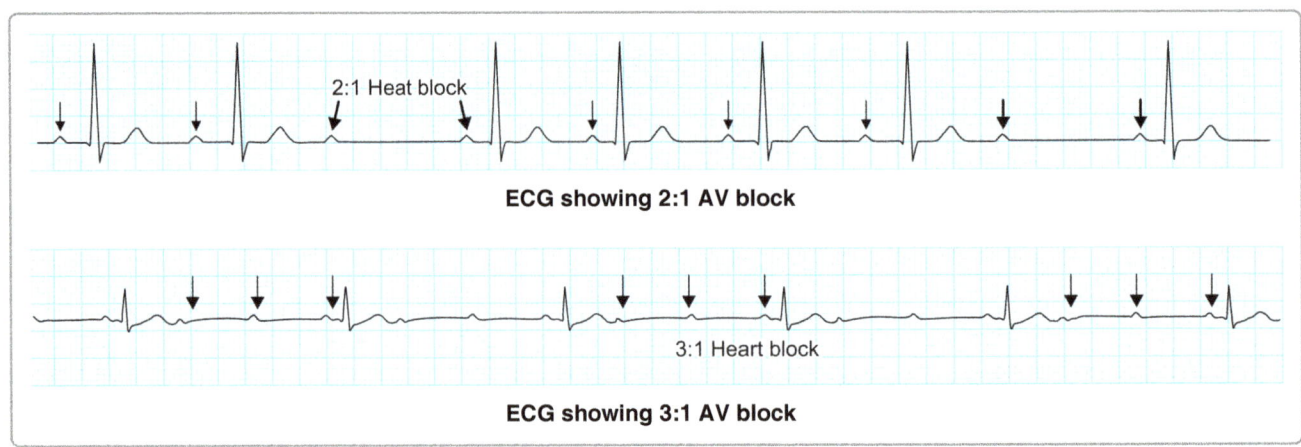

ECG showing 2:1 AV block

ECG showing 3:1 AV block

Ques. What is the prognosis?

Ans. It is more serious than Mobitz type I. There may be:
- Complete heart block
- Stokes–Adams syndrome
- Heart failure

Ques. What is the site of lesion in Mobitz type II AV block?

Ans. Disease of His–Purkinje system.

Ques. What are the causes of Mobitz type II AV block?

Ans. It is commonly seen in acute anterior myocardial infarction (not in digoxin toxicity). Other causes are:
- Idiopathic fibrosis of conductive system
- Electrolytes imbalance (e.g., hyperkalemia)
- Cardiac surgery (e.g., mitral valve repair)
- Drugs, e.g., β-blocker, calcium channel blocker, and amiodarone
- Rarely rheumatic fever, myocarditis, autoimmune disease (SLE and scleroderma), and infiltrative diseases (amyloidosis, hemochromatosis, and sarcoidosis).

Ques. How to treat Mobitz type II AV block?

Ans. As follows:
1. *If associated with inferior myocardial infarction:*
   - If asymptomatic—close monitoring and follow-up.
   - If symptomatic—injection atropine 0.6 mg IV. If fails, temporary pacemaker should be given. Majority will resolve in 7–10 days.
2. *If associated with anterior myocardial infarction:*
   - Usually temporary pacemaker followed by permanent pacemaker is required (because complete heart block may develop).

Ques. What is 2:1 or 3:1 block?

Ans. This type of block occurs when every second or third P wave conducts to the ventricles. This form of second-degree block is neither Mobitz I nor II. Permanent pacemaker is usually indicated in 2:1 block.

COMPLETE HEART BLOCK (3RD DEGREE)

ECG Criteria of Complete Heart Block (Rate is Supposed Here)

- Atrial rate—80/min (PP interval)
- Ventricular rate—35/min (RR interval)
- PP interval—constant
- No relationship between P wave and QRS complex (PR looks variable—a clue for the diagnosis)

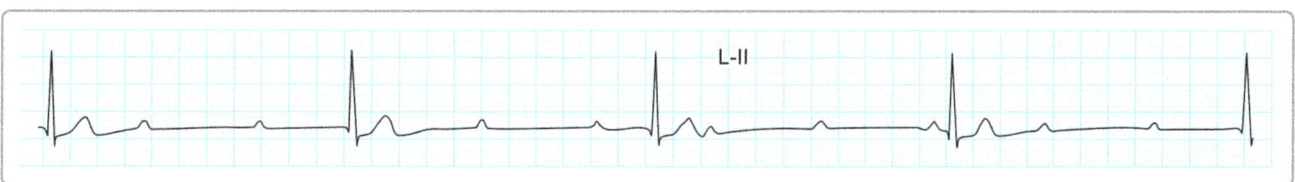

Ques. What is escape rhythm?

Ans. When there is complete dissociation between atria and ventricles, no impulse is transmitted from atria to the ventricle. In that case, ventricular activity is maintained by pacemaker from other site such as AV junctional or ventricular. This is called escape rhythm (it acts as a safety net, otherwise cardiac arrest occurs).

Ques. What are the sites of complete heart block?

Ans. AV block may occur at the level of AV node, bundle of His, bundle branch, and Purkinje system. In most cases, 60% block occurs below the bundle of His.

NB: Remember the following points in complete heart block:

- Ventricular activity is maintained by escape rhythm arising in the AV node or in the bundle of His.
- Narrow complex escape rhythm—this is of junctional origin (more proximally in the AV node or in the bundle of His), QRS is narrow (<0.12 second) and ventricular rate is high (50–60/min). The patient may be asymptomatic.
- Wide complex escape rhythm—it is usually of ventricular origin (distally in His–Purkinje system), QRS complex is wide (>0.12 second), and ventricular rate is slow (15–40/min). The patient is symptomatic (such as dizziness, vertigo, syncope, or blackout).

Ques. What are the causes of complete heart block?

Ans. Common causes are:
1. *Acute complete heart block:*
   - Acute myocardial infarction (commonly inferior)
2. *Chronic complete heart block:*
   - Progressive fibrosis of distal His-Purkinje system (Lev disease) in elderly
   - Progressive fibrosis of proximal His-Purkinje system (Lenègre disease) in younger

Other causes of complete heart block:
- Cardiomyopathy (ischemic or idiopathic dilated)
- Myocarditis
- Drugs (digoxin, β-blocker, and amiodarone)
- Cardiac surgery [aortic valve replacement, VSD repair, and coronary artery bypass surgery (CABG)]
- Radiofrequency AV node ablation.
- Infiltrative disease (sarcoidosis, amyloidosis, and hemochromatosis)
- Infection (infective endocarditis, Chagas disease, and Lyme disease)
- Collagen disease (SLE and rheumatoid arthritis)
- Congenital complete heart block
- Neuromuscular, e.g., Duchenne muscular dystrophy

Congenital complete heart block: It is common in the child of a mother with SLE (due to transplacental transfer of anti-Ro antibody or SS-A). In such case, QRS complex is narrow. Block is at the level of AV node, ventricular pacemaker is proximal to the bifurcation of bundle of His. Heart rate is relatively high, 40–80/min, which increases with exercise and atropine. No treatment is necessary, as most patients are usually asymptomatic.

Ques. What are the signs of complete heart block?

Ans. As follows:
- Pulse—usually bradycardia, 20–40 beats/min (<40 beats/min), high volume, and does not increase by exercise or injection atropine.
- BP—high systolic, normal diastolic, and high pulse pressure.
- Neck vein—cannon waves (large *a* wave) may be present.
- Heart sounds—variable intensity of first heart sound.
- Murmur—systolic flow murmurs (due to increase stroke volume).

Ques. Why variable intensity of first heart sound and systolic flow murmur?

Ans. As follows:
- Variable intensity of first heart sound is due to the loss of AV synchrony.
- Systolic flow murmur is due to increased stroke volume.

Ques. What is the mechanism of cannon wave?

Ans. When the atria contract against the closed tricuspid valve, backward pressure produces cannon wave.

Ques. If the pulse rate is high, what are the likely causes of complete heart block?

Ans. As follows:
- Pulse rate is high in congenital complete heart block. It does not require treatment.
- If the block occurs more proximally in the AV node (narrow complex escape rhythm).

Ques. What are the presentations of complete heart block?

Ans. Dizziness, blackout, or sudden loss of consciousness without warning or syncope (Stokes–Adams attack).

Ques. How to treat chronic complete heart block?

Ans. As follows:
- *If the patient is symptomatic:* Permanent pacemaker should be given.
- Treatment of cause should be done.

Ques. How to treat heart block following acute myocardial infarction?
Ans. As follows:
1. Acute inferior myocardial infarction is often complicated by transient AV block, because the right coronary artery supplies the AV node.
   - *If the patient is asymptomatic*: No treatment is required.
   - *If the patient is symptomatic*: Injection atropine 0.6 mg IV should be given, repeated, if necessary.
   - *If no response*: Temporary pacemaker should be given. AV block is usually resolved in 7–10 days.
2. *Acute anterior myocardial infarction:* Second- or third-degree heart block may occur, which indicates extensive ventricular damage.
   - If second-degree heart block occurs, it may progress to complete heart block. So, a temporary pacemaker should be given, followed by a permanent pacemaker.
   - *If complete heart block occurs*: A temporary pacemaker should be given, followed by a permanent pacemaker.

Ques. What is Stokes–Adams attack?
Ans. It is the brief attack of syncope or blackout in a patient with complete heart block due to ventricular asystole. Stokes–Adams attack may also occur in Mobitz type II heart block, ventricular tachycardia or ventricular fibrillation, or SA diseases.

Ques. What are the clinical features of Stokes–Adams attack?
Ans. As follows:
- Syncope or blackout with or without preceding dizziness
- During attack—the patient is unconscious, looks pale, and there may be convulsion
- If asystole persists—there may be cyanosis, pulse is absent, pupil is fixed and dilated, incontinence of urine, and plantar is extensor.
- Usually, consciousness recovers rapidly followed by flushing

Ques. How to treat Stokes–Adams attack?
Ans. As follows:
- Permanent pacemaker (even after a single syncopal attack)
- During attack, a blow over the cardiac apex and cardiopulmonary resuscitation (CPR) should be done.

ATRIOVENTRICULAR DISSOCIATION

ECG Criteria in AV Dissociation

- Variable PR interval (progressive shortening of P-R is suspicious)
- P may be hidden in T wave or QRS or P may appear after QRS
- Ventricular rate is same as the atrial rate or slightly high

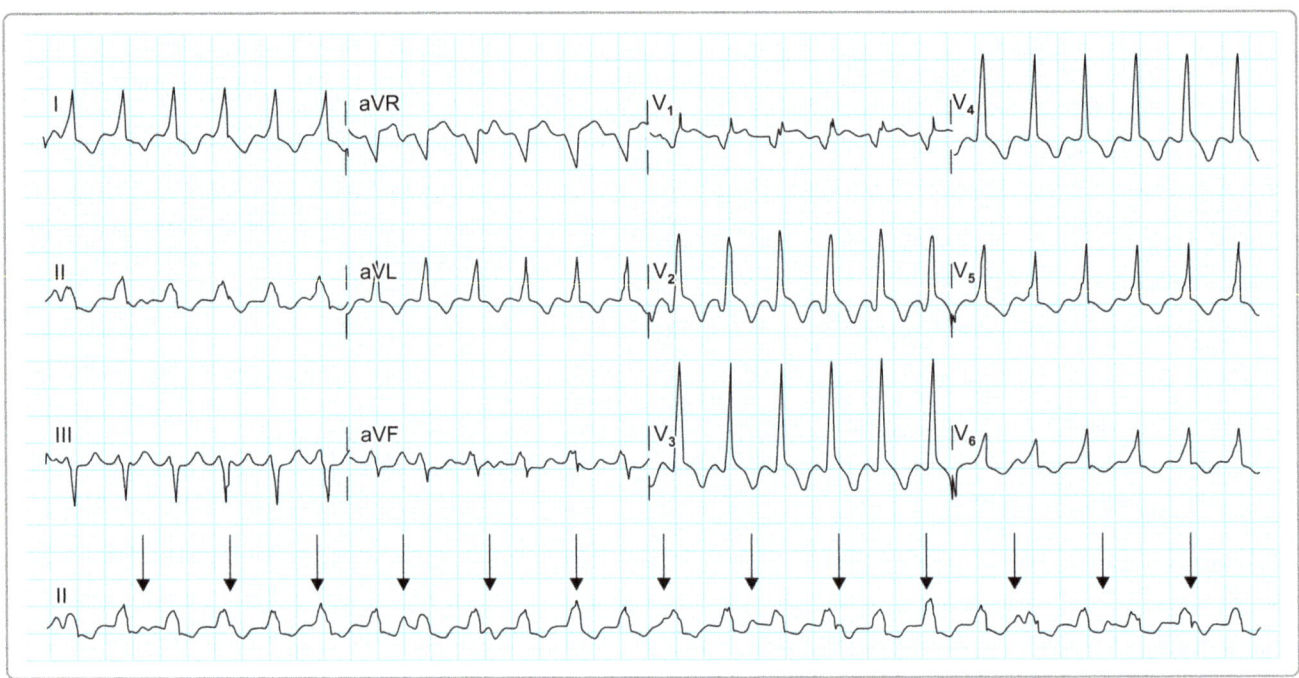

Ques. What is AV dissociation?

Ans. AV dissociation is a type of arrhythmia in which atria and ventricles are activated and contract independently and do not activate in a synchronous fashion. P wave will be unrelated to QRS complex. AV dissociation is a minor, transient arrhythmia.

Atria are activated by SA node and the ventricles are activated by other pacemaker located in AV junction or ventricle. So, atria and ventricle will beat independently of each other.

- P wave is either unrelated to QRS complex or may be buried in the wide QRS complex.
- RR interval is slightly shorter than PP interval. This allows PR interval to progressively shorten, till P wave merges into QRS complex.

Ques. What are the sites of pacemaker in AV dissociation?

Ans. There are two pacemakers in AV dissociation:
- One from the SA node or atria that controls atrial activation
- Another from the AV junction or ventricle that controls ventricular activation

Ques. What are the causes of AV dissociation?

Ans. As follows:
- Acute myocardial infarction
- Digoxin toxicity
- Acute rheumatic carditis
- Myocarditis due to any cause
- Occasionally, in normal people

Ques. How to differentiate between complete heart block with AV dissociation?

Ans. Complete heart block may be confused with AV dissociation. To differentiate between these:
- If P waves are more than QRS, it is highly suggestive of complete heart block.
- If QRS are more than P wave, it is highly suggestive of AV dissociation.

Also to differentiate, AV dissociation from complete heart block:
- In AV dissociation: Ventricular rate is same or slightly higher than the atrial rate.
- In complete heart block: There is a total AV block. So, the ventricular rate is slower than the atrial rate.

Ques. How to treat AV dissociation?

Ans. Treatment of primary cause.

BUNDLE BRANCH BLOCK

It means a delay or block of electrical activity in one of the two branches of the bundle of His, either right or left bundle branch. Right bundle branch contains one fascicle and left bundle branch divides into two fascicles (left anterior fascicle and left posterior fascicle). Bundle branch block is divided into two types: RBBB and LBBB.

Right Bundle Branch Block

It may be complete or incomplete or partial.

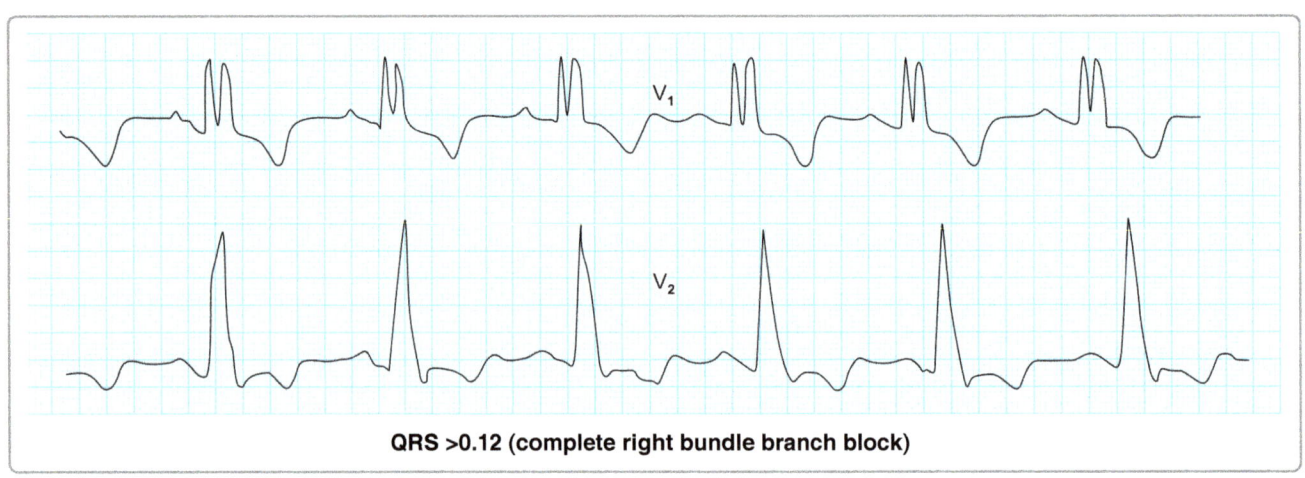

QRS >0.12 (complete right bundle branch block)

ECG Criteria of Complete RBBB

- RSR′—in V_1 and V_2 (M pattern)
- QRS—wide, >0.12 second (>3 small squares)
- qR—in V_1
- Other criteria—broad and deep S in V_5 and V_6 (also in L_1 and aVL)

ECG in Incomplete or Partial RBBB

- Same findings as above and QRS is not wide, <0.12 second (<3 small squares)

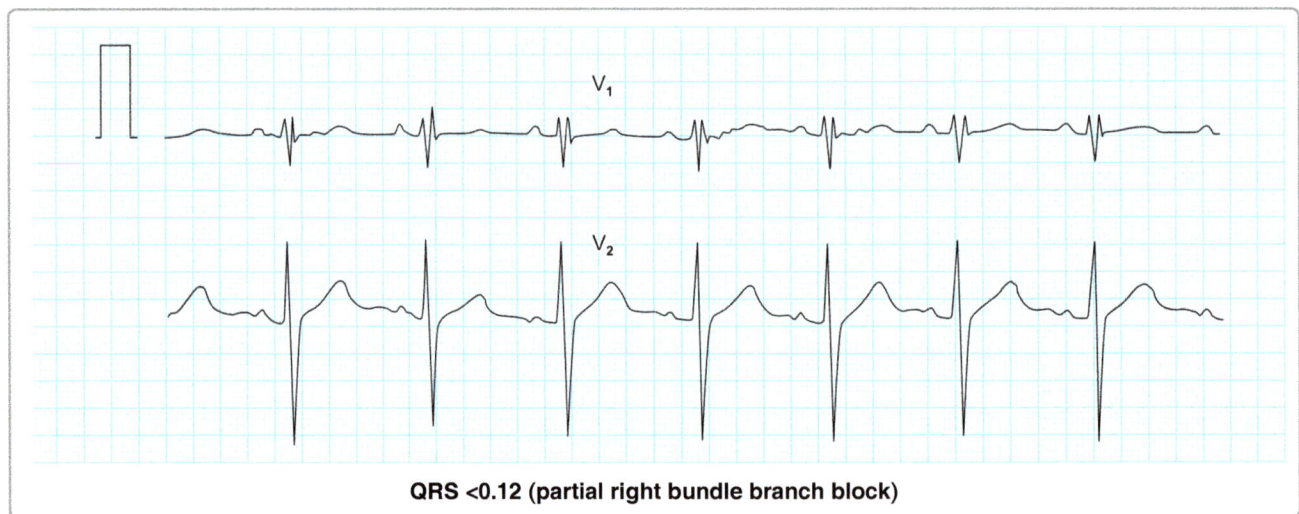

QRS <0.12 (partial right bundle branch block)

Ques. What are the causes of RBBB?

Ans. As follows:
- Isolated congenital anomaly, a normal variant (may be found in 1% young adults and 5% elderly)
- *Cardiac causes*:
  - Acute myocardial infarction
  - Congenital heart disease (such as ASD, tetralogy of Fallot, pulmonary stenosis, and VSD)
  - RVH
  - Cardiomyopathy
  - Conduction system fibrosis
- *Pulmonary causes*:
  - Chronic cor pulmonale with pulmonary hypertension
  - Acute pulmonary embolism

Ques. What is the finding in RBBB, if you examine the heart?

Ans. Wide splitting second heart sound (physiological)

NB: RBBB may occur in healthy people, but LBBB indicates underlying heart disease.

Ques. How to treat RBBB?

Ans. As follows:
- Treatment of primary cause should be done.
- In isolated asymptomatic case, no treatment is necessary. As it may occur in normal healthy person.

FASCICULAR BLOCK (HEMIBLOCK)

Left bundle divides into anterior and posterior fascicles.
- Anterior fascicle spreads in the anterior and the superior part of the left ventricle.
- Posterior fascicle spreads in the posterior and the inferior part of the left ventricle.

Fascicular block is diagnosed by looking at the axis deviation.

Fascicular block are of two types:
- RBBB with left anterior hemiblock (block in anterior fascicle)
- RBBB with left posterior hemiblock (block in posterior fascicle)

ECG in RBBB with Left Anterior Hemiblock

- RBBB with LAD (tall R in L_1 and deep S in aVF)

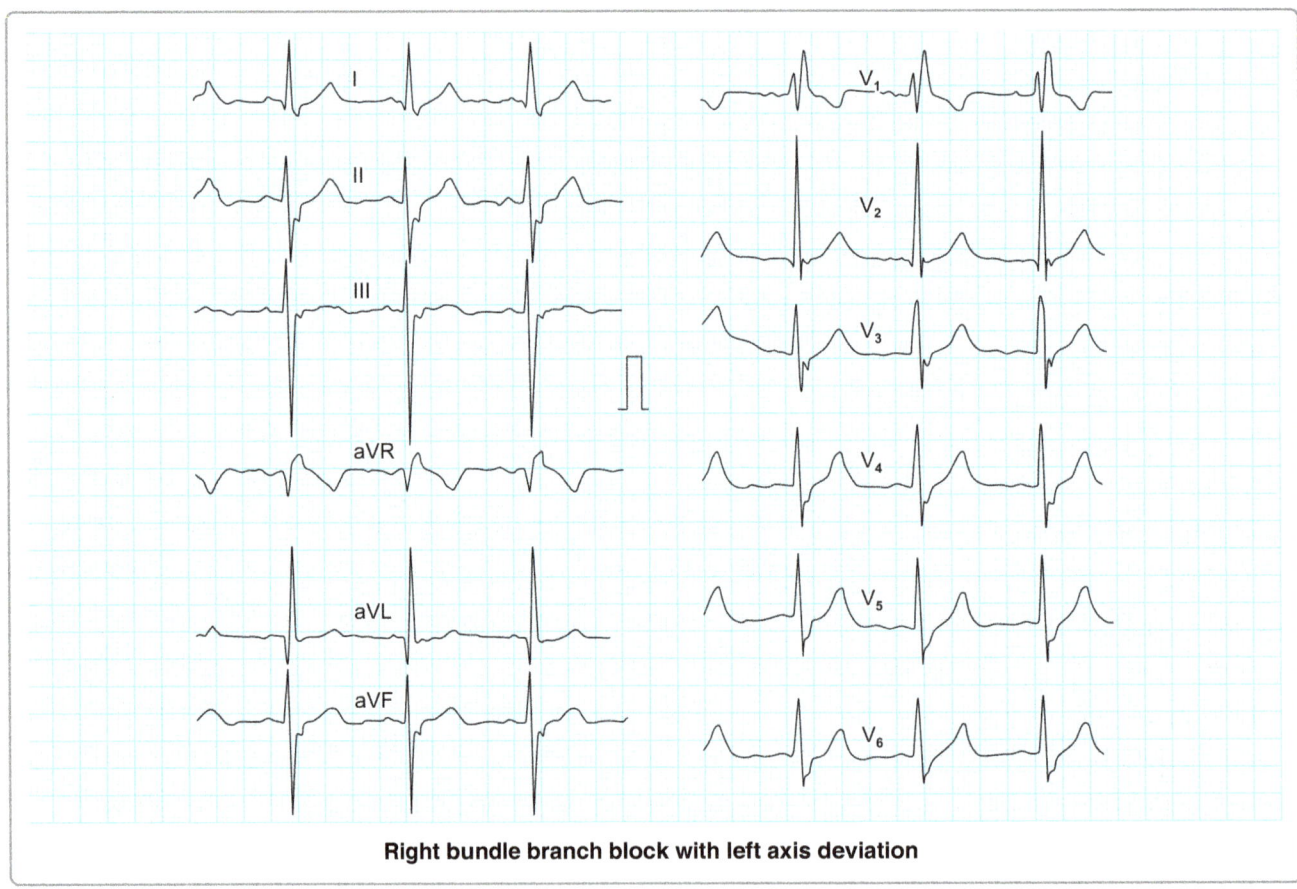

Right bundle branch block with left axis deviation

Ques. What is the cause?
Ans. It may occur in 4% cases of acute myocardial infarction.

Chapter 2: ECG Changes in Different Diseases

ECG in RBBB with Left Posterior Hemiblock

- RBBB with RAD (deep S in L₁ and tall R in aVF)

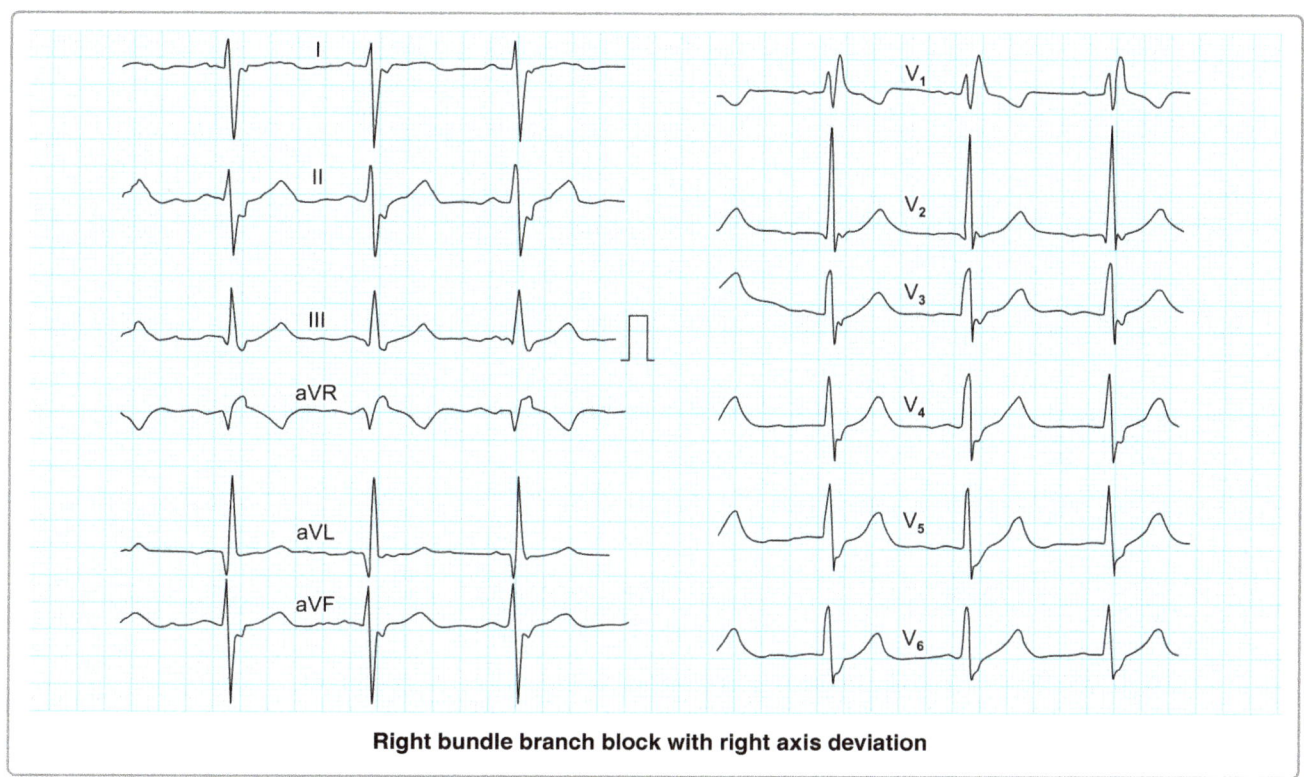

Right bundle branch block with right axis deviation

NB: Remember the following points:

- The combination of RBBB with left anterior or posterior hemiblock is called bifascicular block.
- Left anterior hemiblock is common, left posterior hemiblock is rare.
- Isolated finding of left anterior or left posterior hemiblock does not have any clinical significance.

Ques. What is the most common cause of bifascicular block?

Ans. Coronary artery disease is the most common cause. Other causes are hypertension, acute ST-elevation anterior myocardial infarction, aortic stenosis, and primary degenerative disease of the conductive system (Lenègre–Lev disease).

Ques. How to treat bifascicular block?

Ans. In asymptomatic case—no treatment is necessary.

NB: Complete heart block with acute anterior infarction is sometimes preceded by sudden appearance of bifascicular block. In that case, temporary pacemaker may be needed.

Ques. What is trifascicular block?

Ans. Trifascicular block means when bifascicular block is associated with first-degree AV block. Trifascicular block includes the following:
- RBBB with left anterior hemiblock with first-degree heart block
- RBBB with left posterior hemiblock with first-degree heart block
- Sometimes, bifascicular block with second-degree (2:1) heart block

ECG in Medical Practice

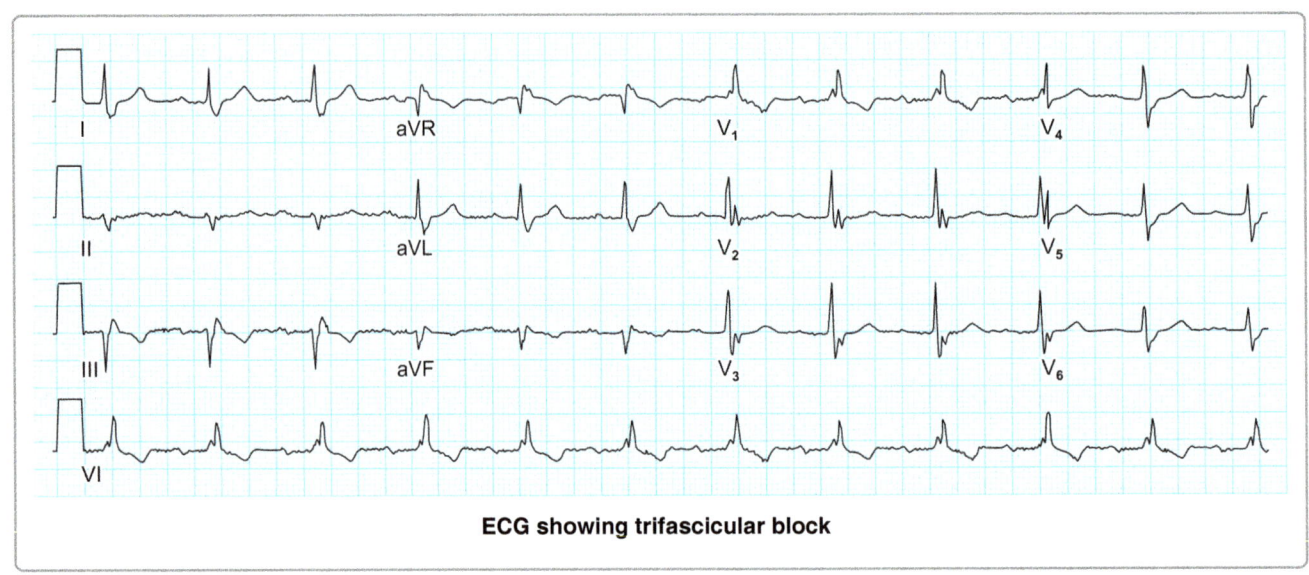

ECG showing trifascicular block

Ques. What are the causes of trifascicular block?

Ans. As follows:
- Ischemic heart disease
- Cardiomyopathy
- Myocarditis
- Electrolyte imbalance (e.g., hypokalemia, hyperkalemia, and hypomagnesemia)
- Digoxin toxicity

Ques. What is the complication of trifascicular block?

Ans. It may turn into complete heart block.

Ques. How to treat?

Ans. Treatment of primary cause. Pacemaker may be necessary.

LEFT BUNDLE BRANCH BLOCK

ECG Criteria of LBBB

- RSR′—in V_5 and V_6, also in L_1 and aVL (M pattern)
- QRS—wide, >0.12 second (>3 small squares)
- Dominant S in V_1 and poor R wave progression in chest lead
- LAD
  (ECG-QRS looks wide from L_1 to all leads—A clue for diagnosis)

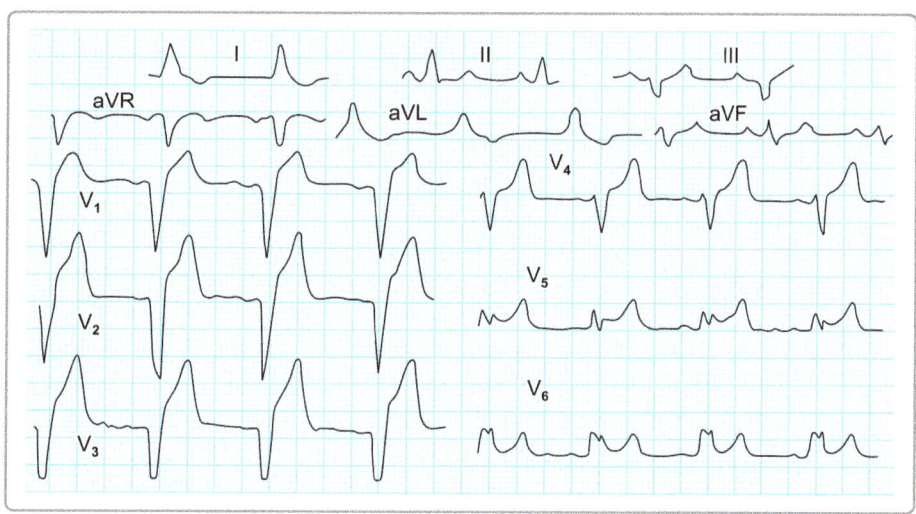

Ques. What are the ECG criteria of incomplete LBBB?

Ans. Typical LBBB morphology but QRS is <0.12 second (<3 small squares).

Ques. What are the causes of LBBB?

Ans. As follows:
- Severe coronary artery disease (two or three vessels disease)
- Acute myocardial infarction
- Cardiomyopathy
- Aortic valve disease (stenosis or regurgitation)
- LVH
- Hypertension
- Myocarditis
- Hyperkalemia
- Primary degenerative disease of the conductive system (Lenègre-Lev disease)

Ques. How to diagnose LBBB clinically?

Ans. On auscultation, there is reverse splitting of second heart sound.

Ques. How to treat LBBB?

Ans. As follows:
- Treatment of primary cause
- In acute myocardial infarction—if there is new LBBB, temporary pacemaker is indicated.

NB: Remember the following points:

- RBBB may be a normal variant, present in healthy persons.
- LBBB is always pathological (it indicates underlying heart disease). Complete LBBB indicates extensive left ventricular disease.
- In the presence of LBBB, acute myocardial infarction is difficult to diagnose.
- When LBBB occurs in acute myocardial infarction, complete heart block may develop.
- Old anterior myocardial infarction may also be difficult to diagnose in the presence of LBBB.
- Small q in V_1 to V_2 may be present normally in LBBB.

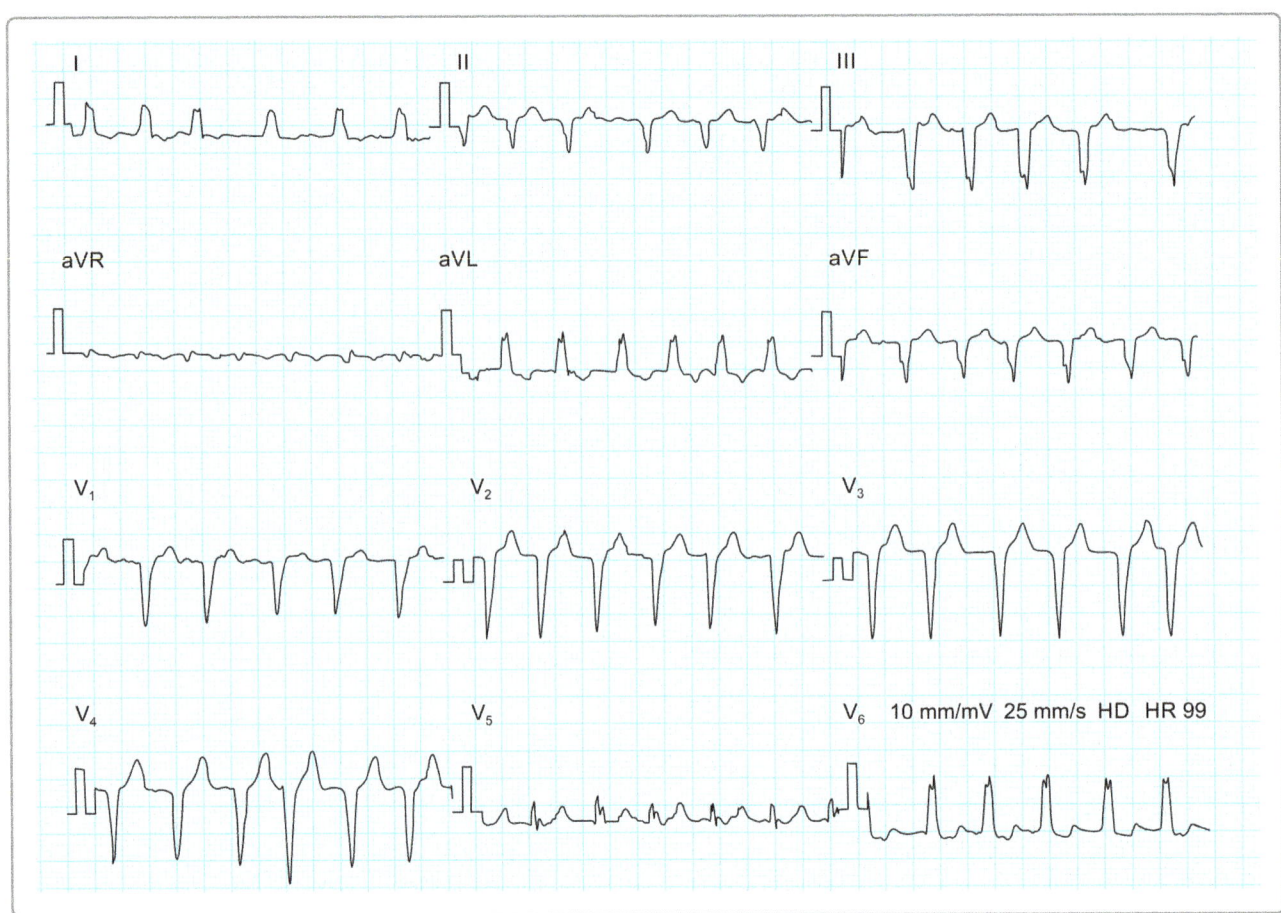

Chapter 2: ECG Changes in Different Diseases

MYOCARDIAL INFARCTION

Before diagnosing myocardial infarction, remember to mention the following points:
- Criteria of infarction (by looking for ST elevation, Q wave, and T inversion)
- Site of infarction (whether anterior, inferior, septal, lateral, and true posterior)
- Recent or old
- STEMI or NSTEMI

Sites of Myocardial Infarction are Detected in Different Leads

Inferior myocardial infarction	L_{III} and aVF (may be in L_{II})
Extensive anterior myocardial infarction	V_1 to V_6
Anteroseptal myocardial infarction	V_1 to V_3 or V_4 (mainly V_2 to V_4)
Lateral myocardial infarction	L_I, aVL, V_5, and V_6
Posterior (true) myocardial infarction	V_1 and V_2 (may be V_1 to V_4)
Subendocardial myocardial infarction (NSTEMI)	Symmetrical T inversion in all chest leads
High lateral myocardial infarction	L_1 and aVL
Anterolateral myocardial infarction	L_1, aVL, V_1 to V_6
Right ventricular infarction	V_3R and V_4R

NB: Remember the following points:
- Once diagnosis is myocardial infarction, be careful to mention whether it is recent or acute and old.
- Whether NSTEMI or STEMI.
- Tell the site always such as inferior, anterior, true posterior, etc.
- Also mention whether it is associated with other findings such as bradycardia, tachycardia, any form of block.

According to duration, myocardial infarction is of three types:
- Hyperacute
- Acute
- Fully evolved phase

Acute myocardial infarction may be of two types:
- STEMI: ST-elevated myocardial infarction
- NSTEMI: Non-ST-elevated myocardial infarction (subendocardial) or non-q wave myocardial infarction

ECG Criteria of Acute Myocardial Infarction (Fully Evolved Case)

- ST elevation (with upward convexity)
- Pathological Q wave
- T inversion

ECG in Medical Practice

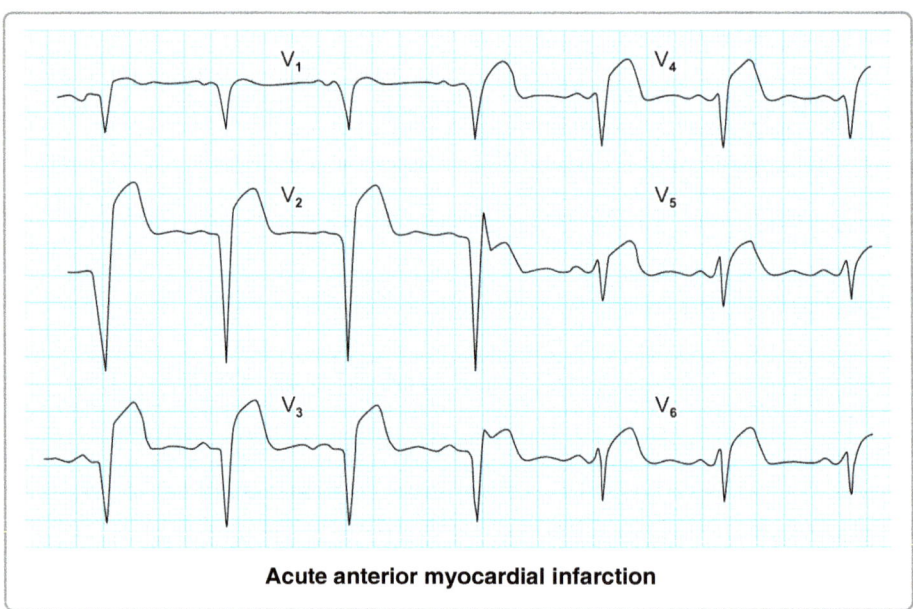

Acute anterior myocardial infarction

Ques. What do the pathological Q, ST elevation, and T inversion signify in myocardial infarction?
Ans. As follows:
- Q wave is due to myocardial necrosis
- ST elevation is due to myocardial injury
- T inversion is due to ischemia

ECG Criteria in Acute STEMI

- ST—elevation with upward convexity

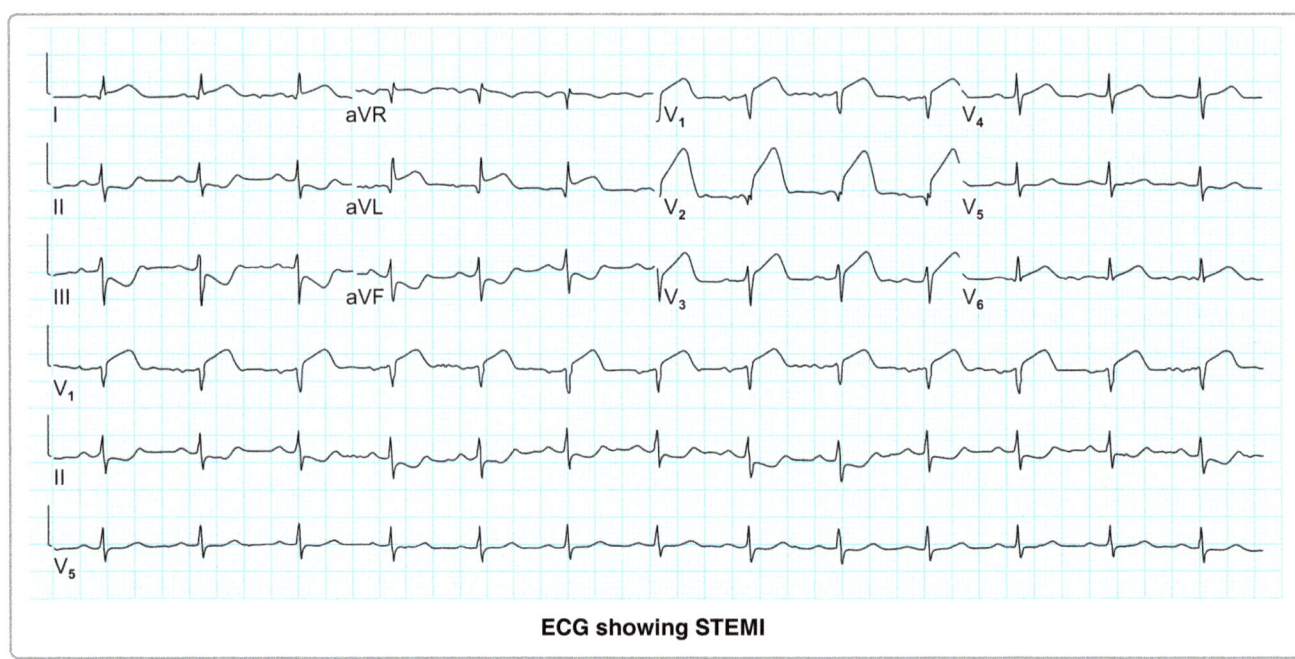

ECG showing STEMI

ECG Criteria in Hyperacute Myocardial Infarction (Within First Few Minutes)

- ST—slope elevation, may be ST depression
- T—tall, pointed and upright, and wide
- R—increased amplitude
- Q—absent
- Ventricular activation time (VAT)—increased

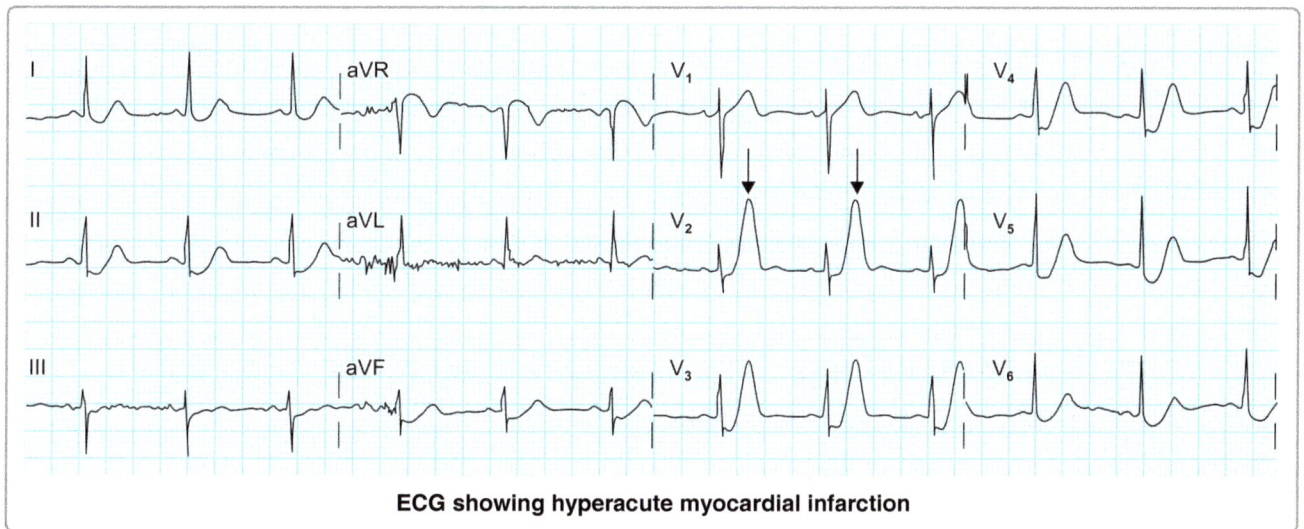

ECG showing hyperacute myocardial infarction

Ques. What is the significance of hyperacute phase?

Ans. It is the most critical phase. Ventricular fibrillation is common in this period. There is myocardial injury, but no infarction or necrosis. This phase may persist for few hours. If treated properly, myocardial blood supply is improved.

Ques. What is the mechanism of tall T in hyperacute myocardial infarction?

Ans. It is due to necrosis of myocardium (myocytes), releasing potassium, which causes localized hyperkalemia, leading to tall T.

Ques. What are the causes of tall T?

Ans. Hyperacute myocardial infarction, hyperkalemia, and Prinzmetal's angina.

Ques. How to differentiate?

Ans. See in T wave abnormality (*Chapter 1*).

ECG Criteria of Old Myocardial Infarction

- Pathological Q wave
- ST—in baseline
- T—normal or inverted

ECG in Medical Practice

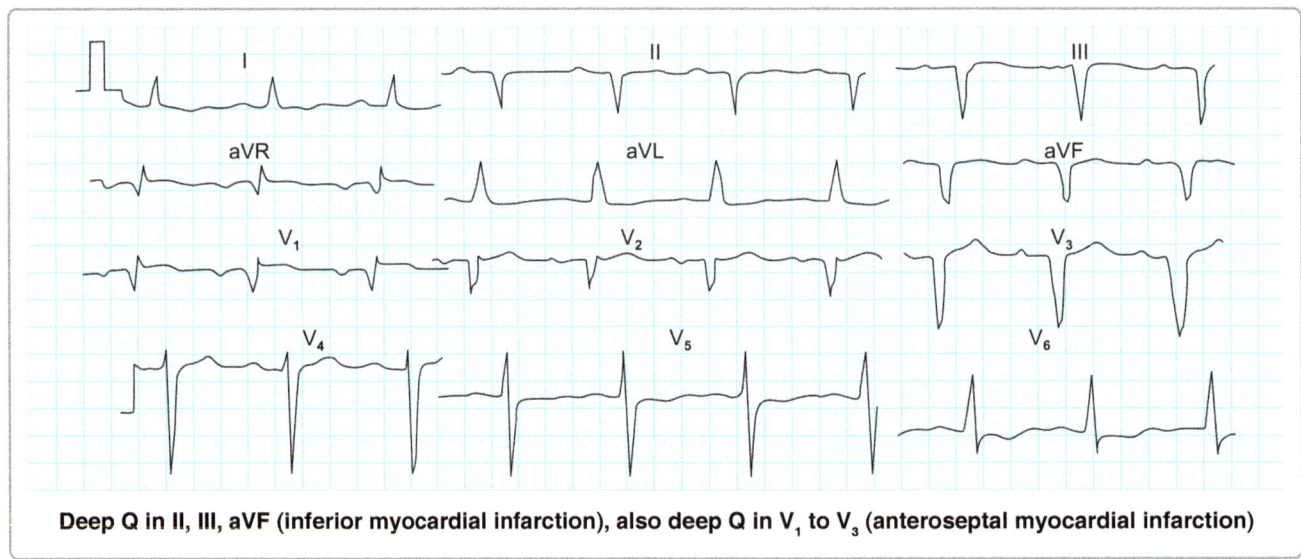

Deep Q in II, III, aVF (inferior myocardial infarction), also deep Q in V$_1$ to V$_3$ (anteroseptal myocardial infarction)

ECG Criteria in NSTEMI (Non-Q Wave Myocardial Infarction or Non-ST Elevation)

- T—deeply inverted in chest leads (usually symmetrical T inversion)
- ST—depression
- Q wave—absent

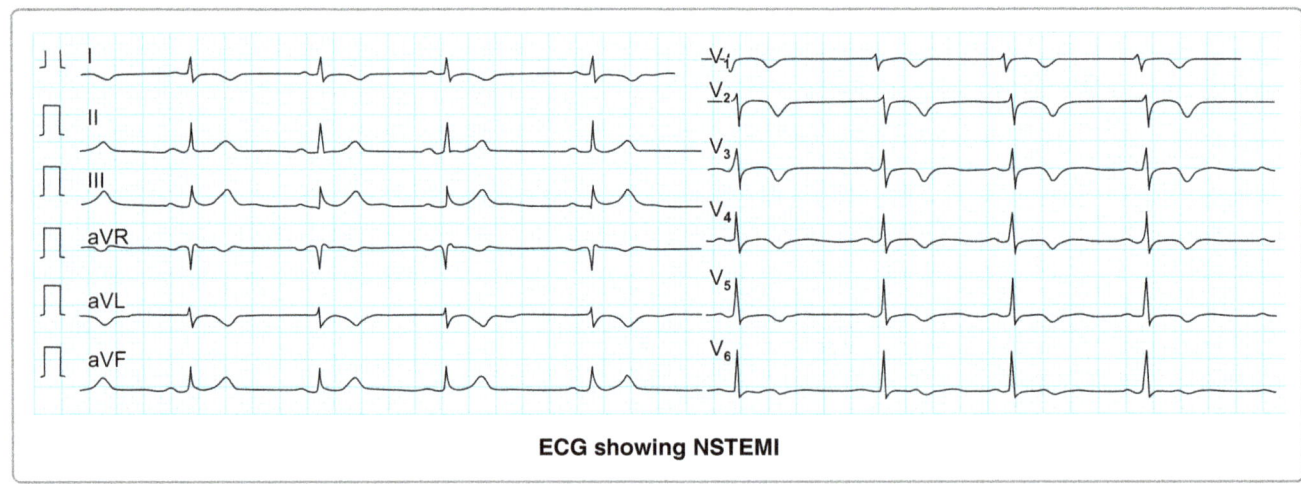

ECG showing NSTEMI

Ques. What are the differences between STEMI (Q wave) and NSTEMI (non-Q wave myocardial infarction)?

Ans. As follows:
- STEMI means infarction of full thickness myocardium (transmural myocardial infarction)
- NSTEMI (Non-Q wave) means infarction of subendocardium (subendocardial myocardial infarction)

Features	STEMI	NSTEMI
1. Prevalence	47%	53%
2. Coronary occlusion	80–90%	15–25%
3. Infarction size	Moderate to large	Small
4. Thrombolysis	Indicated	Not indicated
5. Complication	Common	Uncommon
6. Residual ischemia	10–20%	40–50%
7. Early re-infarction	5–8%	15–25%
8. One month mortality	10–15% (more)	3–5% (less)
9. Two years mortality	30%	30%

Ques. What is the clinical importance of NSTEMI or non-Q wave myocardial infarction?

Ans. As follows:
- There is no evidence that thrombolytic will improve the prognosis. So, thrombolytic therapy is not indicated.
- Complications are uncommon
- Early mortality is less
- They are at higher risk of reinfarction
- Frequent follow-up with adequate preventive measures are required

NB: Remember the following points:
- Myocardial infarction may be STEMI and NSTEMI.
- Fully evolved phase is usually seen after 24 hours.
- ST elevation may not occur before 6 hours.
- Pathological Q is broad >1 mm and deep >2 mm or >25% of amplitude of R wave indicates myocardial infarction.
- Q wave may appear after 8–16 hours (commonly after 24 hours).
- ST segment returns to normal after a few days.
- T wave may remain upright for weeks to months.
- Q wave usually remains permanently in most of the cases (90% cases).
- Acute myocardial infarction may be masked in the presence of LBBB, WPW syndrome, and pacemaker.

ECG Criteria in True Posterior Myocardial Infarction

- R—tall and slightly wide in V_1 to V_2
- T—upright, tall, wide, and symmetrical in V_1 to V_2
- ST—depression
- R/S ratio—in V_1 >1

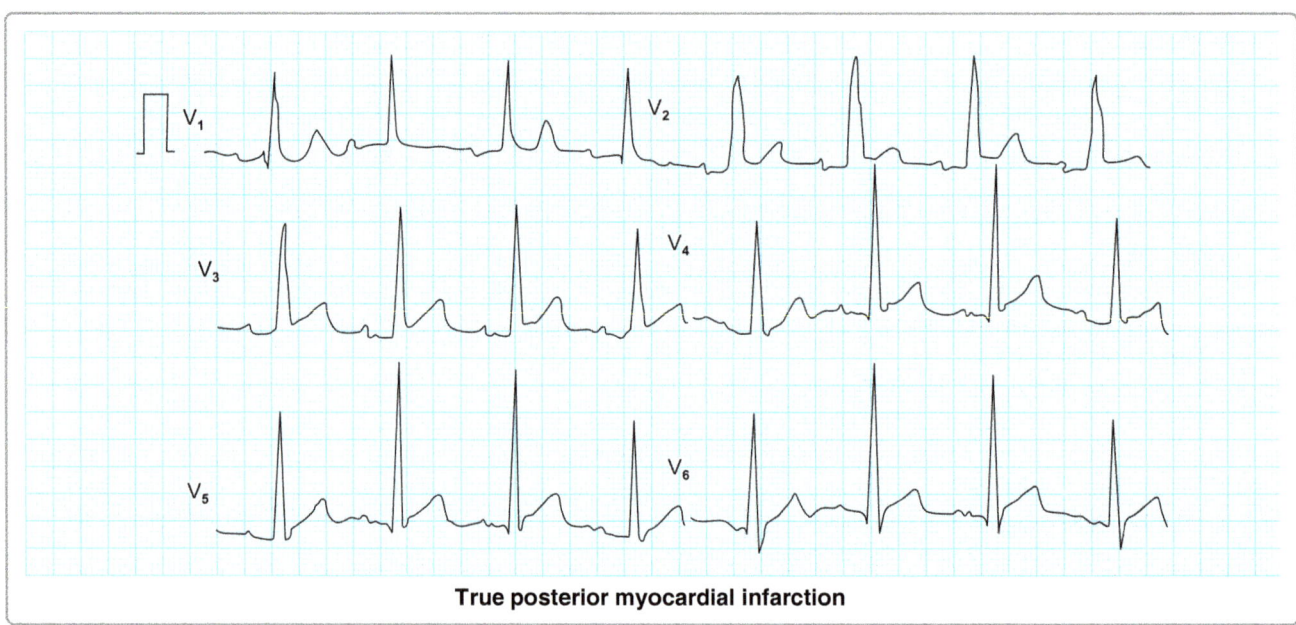

True posterior myocardial infarction

Ques. What are the causes of tall R in V_1?

Ans. As follows:
- Normal variant
- Right ventricular hypertrophy
- True posterior MI
- WPW syndrome (type A)
- Right bundle branch block
- Dextrocardia
- Hypertrophic cardiomyopathy

Ques. How to differentiate between RVH and true posterior myocardial infarction?

Ans. As follows:
- In true posterior myocardial infarction—see the ECG above
- In RVH—tall R in V_1, T inversion, and RAD (may be RAH)

Inferior Myocardial Infarction with Right Ventricular Infarction

In the presence of inferior STEMI, right ventricular infarction is suggested by:
- ST elevation in V_1
- ST elevation in lead III > lead II
- ST elevation in $V_1 > V_2$
- ST elevation in V_1 + ST depression in V_2 (highly specific for right ventricular myocardial infarction)

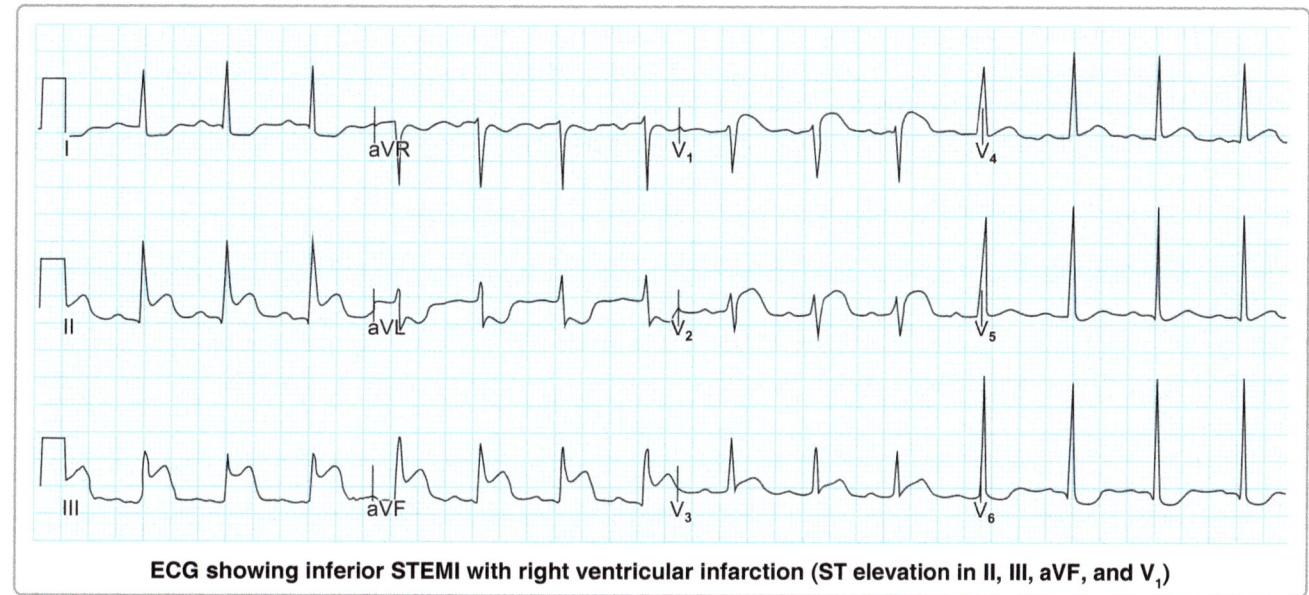

ECG showing inferior STEMI with right ventricular infarction (ST elevation in II, III, aVF, and V_1)

If there is confusion of right ventricular infarction, it is confirmed by ECG of right-sided chest leads which shows:
- ST elevation in V_3R to V_6R.
- Most sensitive is ST elevation >1 mm in V_4R with an upright T wave in that lead.

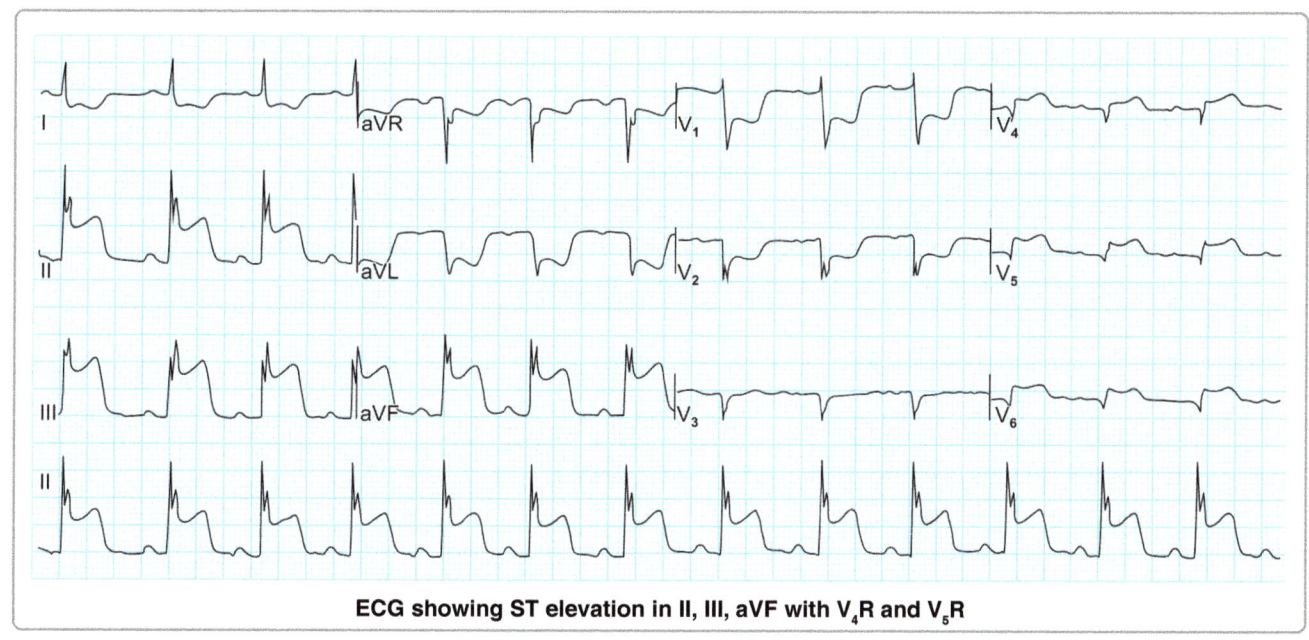

ECG showing ST elevation in II, III, aVF with V_4R and V_5R

Ques. If ST remains elevated after few months of acute myocardial infarction, what is the diagnosis?
Ans. Ventricular aneurysm.

Ques. What are the enzymatic changes of acute myocardial infarction?
Ans. As follows:
- *Troponins*: Troponin I and troponin T are highly specific, rise in 2–4 hours, and persist up to 7 days (may be up to 2 weeks). Minor rise may be seen in unstable angina.
- *Creatine kinase-MB (CK-MB)*: It starts to rise in 4–6 hours and peak in 12 hours. It returns to normal within 48–72 hours. CK-MB is cardiac specific.
- *Aspartate aminotransferase/serum glutamic oxaloacetic transaminase (AST/SGOT)*: It increases after 12 hours, peaks in 24 hours, and returns to normal in 3–4 days.
- *Lactate dehydrogenase (LDH)*: It rises after 12 hours, peaks in 3–4 days, and becomes normal after 7–10 days.

Enzymatic Changes with Time in Acute Myocardial Infarction

Enzyme	Rises (hours)	Peaks at (hours)	Persists for
Troponins I and T	2–4	12–15	7 days (up to 2 weeks)
CK-MB	4–6	12	2–3 days
AST/SGOT	12	24	3–4 days
LDH	12	3–4 days	7–10 days

NB: Remember the following points:
- Troponins I and T, and also CK-MB rise early in acute myocardial infarction.
- If treated with thrombolytic agent, reperfusion is accompanied by rapid rise of CK-MB, due to washout effect.

Ques. What are the complications of myocardial infarction?
Ans. Complications may be *early* and *late*:
1. Early complications:
   - *Arrhythmia*: Ventricular ectopics (common), ventricular fibrillation, ventricular tachycardia, sinus bradycardia (common in inferior myocardial infarction), sinus tachycardia, atrial fibrillation, and heart block
   - Cardiogenic shock
   - Cardiac failure (LVF and biventricular failure)
   - Acute pericarditis (common in second or third day)
   - Thromboembolism (systemic and pulmonary)
   - Rupture of the papillary muscle or chordae tendineae resulting in MR
   - Rupture of interventricular septum causing VSD
   - Rupture of the ventricular wall leading to cardiac tamponade
2. Late complications:
   - Ventricular aneurysm (10%)
   - Postmyocardial infarction syndrome (Dressler syndrome)
   - Frozen shoulder
   - Postinfarct angina (may occur in up to 50% of patients)
   - Ventricular remodeling

Chapter 2: ECG Changes in Different Diseases

Ques. What is postmyocardial infarction syndrome (Dressler syndrome)?

Ans. It is a late complication of myocardial infarction that occurs usually a few weeks or even months (2-10 weeks) after acute myocardial infarction. It is characterized by *(5P's)*:
- **P**ain (chest pain)
- **P**yrexia
- **P**leurisy
- **P**ericarditis (or pericardial effusion)
- **P**neumonitis (or pulmonary infiltrate)

Ques. What is the mechanism of postmyocardial infarction syndrome?

Ans. It is due to autoimmune reaction to necrosed myocardium. Antimyocardial antibody may be found in the blood. Recurrence is common, confuses with new myocardial infarction or unstable angina.

Ques. How to treat postmyocardial infarction syndrome?

Ans. As follows:
- High-dose aspirin (600–900 mg) every 4–6 hours or other nonsteroidal anti-inflammatory drug (NSAID)
- In severe or in recurrent case—corticosteroid may be given
- Anticoagulant should be discontinued (unless strong evidence for high risk of thromboembolism)

Ques. How to treat acute myocardial infarction?

Ans. As follows:
- Admission in critical care unit (CCU)
- Complete bed rest
- High flow O_2 inhalation (60%)—2-4 L/min by nasal cannula
- To relieve pain—IV injection morphine (5-10 mg) or diamorphine (2.5-5 mg) plus antiemetic (cyclizine or metoclopramide). It may be repeated, if necessary.
- Chewable aspirin—300 mg and clopidogrel 300 mg or ticagrelor 180 mg orally.
- Primary percutaneous coronary intervention (PCI), if available.
  - It is indicated when ECG shows new bundle branch block or typical ST elevation in two contiguous leads of 1 mm or more in limbs leads or 2 mm or more in chest leads.
  - It is the treatment of choice in patient presenting with 12 hours of symptoms of onset. Even it can be considered if the patient presents within first 24 hours.
  - After PCI, aspirin with prasugrel or ticagrelor should be continued for 12 months. If aspirin is contraindicated, clopidogrel is a suitable alternative.
- *If PCI is not available and the patient's presentation is delayed*: Thrombolytic therapy such as tenecteplase or reteplase is given as an intravenous bolus, provided there is no contraindication. It is more effective, if started particularly within 12 hours (greatest benefit within first 2 hours).
  - Reperfusion occurs in 50-70% of cases. Only hazard of thrombolytic therapy is bleeding, cerebral hemorrhage causes four extra strokes per 1,000 patients treated and the incidence of other major bleeding is between 0.5 and 1%.
  - If significant risk of bleeding, thrombolytic therapy should be avoided. Again, emergency PCI should be considered.
  - Even where thrombolysis successfully achieves reperfusion, PCI should be considered within 24 hours to prevent recurrent infarction and improve outcome.
- *Other therapy*:
  - β-blocker (if no contraindication)—IV bolus atenolol 5-10 mg or metoprolol 5-15 mg slowly over 5 minutes. Oral atenolol 25-50 mg BD, or bisoprolol 5 mg daily or metoprolol 25-50 mg BD or TDS may be given.
  - Sublingual nitroglycerin—0.3-1 mg (may be repeated)

- *Anticoagulants*: Low-molecular weight heparin (SC enoxaparin, 1 mg/kg body weight 12 hourly) or SC pentasaccharides (fondaparinux 2.5 mg daily) for 8 days.
- Angiotensin-converting enzyme (ACE) inhibitor
- Statin such as atorvastatin or rosuvastatin

Ques. How to treat NSTEMI?

Ans. As follows:

- *High-risk group*: It includes patients with persistent or recurrent angina with ST elevation >2 mm or deep negative T wave changes, clinical signs of heart failure or hemodynamic instability, and life-threatening arrhythmias (ventricular fibrillation and ventricular tachycardia). These groups of patients may develop myocardial infarction or sudden death may occur in these patients. So, coronary angiography and intervention should be done.
- *Low-risk group*: It includes patients with no recurrence of chest pain during observation, no signs of heart failure, normal ECG or minor T wave change on arrival and at 6–12 hours, and normal troponin on initial assays and 6–12 hours postadmission. These patients can be managed with oral aspirin, clopidogrel, β-blocker, and nitrate. An endotracheal intubation should be performed after 6 weeks. If it is negative, it has good prognosis. If it is positive, angiography should be done. If the patient is unable to perform endotracheal intubation, then dobutamine stress echocardiography or myocardial perfusion scintigraphy are recommended.

Ques. What is the role of an anticoagulant in myocardial infarction?

Ans. Anticoagulation can be achieved using unfractionated heparin, fractioned (low molecular weight) heparin, or a pentasaccharide such as subcutaneous fondaparinux (2.5 mg daily). Anticoagulation should be continued for 8 days or until discharge from hospital or coronary revascularization has been completed. After that, warfarin should be considered, if there is persistent atrial fibrillation or extensive anterior myocardial infarction or echocardiography shows mural thrombus.

Ques. What are the contraindications of thrombolytic therapy?

Ans. As follows:

1. *Absolute contraindications*:
   - Hemorrhagic stroke at any time
   - Ischemic stroke in preceding 3 months
   - Central nervous system damage or neoplasm or vascular malformation
   - Recent major trauma, surgery, and head injury (within preceding 3 weeks)
   - Gastrointestinal bleeding within the last month
   - Coagulation or bleeding abnormalities
   - Suspected dissecting aortic aneurysm
   - Diabetic retinopathy (proliferative)
2. *Relative contraindications*:
   - Oral anticoagulant therapy
   - Ischemic stroke >3 months
   - Heavy vaginal bleeding, pregnancy, or puerperal bleeding or within 1 week of postpartum
   - Severe hypertension (malignant hypertension, systolic >180, and diastolic >120)
   - High probability of active peptic ulcer
   - Advanced liver disease
   - Traumatic or prolonged (>10 minutes) CPR or major surgery (< 3 weeks)

NB: Streptokinase is avoided, if the patient received it within 5 days to 5 years. Circulating neutralizing antibody is produced. In such case, alteplase or tissue plasminogen activator (tPA) or other thrombolytic drugs, tenecteplase and reteplase, may be used.

Ques. How would you follow-up a patient after acute myocardial infarction?

Ans. The patient should be reviewed after 6–8 weeks. Risk factors should be reviewed and modified accordingly:
- Lifestyle modification (avoid stress, heavy work, etc.)
- Smoking should be stopped
- Regular exercise
- Diet (weight control and lipid-lowering)
- Good control of hypertension (BP <140/85 mm Hg) and diabetes mellitus
- Dual antiplatelet (aspirin with ticagrelor or prasugrel) should be continued for 12 months.
- β-blocker (for long time), may be discontinued after 3 years in low-risk, normotensive patient.
- ACE inhibitor should be continued indefinitely in patient with persistent left ventricular dysfunction (EF < 40%).
- Lipid-lowering agents (target total cholesterol <5.0 mmol/L and/or LDL <3.0 mmol/L)
- Rehabilitation

NB: Remember: Myocardial infarction may be difficult to diagnose in presence of the following diseases:

- WPW syndrome
- LBBB
- LVH cardiomyopathy
- Hyperkalemia
- COPD with RVH
- Chest deformity

MYOCARDIAL ISCHEMIA

Myocardial ischemia includes stable angina and acute coronary syndrome.

ECG Criteria of Stable Angina

- Resting ECG may be normal
- There may be ST depression or T inversion or both
- ECG during chest pain may show ST depression

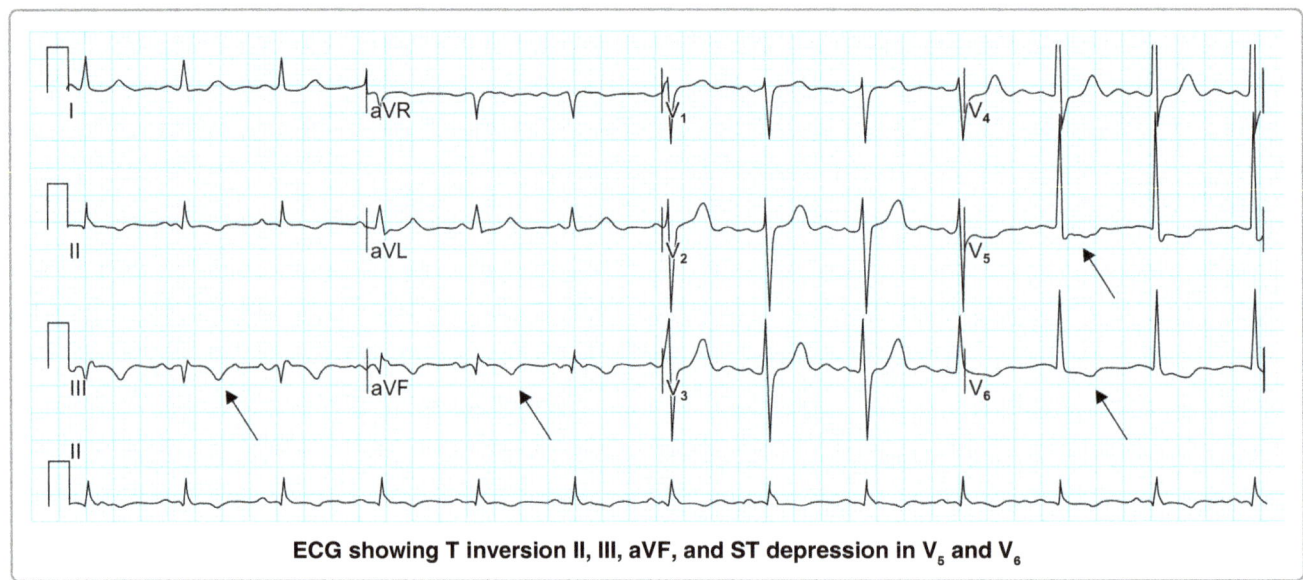

ECG showing T inversion II, III, aVF, and ST depression in V_5 and V_6

Ques. What are the types of angina?

Ans. As follows:
- Stable angina or angina pectoris
- *Unstable angina*: It is characterized by angina of new onset or rapidly worsening angina, angina at rest, or minimal activity. It is more severe, lasting for longer duration, occurs more frequently, not improved by rest or nitroglycerine. Unstable angina is due to rupture, fissuring, or ulceration of an atherosclerotic plaque or thrombus. ECG shows transient ST segment depression and T wave changes (depression) but enzymes are normal. It may cause myocardial infarction in 10–20% cases.
- *Prinzmetal's angina*: It occurs at rest without any provoking factor, usually in the early morning. It is more common in female. It occurs due to coronary artery spasm. ECG shows transient ST elevation, similar to STEMI. However, in Prinzmetal's angina, ST elevation is transient, resolves spontaneously, or with nitroglycerine during pain. Enzymes are normal.
- *Decubitus angina*: It occurs when patient lies down. It is due to impaired left ventricular function.

Ques. What is angina pectoris?

Ans. Angina pectoris is a symptom complex caused by transient myocardial ischemia, which occurs when there is an imbalance between myocardial oxygen supply and demand.

Ques. **What is the presentation of angina pectoris?**
Ans. Main symptom is chest pain, which is characterized by:
- Site—central, retrosternal chest
- Character—stabbing or squeezing or constricting
- Duration—5–10 minutes
- Radiation—lower jaw, neck, and inner side of the left arm up to the finger
- Precipitated by exertion, eating, or emotion (3E)
- Relieved by rest and nitroglycerine

Ques. **How to investigate?**
Ans. As follows:
- ECG is often normal. During attack, there is ST-depression and T-inversion.
- CXR
- Echocardiography
- Endotracheal intubation
- Coronary arteriography
- *Other stress tests*: Myocardial perfusion scan, stress echocardiography, and transthoracic echocardiography.
- *For risk factor*: Fasting lipid profile and blood sugar, thyroid function test (according to history).

Treatment

During Acute Attack

- Sublingual glyceryl trinitrate (GTN), given from a metered-dose aerosol or as tablet which is allowed to dissolve under the tongue and retained in the mouth. It usually relieves angina in 2–3 minutes.
- If no response, it can be repeated. But if still no response, myocardial infarction should be excluded.

Prevention of Further Attack

1. *Antiplatelet therapy*: Low dose aspirin (75–150 mg) and clopidogrel (75 mg daily).
2. *Antianginal drugs*:
   To prevent angina pain: Oral nitrates, such as GTN 2.6 mg twice daily or isosorbide dinitrate (10–20 mg 8 hourly) and isosorbide mononitrate (20–60 mg once or twice a day) can be given by mouth.
   - *Other drugs*: β-blocker (atenolol, metoprolol, and bisoprolol). Calcium antagonists (nifedipine, nicardipine, verapamil, and diltiazem) and potassium channel activators such as nicorandil may be used.
   - *If recurrent or persistent pain*: Coronary angiogram should be done. If coronary artery blockage, then stenting or CABG may be required.
3. *Risk Factors should be Controlled*:
   - Smoking must be stopped
   - Reduction of weight, if obese
   - Regular exercise, at least for 30 minutes daily
   - Avoid alcohol intake
   - Control of hypertension and diabetes mellitus
   - Lipid-lowering drugs such as atorvastatin and rosuvastatin
   - Avoidance of anxiety, tension, and depression
   - Lifestyle modification

Acute coronary syndrome

It is used to describe the spectrum of syndrome that includes the following:
- Unstable angina
- STEMI (described before)
- NSTEMI (described before)

ECG Criteria in Unstable Angina

- ST segment depression
- T inversion

It may be confused with NSTEMI. To differentiate cardiac enzymes should be done (troponin and CK-MB).
- *If enzymes are elevated*: It indicates NSTEMI.
- *If enzymes are not elevated*: It indicates unstable angina.

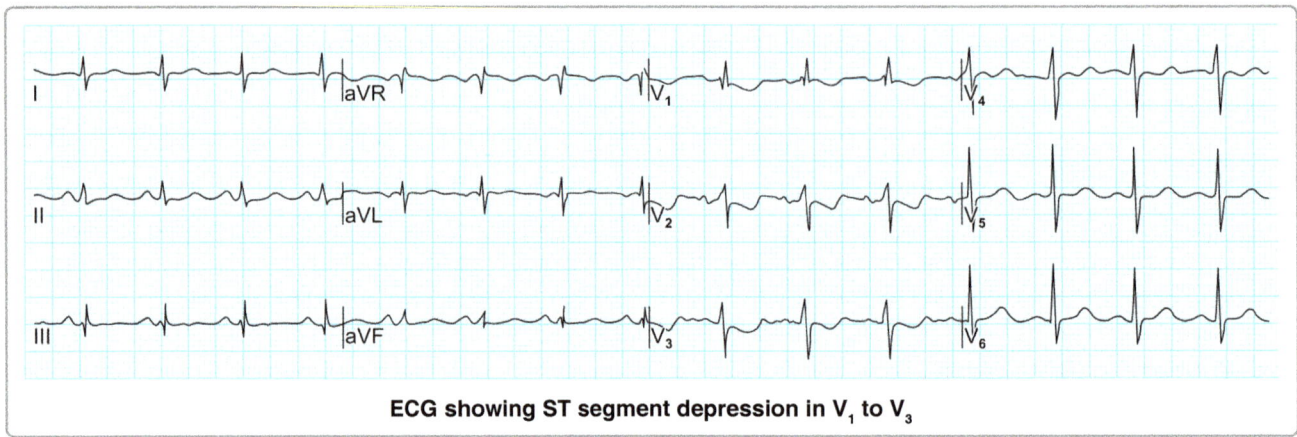

ECG showing ST segment depression in V_1 to V_3

VENTRICULAR ANEURYSM

ECG Criteria of Ventricular Aneurysm

- Persistent ST elevation (after myocardial infarction)

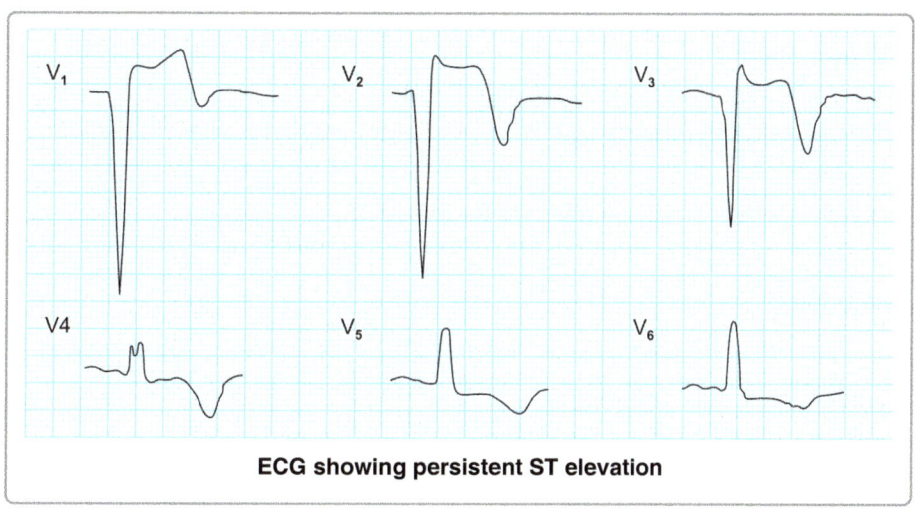

ECG showing persistent ST elevation

Ques. How to diagnose ventricular aneurysm?

Ans. As follows:
- History of myocardial infarction
- Double apex beat shows paradoxical movement (called see-saw movement)
- Heart may be enlarged
- ECG—persistent ST elevation in repeated ECG
- CXR—heart enlarged, with a bulged or rounded protrusion from the left ventricular wall, calcification may occur at the wall of aneurysm
- Paradoxical movement on fluoroscopy
- Confirmed by echocardiogram
- Left ventriculography
- Radionuclide study may be done

Ques. What are the likely cause of ventricular aneurysm?

Ans. It is usually 6 weeks after transmural myocardial infarction (usually anterior myocardial infarction). Site of ventricular aneurysm are
- Anterior or apical aneurysm—persistent ST elevation in V_1 to V_6
- In inferior aneurysm—persistent ST elevation in lead II, III and aVF

Ques. What are the complications of ventricular aneurysm?

Ans. As follows:
- Heart failure
- Arrhythmia (ectopic, atrial fibrillation, occasionally, serious ventricular arrhythmia, etc.)
- Systemic embolism from mural thrombus

Ques. How to treat ventricular aneurysm?

Ans. As follows:
1. *Symptomatic treatment*:
   - If heart failure—diuretic, ACE inhibitor, and digoxin
   - If arrhythmia—antiarrhythmic drugs
   - Aspirin in low dose
   - Treatment for embolism (anticoagulant and aspirin)
2. If difficult to control, surgery is indicated (aneurysmectomy may be done, but mortality is very high).

NB: Remember the following points:
- 3.5–20% develop aneurysm following acute myocardial infarction. It is usually a late complication following myocardial infarction.
- Calcification of aneurysmal wall may develop which indicates long-standing case.
- Shape of ST elevation is relatively unique and coving.

ACUTE PERICARDITIS

ECG Criteria of Acute Pericarditis

- ST elevated with upward concavity (chair-shaped or saddle-shaped): Better seen in L_I, L_{II}, aVL, aVF, V_4 to V_6
- T upright in acute phase
- PR depression (very specific indicators of acute pericarditis)

Subsequent ECG changes:
- ST returns to baseline
- T inversion that remains for weeks to months

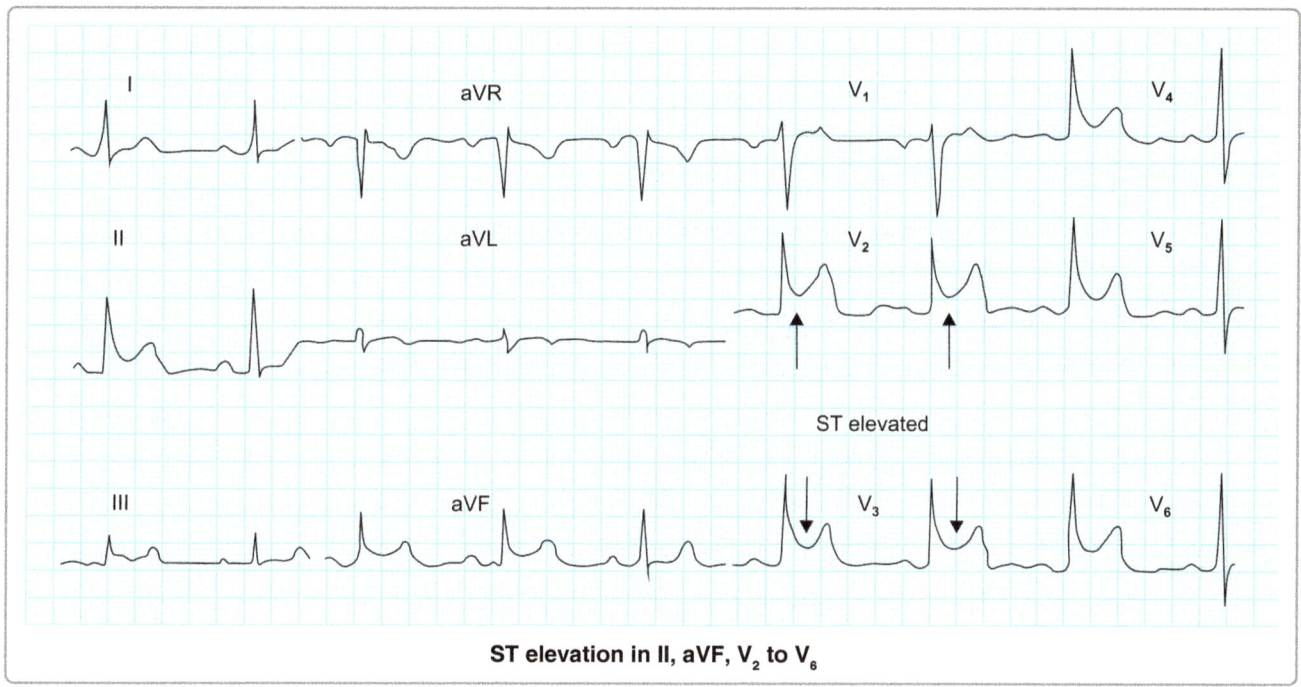

ST elevation in II, aVF, V_2 to V_6

Ques. How to differentiate acute pericarditis from acute myocardial infarction by ECG?

Ans. As follows:
- In myocardial infarction—ST elevation with upward convexity
- In pericarditis—ST elevation with upward concavity (pericardium envelops the heart, so ST changes are more generalized and seen in most leads)

Ques. What is the clinical finding in acute pericarditis?

Ans. Pericardial rub. Features are:
- It is a high-pitched, harsh, scratching, grating, leathery sound, to and fro in quality
- Better heard over the left lower parasternal area with the patient leaning forward (bare area of heart—it is the part of heart, which is not covered by lung)
- Augmented by pressing the stethoscope
- It is usually heard in systole, but may be present in diastole
- It is present after holding the breath (to differentiate from pleural rub)

Ques. What are the presentations of acute pericarditis?

Ans. As follows:
- Chest pain which is retrosternal. It is usually sharp or stabbing in nature, may radiate to the shoulder and neck.
- Pain is aggravated by movement, lying down and deep breathing, exercise, and swallowing.
- Pain may be relieved by sitting or bending forward.

Ques. What investigations are done in acute pericarditis?

Ans. As follows:
- ECG
- CXR PA view
- Echocardiography
- Computed tomography (CT) and cardiac MR may be done in some cases
- Other investigations according to suspicion of cause

Ques. What are the causes of acute pericarditis?

Ans. As follows:
- Following acute myocardial infarction (usually in second or third day)
- Viral (coxsackie B and echovirus): A common cause
- Acute rheumatic fever
- Bacterial (such as *Staphylococcus aureus* and *Haemophilus influenzae*)
- Tuberculous pericarditis
- Fungal (such as histoplasmosis and coccidioidomycosis)
- Uremia (an indication of urgent dialysis)
- Malignancy (from carcinoma of bronchus, breast, lymphoma, and leukemia)
- Trauma
- Radiation
- Drugs (doxorubicin and cyclophosphamide)
- Collagen disease (SLE and scleroderma)

Ques. How would you treat acute pericarditis?

Ans. As follows:
- To relieve pain—NSAID (indomethacin or ibuprofen or aspirin)
- In severe or recurrent case—corticosteroid should be given
- If no response to steroid—azathioprine or colchicine may be given
- If recurrence with no response to medical treatment—pericardiotomy may be done
- Treatment of primary cause such as antibiotic, if bacterial infection. Anti-Koch's, if tuberculosis is suspected

Ques. What are the features of postmyocardial infarction pericarditis?

Ans. As follows:
- It occurs in 20% of patients in the first few days following myocardial infarction, more commonly anterior myocardial infarction and STEMI with high serum cardiac enzymes.
- Incidence is <5–6% with thrombolysis.
- Pericarditis may occur as Dressler syndrome, 2–10 weeks after infarction.

PERICARDIAL EFFUSION

ECG Criteria of Pericardial Effusion

- Low-voltage tracing
- T inversion
- Sinus tachycardia
- PR segment depression
  (There may be electrical alternans, in which height QRS complex may alternate from beat to beat. The combination of small QRS, tachycardia, and electrical alternans is highly suggestive of pericardial effusion).

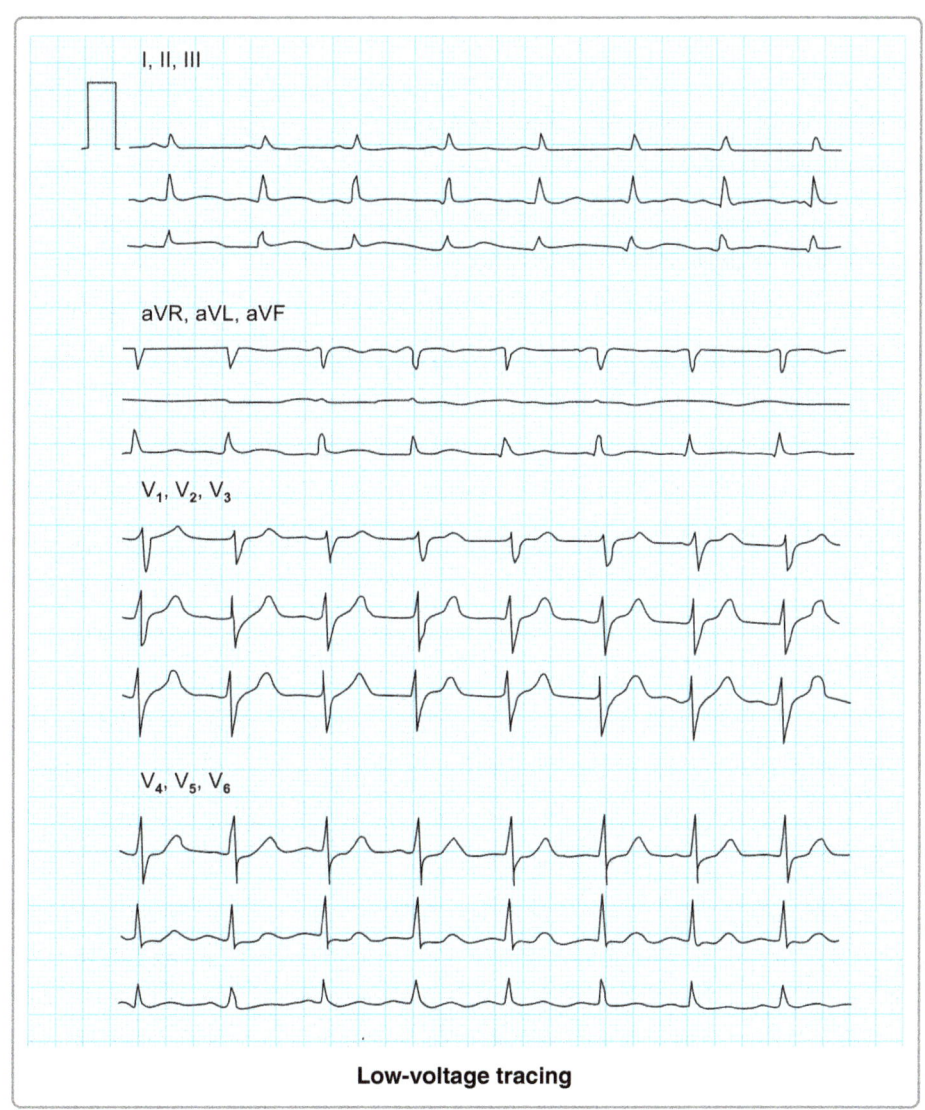

Low-voltage tracing

ECG in Medical Practice

Ques. What investigation should be done in pericardial effusion?

Ans. As follows:
- ECG
- Echocardiogram (2D or M-mode)
- CXR PA view
- CT or MRI (magnetic resonance imaging) of chest

Ques. What is cardiac tamponade?

Ans. It is a state of compression of heart in rapidly developing pericardial effusion. It interferes with the diastolic filling of heart and the patient develops features of shock.

Ques. What are the ECG changes in cardiac tamponade?

Ans. ECG findings are same as in pericardial effusion. Sinus tachycardia and electrical alternans are specific but not sensitive sign of cardiac tamponade.

Ques. What are the causes of cardiac tamponade?

Ans. As follows:
- Trauma or cardiac surgery (causing hemopericardium)
- Malignancy (repeated effusion may occur)
- Myocardial rupture
- Dissecting aortic aneurysm
- Sometimes, any cause of pericardial effusion can cause

Ques. How to treat?

Ans. As follows:
- It is a medical emergency. Pericardiocentesis should be done
- Treatment of primary cause

WOLFF–PARKINSON–WHITE SYNDROME

ECG Criteria of WPW Syndrome

- PR—short <0.12 second
- QRS—wide
- Delta wave—in the upstroke of QRS (slurred QRS)
- Q wave—may be present in lead II, III and aVF (confused with inferior myocardial infarction).

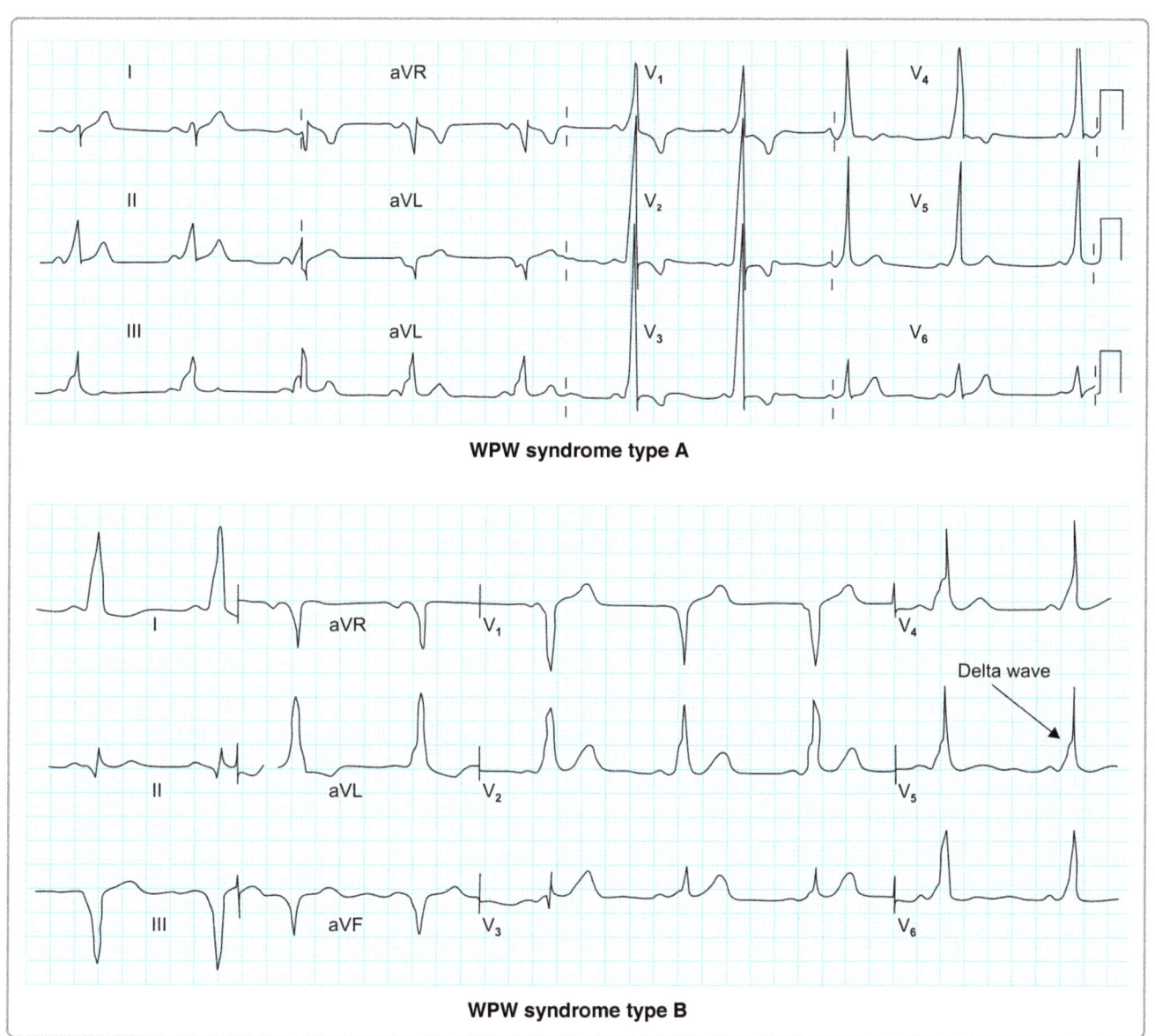

WPW syndrome type A

WPW syndrome type B

Ques. What is WPW syndrome?

Ans. It is a syndrome in which there is an accessory pathway that bypasses the AV node and connects the atrium and the ventricle (by bundles of Kent). It may be associated with other congenital anomaly, commonly Ebstein anomaly.

Ques. What are the types of WPW syndrome?

Ans. It is of two types:
- Type A: Accessory pathway on the left side.
- Type B: Accessory pathway on the right side.

(The accessory pathway is called the bundle of Kent).

NB: To find the type, look at V_1: Type A (deflection—above) and type B (deflection—below).

Ques. What are the ECG changes in different types of WPW syndrome?

Ans. As follows:
- Type A: Tall R in V_1 and V_2.
- Type B: Deep Q in V_1 and V_2 (also Q in L_{III} and aVF).

Ques. How to locate the aberrant pathway of WPW syndrome?

Ans. By electrophysiological study.

Ques. What investigations should be done in WPW syndrome?

Ans. As follows:
- ECG
- Electrophysiological study
- Echocardiogram to exclude other disease

Ques. How to treat WPW syndrome?

Ans. As follows:
- *If asymptomatic*: No treatment is required
- *If symptomatic*:
  - Transvenous radiofrequency catheter ablation of accessory pathway is the specific treatment.
  - If this is not available—prophylactic antiarrhythmic drug should be given (β-blocker, amiodarone, flecainide, and propafenone). These drugs prolong refractory period of accessory pathway.
  - Previously, surgical resection of accessory pathway used to be done.

Ques. What are the presentations of WPW syndrome?

Ans. As follows:
- May be asymptomatic and may present with palpitation
- Paroxysmal attack of atrial or supraventricular tachycardia (common) due to reentry circuit.
- Atrial fibrillation
- Syncope
- Sudden death (due to atrial fibrillation)
- Rarely—ventricular tachycardia and ventricular fibrillation

Ques. What is the definite treatment of WPW syndrome?

Ans. Catheter ablation is the definite treatment.

Ques. What is the prophylactic treatment of WPW syndrome?
Ans. β-blocker, flecainide, propafenone, or amiodarone.

Ques. Why digoxin is avoided in WPW syndrome?
Ans. Digoxin blocks the AV node and increases the conduction through the accessory pathway. So, it increases the heart rate (verapamil may cause same effect). It may precipitate ventricular fibrillation.

Ques. What are the drugs contraindicated in WPW syndrome?
Ans. Digoxin and IV verapamil. These drugs shorten the refractory period of accessory pathway and also increase the conduction through the accessory pathway.

Ques. What are the types of accessory pathways?
Ans. There are three types:
- *Bundles of Kent*: It is the accessory pathway that bypasses the AV node and connects the atrium and ventricular myocardium. It is typical in WPW syndrome.
- *James bypass tract*: It is the accessory pathway that connects the atrium to the bundle of His. It is typical in Lown-Ganong-Levine (LGL) syndrome.
- *Mahaim fiber*: It is the accessory pathway that connects the atrium, the AV node, or the bundle of His to the distal Purkinje fibers or ventricular myocardium. ECG shows normal PR, but abnormally wide QRS with delta wave (which may be intermittent).

Ques. Why PR interval is short and what is the mechanism of delta wave?
Ans. As follows:
- *Short PR interval*: Impulse is conducted rapidly from the atria to the ventricles through the accessory pathway, causing early ventricular depolarization. So, PR interval is short.
- *Delta wave*: The accessory pathway causes early depolarization of part of the ventricle, giving rise to slow upstroke (delta wave—first portion of QRS complex). Then, the normally conducted impulse through the AV node causes depolarization of the rest of ventricle, giving rise to the rest of QRS complex.
- Delta wave is absent, if there is tachycardia, as the ventricle is excited by normal pathway.

NB: Remember the following points:
- Hallmark of WPW syndrome in ECG is delta wave.
- When WPW syndrome is associated with tachycardia, it may be confused with ventricular tachycardia.
- Digoxin and verapamil may increase the heart rate. These drugs may precipitate ventricular tachycardia and ventricular fibrillation.
- In about 50% cases of WPW syndrome, the accessory pathway only conducts in the retrograde pathway from ventricles to atria and so, does not alter ECG in sinus rhythms. This is called concealed accessory pathway.

Ques. What are the ECG changes in atrial fibrillation in the presence of WPW syndrome?
Ans. ECG changes in such cases are as follows:
- Irregular rapid ventricular response due to atrial fibrillation.
- Rapid heart rate due to conduction through accessory pathway.
- Wide and variable QRS morphology.

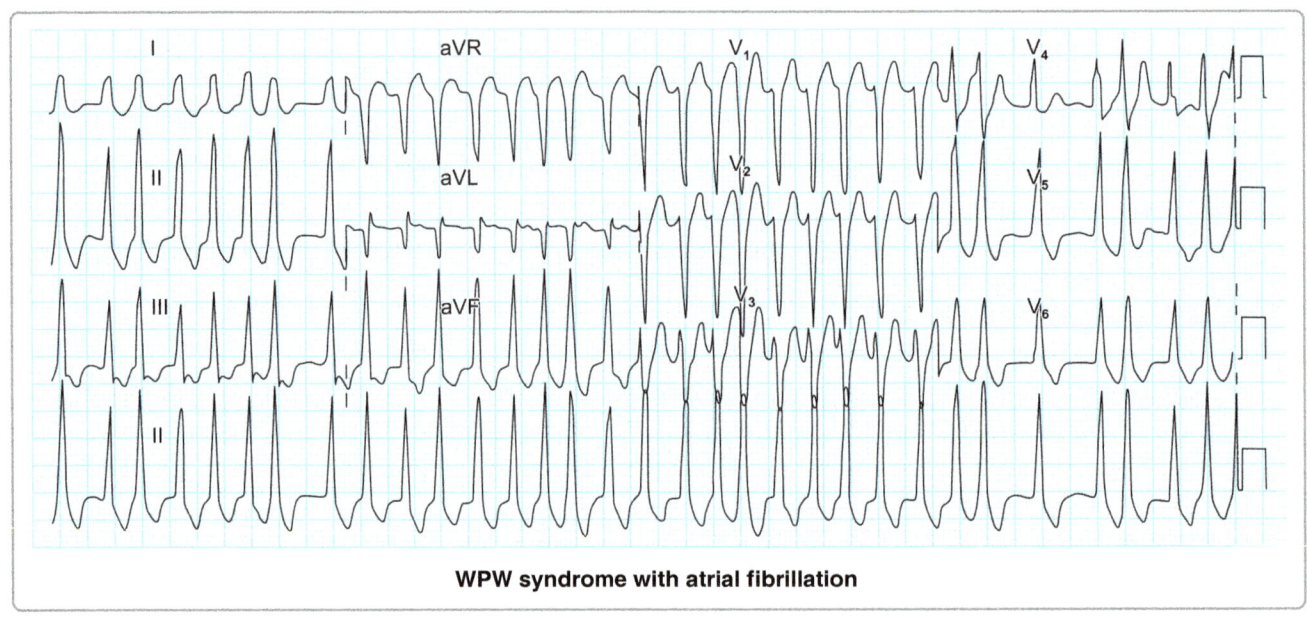

WPW syndrome with atrial fibrillation

Ques. How to treat atrial fibrillation with WPW syndrome?

Ans. It is a medical emergency. Sudden death may occur. Treatment is as follows:
- If troublesome symptoms—DC shock should be given. If not available, IV flecainide.
- Radiofrequency ablation of abnormal pathway.
- Drugs that slow the conduction of accessory pathway may be used—amiodarone, flecainide, disopyramide, sotalol, etc.

Ques. What diseases are difficult to diagnose in the presence of WPW syndrome?

Ans. As follows:

Type A confuses with:
- RBBB
- RVH
- True posterior myocardial infarction.

Type B confuses with:
- LBBB
- LVH
- Inferior myocardial infarction.

LOWN–GANONG–LEVINE SYNDROME

ECG Criteria of LGL Syndrome

- PR interval—short
- QRS—normal (no delta wave)

Ques. What is LGL syndrome?

Ans. It is a syndrome in which there is a congenital accessory pathway (James bypass tract) that joins the atrium to the common bundle of His.

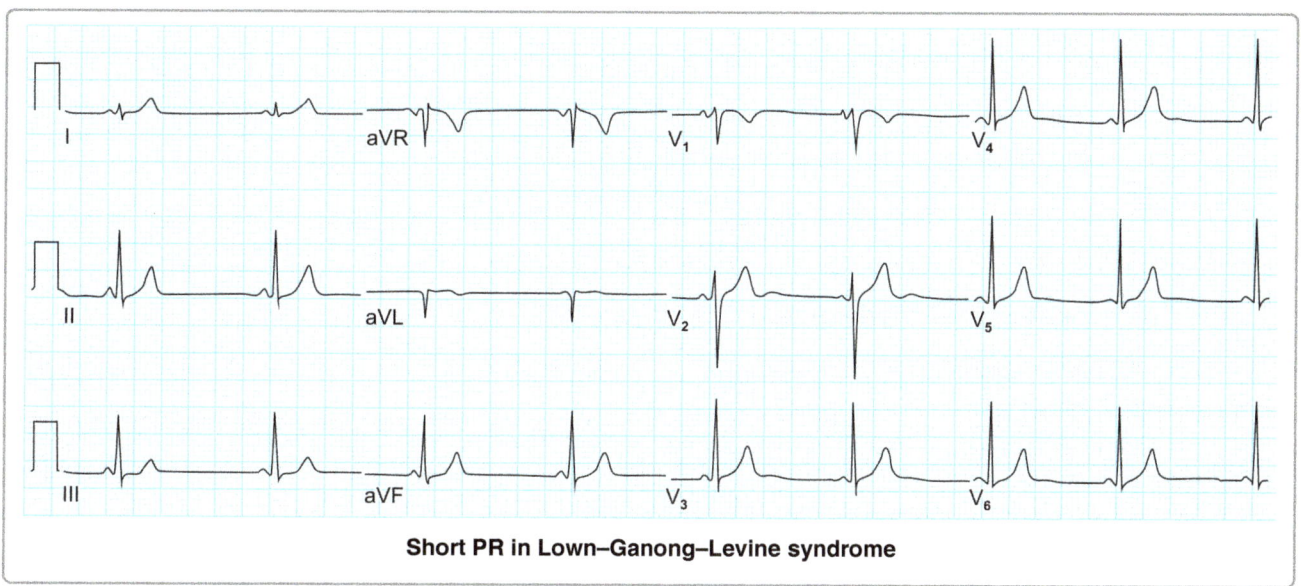

Short PR in Lown–Ganong–Levine syndrome

Ques. Why QRS is normal in LGL syndrome?

Ans. The accessory pathway simply connects the atrium to the common bundle of His. It does not activate the ventricle directly. So, PR is short, but no delta wave and QRS are normal.

Ques. What are the causes of short PR interval?

Ans. As follows:
- WPW syndrome
- LGL syndrome

Ques. How to differentiate between these two?

Ans. As follows:
- In WPW syndrome, there is delta wave.
- In LGL syndrome, there is no delta wave.

Ques. What is the presentation of LGL syndrome?

Ans. Asymptomatic usually. Sometimes may present with paroxysm of tachycardia.

Ques. What is the prognosis of LGL syndrome?

Ans. Good prognosis.

Ques. How to treat LGL syndrome?

Ans. No treatment is necessary. Symptomatic treatment for tachycardia may be needed.

PACEMAKER

ECG Criteria of Atrial Pacing

- There is a spike followed by P wave.
- QRS—normal

In atrial pacing (AAI), the atrium is both paced and sensed. This type of pacing is useful when there is only sinus node dysfunction and AV conduction is intact.

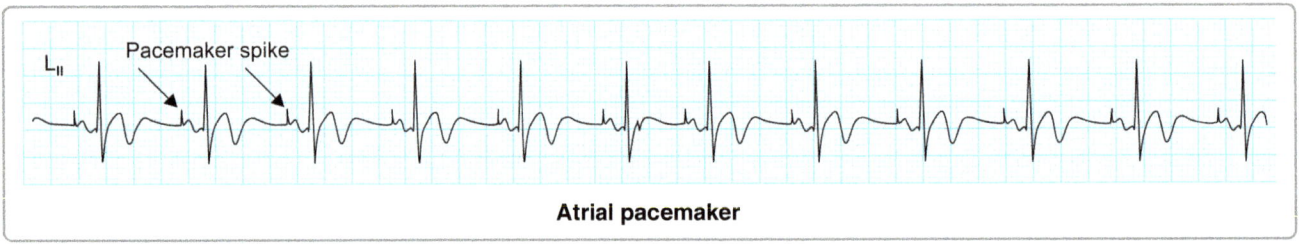

Atrial pacemaker

ECG Criteria of Ventricular Pacing

- There is a spike followed by QRS
- QRS—wide (looks like LBBB)

In ventricular pacing (VVI), the ventricle is both paced and sensed. This type of pacing is useful when there is only AV block, but sinus node function is intact.

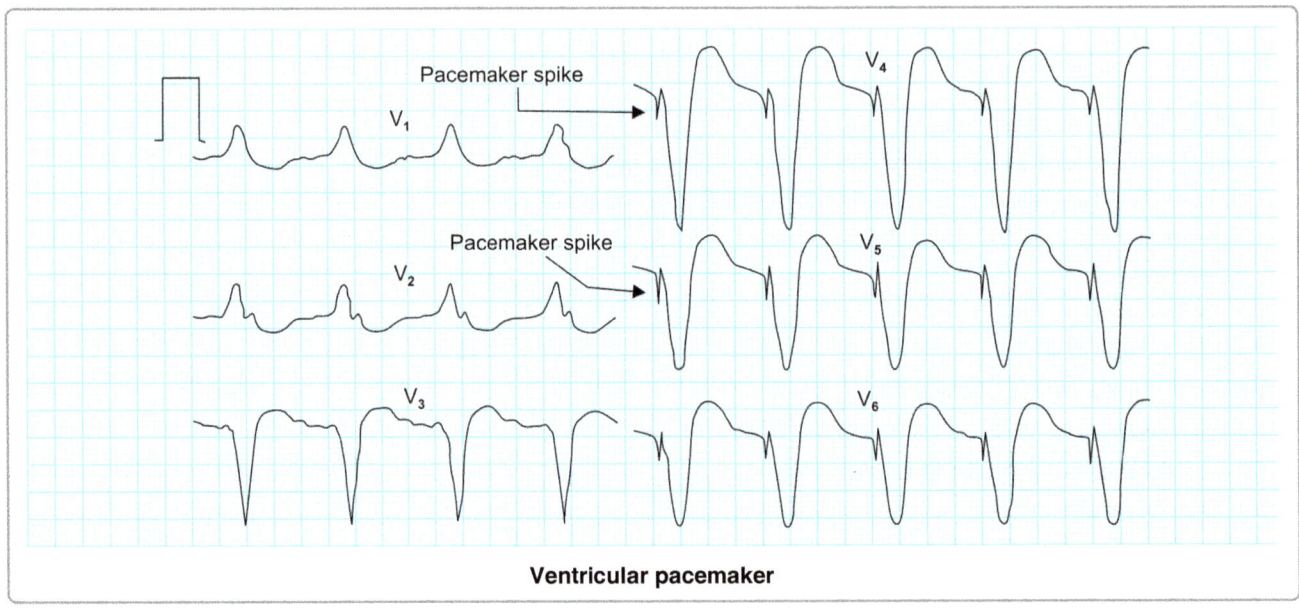

Ventricular pacemaker

Chapter 2: ECG Changes in Different Diseases

ECG Criteria of Dual Chamber (Atrial and Ventricular) Pacing

- There is a spike followed by P wave.
- There is another spike followed by QRS.

In dual chamber pacing (DDD), both the atrium and ventricle are paced and sensed. This type of pacemaker maintains AV synchrony.

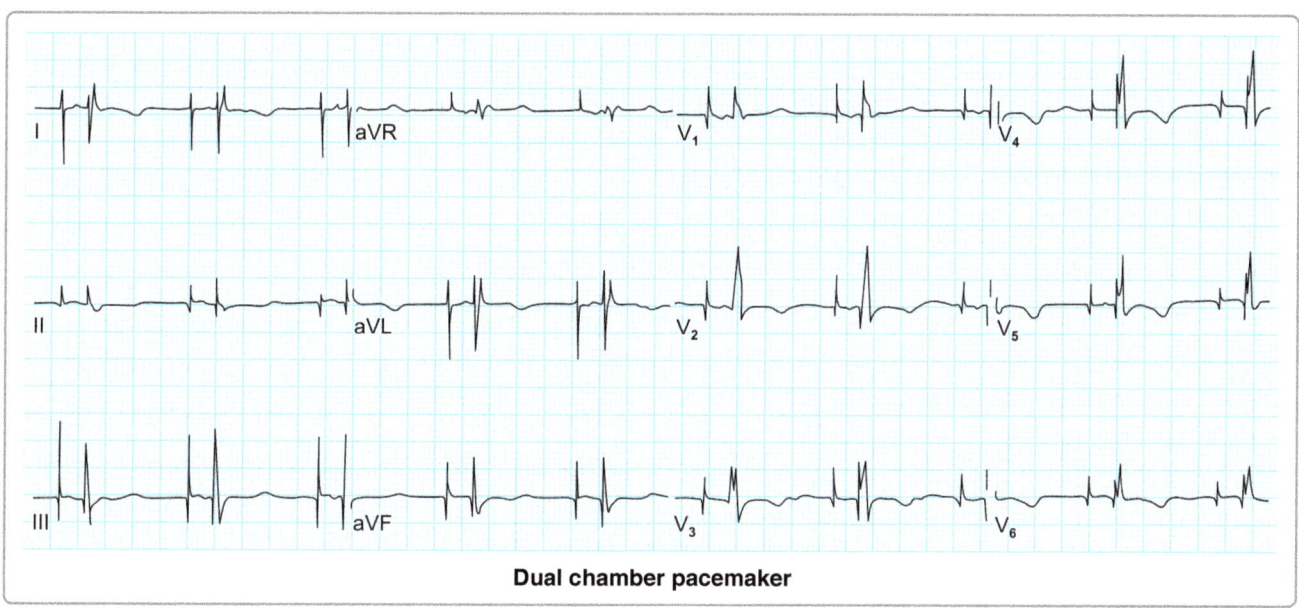

Dual chamber pacemaker

NB: Remember the following points:

- In atrial pacing: Spike is followed by P and normal QRS.
- In dual chamber pacing: One spike is followed by P and another is followed by wide QRS.
- In right ventricular pacing: Wide QRS looks like LBBB pattern.
- In atrial or ventricular pacing: Spike may not be seen (in demand pacemaker).
- Diagnosis of myocardial infarction may be difficult in presence of pacemaker.

Ques. What are the indications of permanent pacemaker?

Ans. Most common—complete heart block with syncope or Stokes–Adams syndrome and sick sinus syndrome.

Other indications:
- Symptomatic or asymptomatic Mobitz type 2 second-degree AV block.
- Symptomatic Mobitz type 1 second-degree AV block.
- Bifascicular or trifascicular block with syncope.
- Carotid sinus syndrome with bradycardia.
- Repeated vasovagal syndrome with bradycardia.
- In some cases of permanent atrial fibrillation (when other treatment fails, radiofrequency ablation followed by permanent pacemaker).

NB: After myocardial infarction, permanent pacemaker is indicated in the following cases:

- Inferior infarction with complete heart block persisting over 2 weeks.
- Anterior infarction with persistent type 2 or complete heart block or newly acquired bundle branch or bifascicular block with transient type 2 second-degree heart block or complete heart block.

Indications of Temporary Pacemaker

- Acute inferior myocardial infarction with second- or third-degree AV block or severe bradycardia with hemodynamic change.
- Acute extensive anterior myocardial infarction with second- or third-degree AV block or new bifascicular block (LBBB or RBBB with left anterior hemiblock and RBBB with left posterior hemiblock).
- Patient awaiting for permanent pacing
- Some tachycardias, such as AV reentry tachycardia and ventricular tachycardia, can be terminated by overdrive pacing.
- After open heart surgery
- Some cases of cardiac arrest
- Severe digoxin toxicity

Brief Notes About Pacemaker

Pacemaker is an artificial device used to stimulate the heart electrically. It is composed of two parts:

- Battery-powered generator
- Wire electrode, which is attached to the heart chamber to be stimulated (atrium or ventricle or both)

There are two types of pacemaker—temporary and permanent.

Temporary pacemaker: They are two types:

- *Transcutaneous pacing*: Administered by delivering an electrical stimulus sufficient to induce cardiac contraction through two large adhesive gel pad electrodes placed over the apex and upper right sternal edge or over the precordium and back. It is easy and quick to set-up, but causes significant discomfort, because it induces forceful pectoral and intercostal muscle contraction. It is the preferred method in selected patients with asymptomatic bradycardia or conduction abnormality. It may be life-saving for a patient in whom cardiac arrest is precipitated by bradycardia.
- *Transvenous pacing*: The pacing wire is introduced through a peripheral vein (internal jugular, or antecubital, or subclavian, or femoral) and placed in the apex of right ventricle, under fluoroscopic imaging. The electrode is connected to a portable battery-operated external pulse generator. It is withdrawn when cardiac function is improved (usually after 7–10 days). It is the preferred method in patients with symptomatic bradycardia. A temporary pacemaker is always set to work "on demand"; the usual rate is 60–80/minute.
- *Complications of temporary pacing*:
  - Pneumothorax
  - Brachial plexus or subclavian artery injury
  - Local infection or septicemia *(by Staphylococcus aureus)* and pericarditis.

Permanent pacemaker: The battery-powered generator is placed subcutaneously in the chest wall or axillary region and the electrode is placed through a vein in the cardiac chamber. They are two types—dual-chambered or single-chambered (atrial or ventricular).

There are two modes of pacemaker function:

- *Fixed rate*: It fires specific preset rate, regardless of patient's own heart rate.
- *Demand pacemaker*: It works when the patient's heart rate falls below a preset rate. Currently, all pacemakers that are used are demand type.

Demand pacemaker has two components:
- *A sensing mechanism*: It is designed so that the pacemaker will be inhibited, when the heart rate is adequate.
- *A pacing mechanism*: It is designed to trigger the pacemaker when no intrinsic QRS complex occurs within a predetermined time period.

There is commonly a 3-letter code that describes pacemaker function, designated as:
- *First*: Chamber paced
- *Second*: Chamber sensed
- *Third*: Mode of response

Letter code of pacing modes and functions

First: Chamber paced	Second: Chamber sensed	Third: Mode of response
V = Ventricle	V = Ventricle	T = Triggered
A = Atrium	A = Atrium	I = Inhibited
D = Double	D = Double	D = Double
O = None	O = None	O = None

Single Chamber Pacing (AAI and VVI)

VVI is commonly used. Ventricular pacing is only suitable for patients with continuous atrial fibrillation and bradycardia. AAI is less reliable, but it is commonly used in SA disease (sick sinus syndrome) with intact AV conduction. Tip of the electrode is placed in the right ventricle or atrium. Main problems are:
- It is unable to maintain normal pacemaker function, as the rate of pacemaker is fixed.
- It cannot adapt the different need of rate during exercise.
- Also, the normal sequence of atrial and ventricular contraction is lost, i.e., AV synchrony is not maintained.
- VVI pacemaker may be associated with pacemaker syndrome.

Dual Chamber Pacing (DDD)

One electrode is placed in the right atrium and one is placed in the right ventricle. It has some advantages:
- It maintains the AV synchrony. So, there is improved exercise performance of the patient.
- It prevents pacemaker syndrome, which is common in a single chamber pacing.
- There is also lower incidence of atrial arrhythmia in a patient with SA disease.

Main problems of DDD:
- If sinus node function is abnormal—the paced rate does not increase with activity.
- *Pacemaker-mediated tachycardia*: If they sense a retrogradely conducted P wave after ventricular depolarization, they trigger another ventricular beat, which may in turn cause another retrogradely conducted P wave. It leads to pacemaker-mediated tachycardia. This can be overcome by reprogramming atrial refractory period (by increasing refractory period or by shortening AV delay).

Ques. What are the complications of pacemaker?

Ans. There may be early and late complications:
A. Early complications:
   - Pneumothorax
   - Infection
   - Lead displacement
   - Cardiac tamponade
   - Pocket hematoma

ECG in Medical Practice

B. Late complications:
- Infection
- Erosion of generator or lead
- Chronic pain at implant site
- Lead fracture
- Malfunction
- Perforation of ventricular wall
- Ventricular arrhythmia (such as PVC)
- Electromagnetic interference
- Pacemaker failure
- Pacemaker-mediated tachycardia (by dual chamber pacing).
- Pacemaker syndrome (by single chamberpacing).

Pacemaker Malfunction

Pacemaker malfunction may occur due to:
- Dislodgement of pacemaker wire.
- By fibrosis around the tip of pacemaker wire.

ECG Changes in Pacemaker Malfunction

- ECG shows pacemaker spikes, but no QRS.
- In other case (especially with a broken electrode wire or a short circuit in pacing circuit or electrical interference from muscles of chest wall), no pacemaker spike is seen in ECG. Failure to sense may occur in which pacemaker spike is inappropriate that may fall on T wave.

NB: If there is malfunction in temporary pacemaker, always search for loose connection between the battery and pacing wire. There may be faulty battery or dislodged wire.

Ques. What is pacemaker syndrome?

Ans. It is a disorder characterized by transient hypotension, fatigue, dizziness, syncope, and distressing pulsation in the neck and chest. This occurs at the onset of ventricular contraction due to the loss of AV synchrony. It occurs in single chamber pacing, which can be prevented by dual chamber pacing or by reducing the pacemaker rate so that the sinus rhythm predominates.

DIGOXIN EFFECT

ECG Criteria of Digoxin Effect

- ST—depression (sloping or scooping depression, reverse tick mark, may be rounded concave that looks like thumb impression, mostly in V_4 to V_6).
- QT—short

NB: This effect is not due to digoxin toxicity, rather indicates digoxin effect.

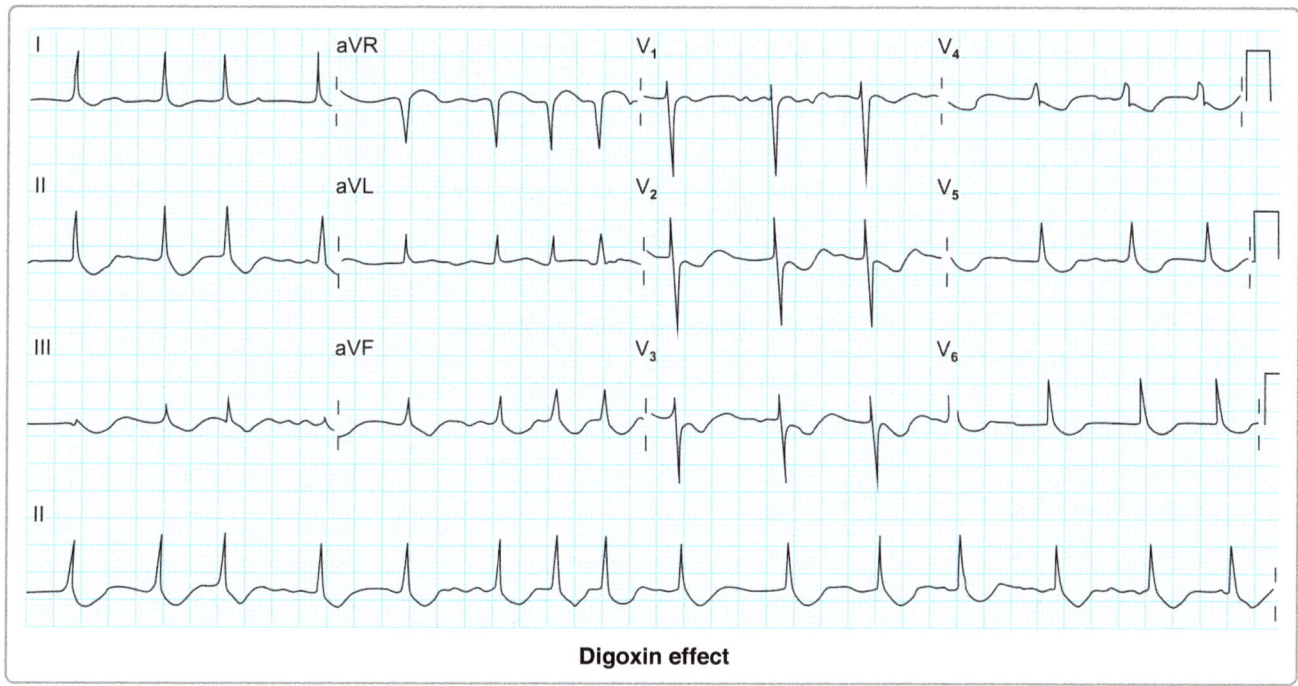

Digoxin effect

Ques. What are the toxicities of digoxin?

Ans. As follows:
- *Extracardiac*:
  - Anorexia, nausea, vomiting, diarrhea, and abdominal pain
  - Visual disturbance, drowsiness, confusion, delirium, depression, hallucination, and gynecomastia.
- *Cardiac*:
  - Any arrhythmia—ventricular ectopic, ventricular bigeminy, PAT with AV block, sinus bradycardia, and nodal rhythm.
  - All types of heart block (first-degree, second-degree, and complete heart block) and bidirectional ventricular tachycardia (successive QRS alternate in direction—one upward and one downward).
  - Atrial fibrillation and atrial flutter rarely occur

NB: Digoxin poisoning can cause hyperkalemia due to inhibition of sodium–potassium activated adenosine triphosphatase (ATPase) pump.

ECG in Medical Practice

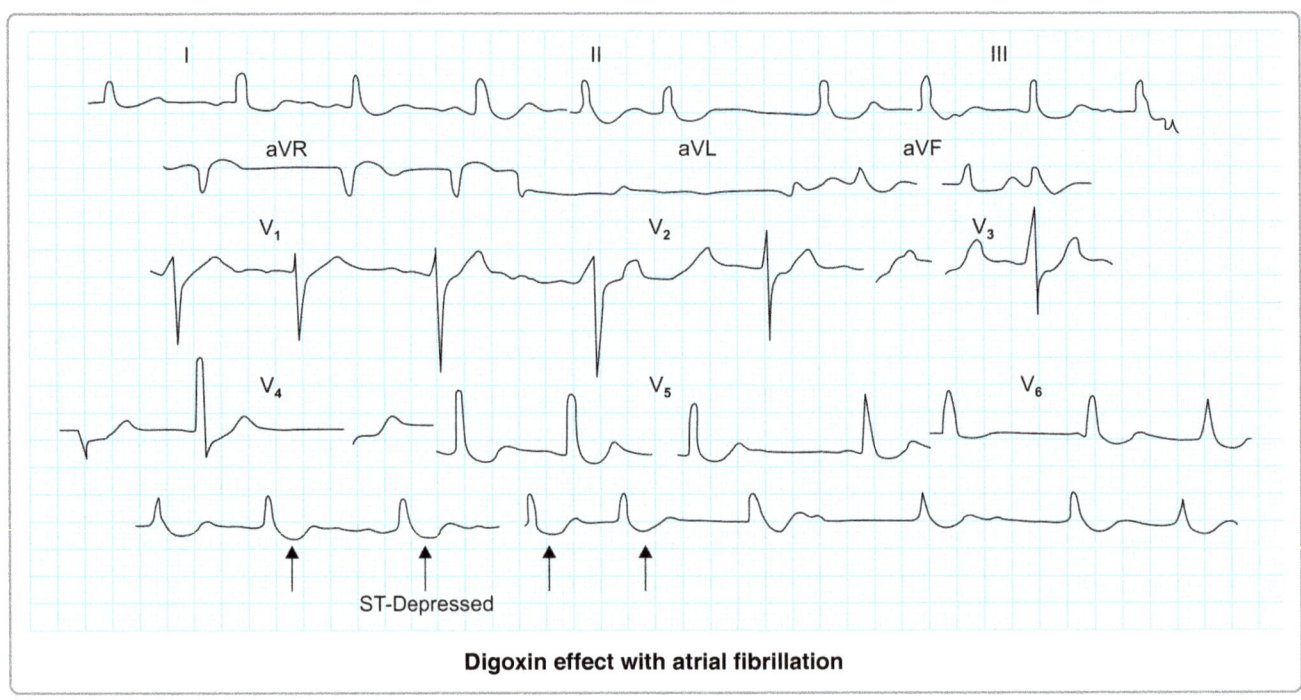

Digoxin effect with atrial fibrillation

Ques. What investigations should be done in digoxin toxicity?

Ans. As follows:
- Serum electrolytes
- Serum digoxin level

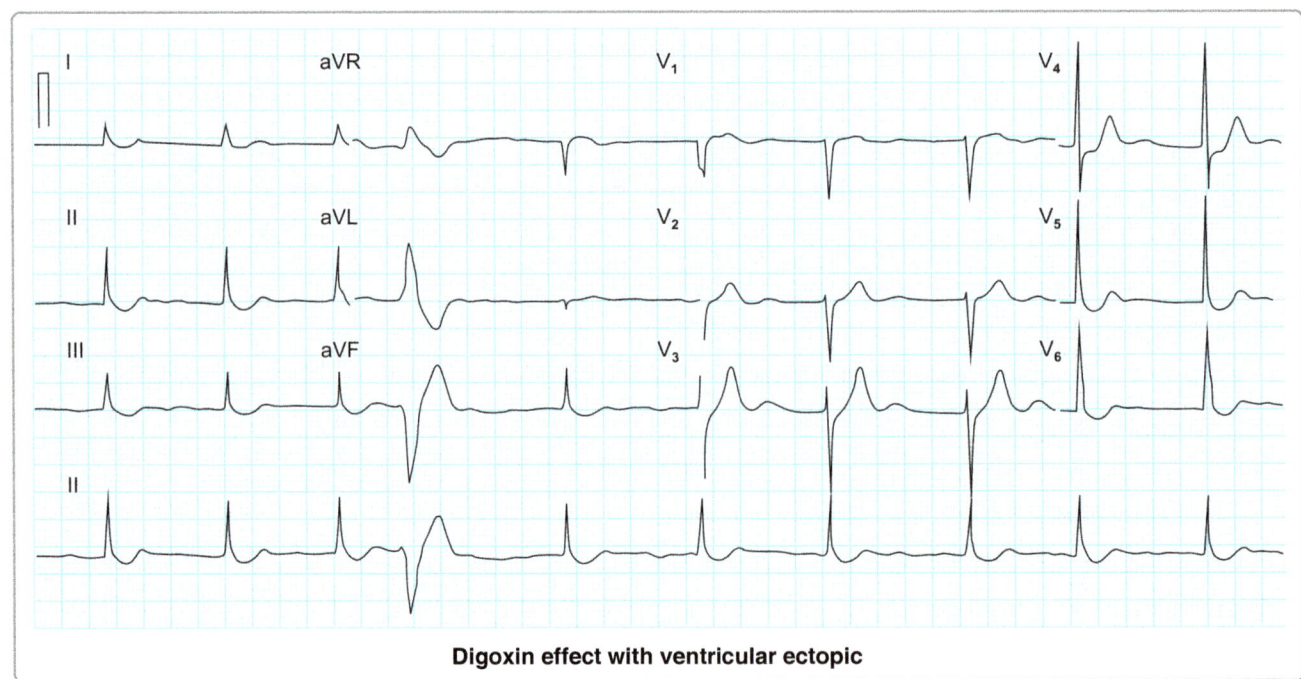

Digoxin effect with ventricular ectopic

Ques. What is the normal value of digoxin in plasma?

Ans. 1–2 μg/L (value above >4 μg/L is associated with toxicity).

Ques. How to treat digoxin toxicity?

Ans. As follows:
- Digoxin should be stopped
- Correction of electrolyte imbalance, especially hypokalemia
- Treatment of underlying arrhythmia or any other cause
- In severe bradycardia or complete heart block with hemodynamic change—injection atropine 1.2–2.4 mg IV may be given. If no response, temporary pacemaker may be needed.
- In severe life-threatening case or in digoxin poisoning with compromised cardiac output—digoxin-specific antibody (Digoxin-Fab) may be given.

HYPOKALEMIA

ECG Criteria of Hypokalemia

- U wave—prominent in chest leads (most common).
- Others—ST depression, T is small or inverted, and prolonged PR interval.

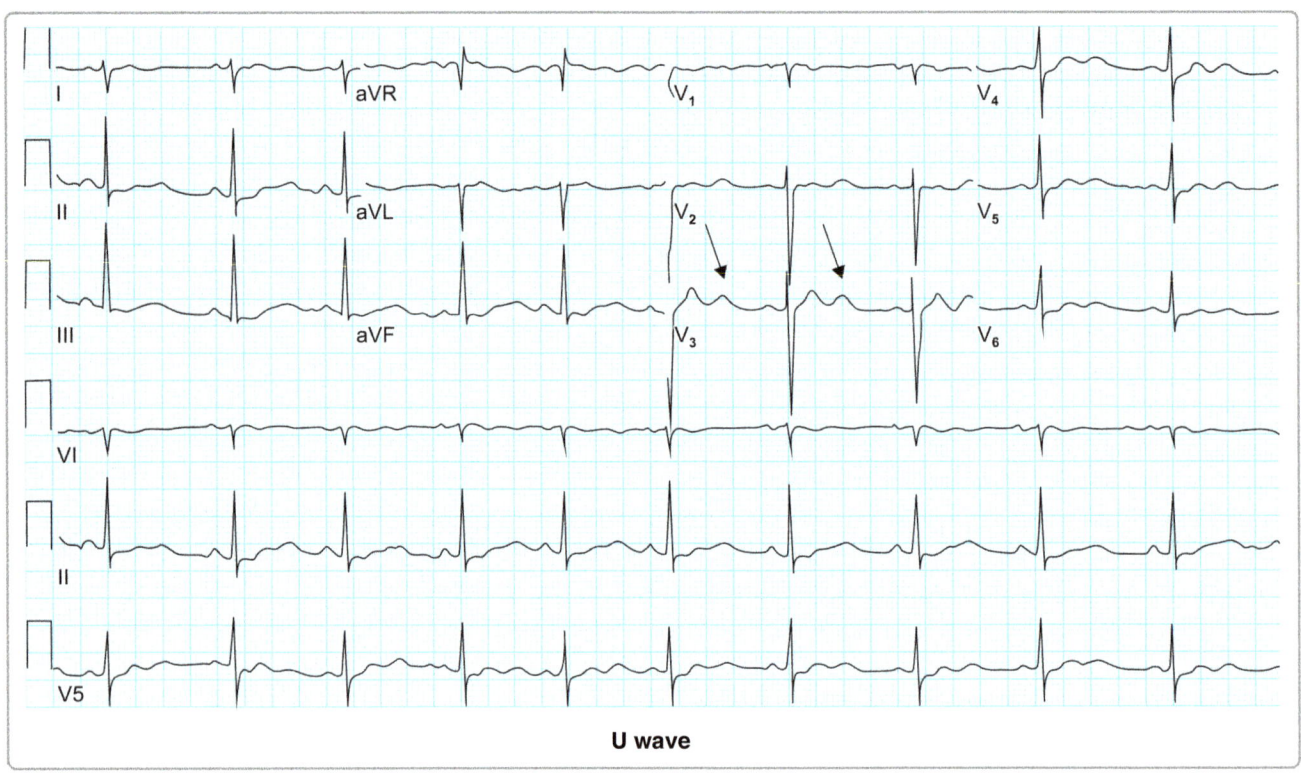

U wave

Ques. What are the effects of hypokalemia on heart?

Ans. As follows:
- Arrhythmia—atrial and ventricular including ventricular tachycardia and ventricular fibrillation.
- Aggravates digoxin toxicity
- Cardiac arrest (in diastole)

Ques. How to treat hypokalemia?

Ans. As follows:
- If serum potassium is >2.5 mmol/L—oral potassium therapy. Also, fruits, fruit juice, and green coconut water.
- If severe or serum potassium is <2.5 mmol/L—potassium is given in infusion (mixed with normal saline).
- Treatment of primary cause. If the patient is on diuretic (such as frusemide and thiazide), it should be stopped.
- Potassium-spearing diuretic such as spironolactone may be given, if there is persistent hypokalemia.

NB: Potassium should never be given intravenously directly. Failure to correct hypokalemia may be due to concurrent hypomagnesemia. So, it should be measured and corrected.

Ques. **What are the causes of hypokalemia?**

Ans. As follows:
- Diuretics (especially thiazide and frusemide)—common cause.
- Gastrointestinal loss—diarrhea, vomiting, purgative abuse, villous adenoma, and ileostomy.
- Renal loss—RTA types I and II, renal tubular necrosis (diuretic phase), Bartter syndrome, Liddle syndrome, and Gitelman syndrome.
- Endocrine cause—Cushing's syndrome and Conn's syndrome.
- Others—heart failure, liver failure, nephrotic syndrome, drugs (salbutamol and fenoterol), insulin therapy [in diabetic ketoacidosis (DKA)], alkalosis, hypokalemic periodic paralysis, and chronic hypokalemia are associated with interstitial renal disease.

Ques. **What are the effects of hypokalemia?**

Ans. As follows:
- It may be asymptomatic (if serum potassium >2.5 mmol/L).
- If severe hypokalemia (if serum potassium <2.5 mmol/L)—muscular weakness, paralysis, loss of tendon reflex, paralytic ileus, arrhythmia, increase digoxin toxicity, and cardiac arrest.

HYPERKALEMIA

ECG Criteria of Hyperkalemia

- T—tall, peaked, and tented (in chest leads)
- P—wide, small, and ultimately absent
- PR interval—prolonged
- QRS—wide, slurred, and bizarre

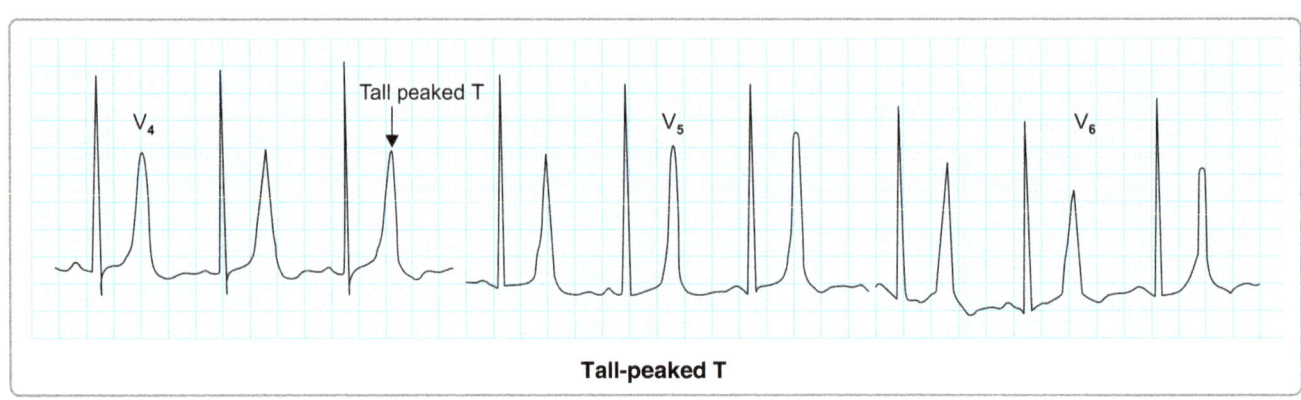

Tall-peaked T

Ques. What are the causes of hyperkalemia?

Ans. As follows:
- High potassium intake (oral or IV fluid with potassium, food or drugs containing potassium).
- *Renal diseases*:
  – Acute and chronic renal failure
  – Impaired tubular secretion of K^+ (renal lupus, amyloidosis, and transplanted kidney)
- *Endocrine diseases*:
  – Addison's disease
  – DKA
  – Primary hypoaldosteronism
- *Drugs*:
  – Potassium-sparing diuretics (spironolactone, amiloride, and triamterene)
  – ACE inhibitor
  – NSAID
  – Cyclosporine

NB: Combination of ACE inhibitor and K^+-sparing diuretic or NSAID is dangerous.

- Pseudohyperkalemia (due to abnormal release of K^+ from abnormal or damaged cells), also called spurious hyperkalemia, causes of which are:
  – Blood kept at room temperature for a long time before analysis
  – Acute leukemia
  – Hemolysis
  – Thrombocytosis
  – Infectious mononucleosis

- *Miscellaneous*:
  - Acidosis
  - Rhabdomyolysis
  - Tumor lysis syndrome
  - Digoxin poisoning
  - Vigorous exercise
  - Hyperkalemic periodic paralysis
  - Hyporeninemic hypoaldosteronism (Type IV RTA)
  - Gordon syndrome
  - Transfusion of stored blood

Ques. What are the effects of hyperkalemia on heart?

Ans. As follows:
- Any arrhythmia, even ventricular tachycardia and ventricular fibrillation.
- Hyperkalemia causes hyperpolarization of cell membranes, leading to decreased cardiac excitability, hypotension, bradycardia, and eventual asystole or cardiac arrest.

Ques. What are the features of hyperkalemia?

Ans. As follows:
- May be asymptomatic
- Muscular weakness, which may be severe causing flaccid paralysis and loss of tendon jerk
- Paralytic ileus (abdomen may be distended)
- Tingling around the lip or finger
- Sudden death due to cardiac arrest or arrhythmia

Ques. How to treat hyperkalemia?

Ans. As follows:
- Withdrawal of potassium, potassium-containing food, and offending drug
- Injection 10% calcium gluconate 10–20 cc IV slowly over 10 minutes. It may be repeated (it has membrane-stabilizing effect, it protects the myocardium, and it also reduces the risk of cardiac arrest).
- Injection 50 mL of 50% glucose IV + injection insulin 10 units (especially if there is hyperglycemia). This can be repeated if necessary (glucose can be given without insulin, it stimulates endogenous insulin secretion).
- Nebulized salbutamol may be given, it increases urinary excretion of potassium by increasing Na-K-ATPase pump activity.
- Correction of acidosis—by IV sodibicarb (1.26%), 500 mL 6–8 hourly (until serum HCO_3 is normal)
- Treatment of primary causes
- In some cases, exchange resins (calcium resonium 15–30 g orally)
- If all fail—hemodialysis or peritoneal dialysis may be needed

NB: Hyperkalemia is dangerous, if K^+ is >7 mmol/L. It may cause cardiac arrest in systole.

ECG in Medical Practice

ECG of Severe Hyperkalemia (K⁺ is >7 mmol/L)

- Bizarre QRS widening
- P is absent, bradycardia
- QRS is wide with merging with T wave creating a sine wave appearance

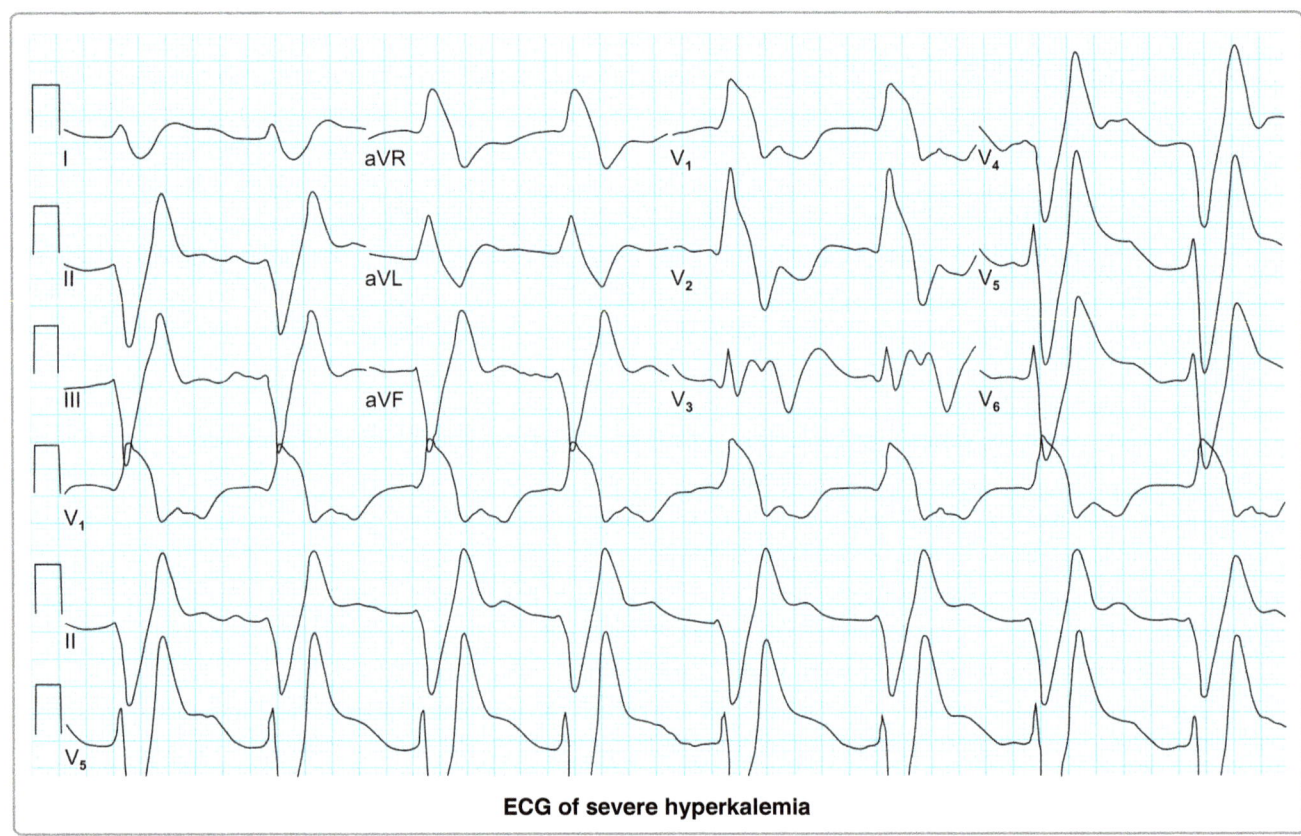

ECG of severe hyperkalemia

HYPERMAGNESEMIA

ECG Criteria of Hypermagnesemia

- It looks like ECG change of hyperkalemia
- *Other ECG changes may be*: Prolongation of PR interval, prolonged QT interval, widening of QRS complex, and increased amplitude of T wave.

Ques. What are causes of hypermagnesemia?

Ans. As follows:
- Acute or chronic renal failure
- *Increase intake*: Magnesium infusion and oral ingestion (antacid and magnesium enemas)
- *Miscellaneous*: Mild hypermagnesemia can occur in following conditions—
  - Primary hyperparathyroidism
  - Familial hypocalciuric hypercalcemia
  - DKA
  - Hypercatabolic states, such as tumor lysis syndrome
  - Adrenal insufficiency

Ques. What are the cardiac effects of hypermagnesemia?

Ans. Severe hypermagnesemia may cause: (>5 mmol/L)
- Complete AV block
- Cardiac arrest

Ques. How to treat hypermagnesemia?

Ans. As follows:
- IV loop diuretics and intravenous hydration
- Calcium gluconate may be given to reduce cardiac effects. In severe case, dialysis may be necessary.

HYPOMAGNESEMIA

ECG Criteria of Hypomagnesemia

- It looks like ECG change in hypokalemia
- *Other ECG changes may be*: Prolongation of PR interval, prolonged QT interval, widening of QRS complex, and diminished amplitude of T wave.

Ques. What are the causes of hypomagnesemia?

Ans. As follows:
- Less intake such as starvation and malnutrition (also in chronic alcoholism and parenteral nutrition)
- Excessive loss
    - *Gastrointestinal tract (GIT)*: Prolonged vomiting. Nasogastric (NG) suction, chronic diarrhea or laxatives abuse, and malabsorption syndrome. Small bowel bypass surgery and intestinal fistula.
    - *Renal loss*: Diuretics therapy, nephrotoxic drug (e.g., gentamicin and cisplatin), DKA, Bartter and Gitelman syndromes, and primary renal magnesium wasting.
- *Others*: Acute pancreatitis and Hungry bone syndrome

Ques. What are the cardiac effects of hypomagnesemia?

Ans. Severe hypermagnesemia may cause: (<1.5 mmol/L).
- Atrial and ventricular ectopics
- Atrial tachyarrhythmia
- Torsades de pointes

Ques. How to treat hypomagnesemia?

Ans. As follows:
- *In mild case*: Oral therapy (may cause diarrhea)
- *In severe case*: IV magnesium chloride 0.5 mmol/kg in first 24 hours. Repeated, if necessary.
- If hypomagnesemia is due to diuretic therapy, adjuvant use of potassium-sparing agent may reduce magnesium loss by kidney.
- Treatment of primary cause

HYPOCALCEMIA

ECG Criteria of Hypocalcemia

- Prolongation of QT interval
- Prolongation of ST segment

NB: Hypocalcemia may cause atrial or ventricular arrhythmia, even torsades de pointes.

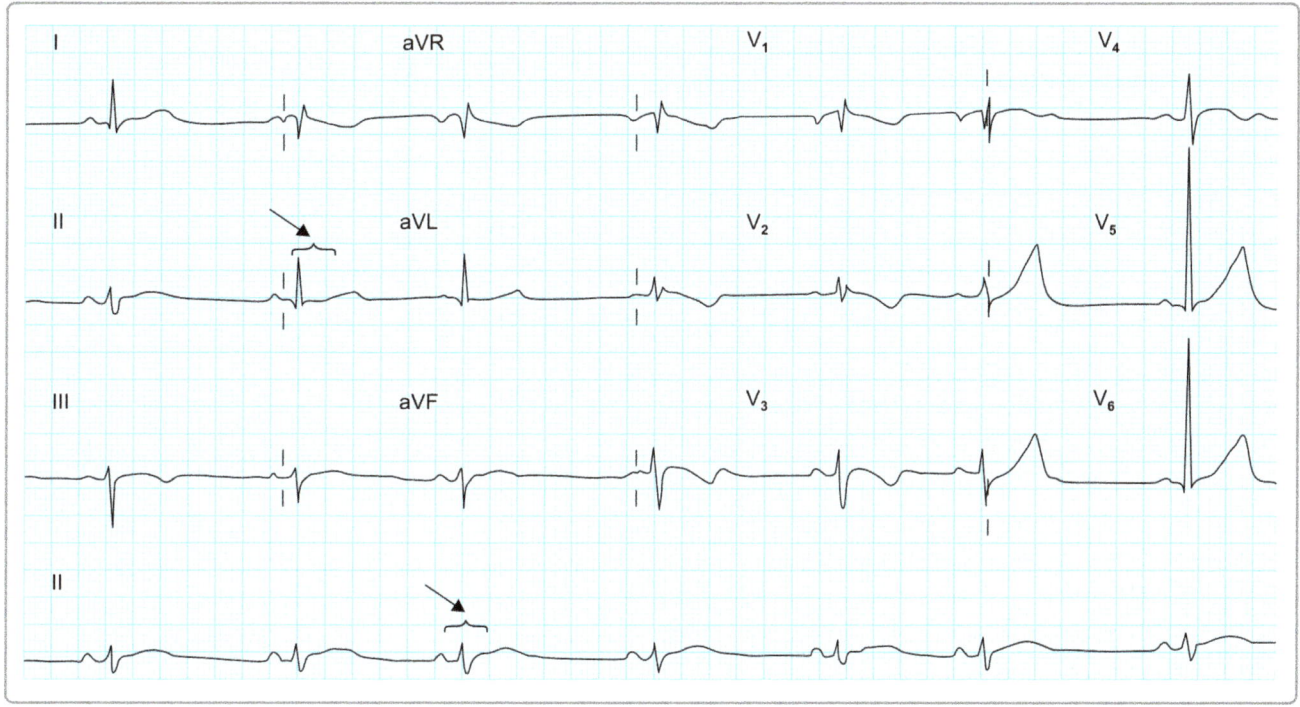

Ques. What are the causes of hypocalcemia?

Ans. As follows:
- Hypoalbuminemia
- Vitamin D deficiency
- Hypoparathyroidism
- Pseudo and pseudopseudohypoparathyroidism
- Acute pancreatitis
- Alkalosis
- *Drugs*: Bisphosphonate, citrate, lactate, foscarnet, and sodium ethylenediaminetetraacetic acid (EDTA).

Ques. What cardiac complications may occur with hypocalcemia?

Ans. As follows:
- Torsades de pointes
- Rarely, ventricular fibrillation

Ques. **What are the features of hypocalcemia?**

Ans. As follows:
- *In mild case*: It may be asymptomatic.
- *In severe case*: May be tetany characterized by carpopedal spasm, stridor, and convulsion.
- Hypocalcemia due to vitamin D deficiency causes rickets in children and osteomalacia in adult.
- Prolonged hypocalcemia can cause calcification of basal ganglia, grand mal epilepsy, psychosis, and cataract.

Ques. **How to treat hypocalcemia?**

Ans. As follows:
- *In severe case*: IV calcium gluconate. Repeated, if necessary
- Oral supplementation
- Vitamin D therapy, if there is deficiency
- Treatment of cause, if any

Chapter 2: ECG Changes in Different Diseases

HYPERCALCEMIA

ECG Criteria in Hypercalcemia

- Short QT interval
- May be prominent U wave
- Shortening of ST segment
- May be prolongation of PR interval and QRS complex

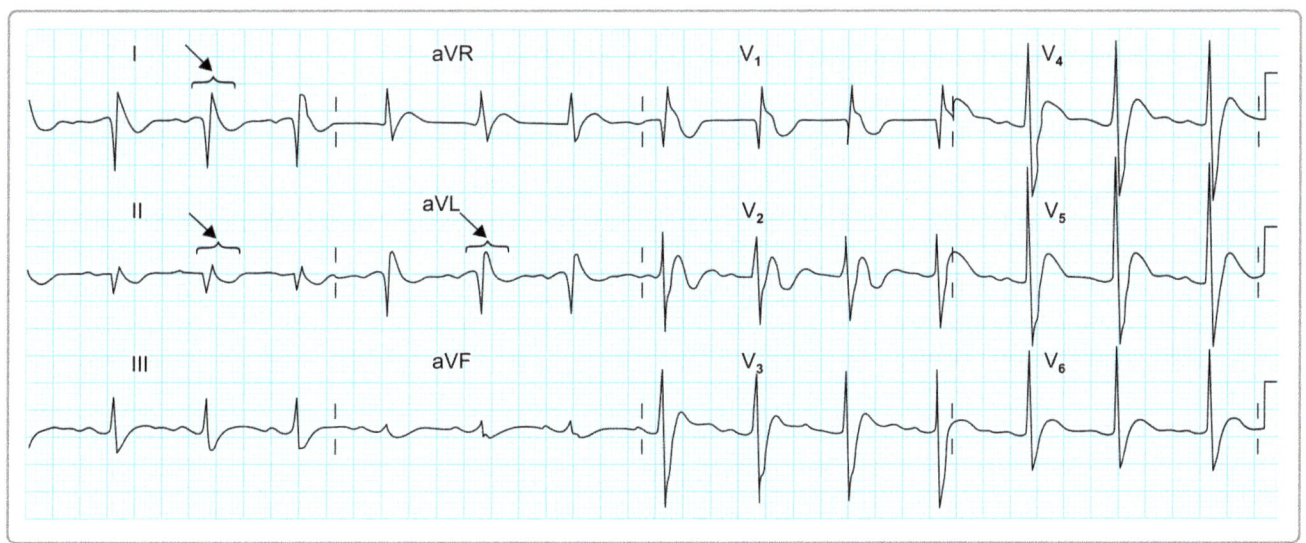

Ques. What are the causes of hypercalcemia?

Ans. As follows:
- Primary or tertiary hyperparathyroidism
- Secondary deposit in the bone marrow
- Multiple myeloma
- Sarcoidosis
- Hypervitaminosis D
- Endocrine disease (e.g., thyrotoxicosis and Addison's disease)
- Paget's disease with immobilization
- Milk alkali syndrome
- Drug (e.g., thiazide diuretics and lithium intoxication)

Ques. What are the cardiac effects in hypercalcemia?

Ans. As follows:
- Hypercalcemia may cause atrial or ventricular arrhythmia, especially if the patient is taking digoxin.
- Severe hypercalcemia may cause significant ST elevation, mimicking acute myocardial infarction.

Ques. What are the clinical features of hypercalcemia?

Ans. It may be asymptomatic. Other features are:
- Anorexia, nausea, vomiting, and dyspepsia
- Weakness and lethargy
- Constipation
- Polyuria and polydipsia
- Poor concentration, drowsiness, dizziness, and depression
- Peptic ulcer
- Renal colic

Ques. How to treat?

Ans. As follows:
- Rehydration—infusion of normal saline, 4–6 L daily for 2–3 days.
- *Calcium-lowering drugs*:
  - IV bisphosphonate—disodium pamidronate (90 mg IV over 4 hours with 0.9% saline) or zoledronic acid 4 mg IV.
  - Calcitonin—100 units 8 hourly IM or SC for 24–48 hours in severe case
  - Prednisolone (30–60 mg daily, in hypercalcemia due to sarcoidosis, hypervitaminosis D, and multiple myeloma).
- Forced diuresis by IV frusemide along with saline
- If all fail, then hemodialysis
- Treatment of primary cause

PULMONARY EMBOLISM

ECG Criteria of Pulmonary Embolism

- Sinus tachycardia (common)
- P pulmonale (tall P wave in L_{II}, L_{III}, and aVF)
- RBBB (incomplete or complete)
- ST depression and T wave inversion in right precordial leads (V_1 and V_2)
- RAD
- S_I, Q_{III}, and T_{III} patterns (S in L_I, Q and T inversion in L_{III}). This is the classic combination of ECG findings in pulmonary embolism.

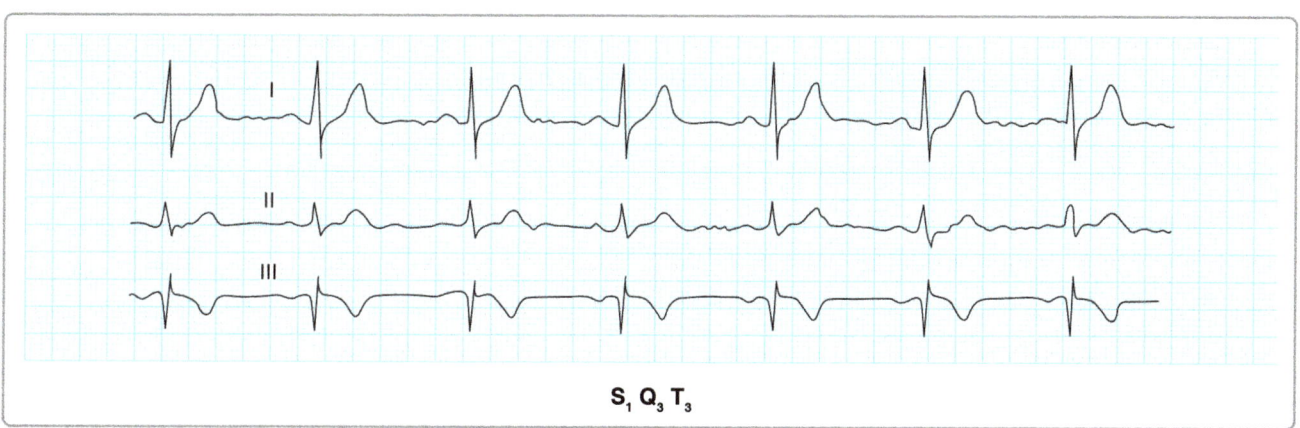

$S_1 Q_3 T_3$

Ques. What are the arrhythmias that may be found in pulmonary embolism?

Ans. As follows:
- Sinus tachycardia (common)
- Atrial fibrillation
- Atrial flutter
- Ventricular ectopics

Ques. What are the features of acute massive pulmonary embolism?

Ans. As follows:
- Severe central chest pain
- Severe dyspnea
- Faintness or syncope
- *On examination*:
  - Tachycardia
  - Tachypnea
  - Cyanosis
  - Wide splitting of second heart sound.
  - Right ventricular gallop
  - Features of shock

Ques. What are the types of pulmonary embolism?

Ans. There are three types:
- Acute massive pulmonary embolism
- Acute small or medium pulmonary embolism
- Chronic pulmonary embolism

Ques. What are the causes of pulmonary embolism?

Ans. As follows:
- Deep vain thrombosis
- Septic emboli
- Malignancy
- Fat following fracture of long bone like the femur
- Air embolism
- Amniotic fluid

Ques. What are the poor prognostic factors of pulmonary embolism in ECG?

Ans. The following ECG abnormalities are associated with a poor prognosis:
- Atrial arrhythmias
- RBBB
- Inferior Q waves
- Precordial T wave inversion and ST-segment changes

Ques. What investigations are done to diagnose pulmonary embolism?

Ans. As follows:
- CXR PA view (oligemic lung fields, enlarged pulmonary artery, and wedge-shaped opacity due to pulmonary infarction, linear atelectasis, focal infiltration, raised hemidiaphragm, and pleural effusion, usually blood-stained. It may be a normal X-ray in many cases).
- ECG—see above
- Blood gas analysis—low PaO_2 and low $PaCO_2$.
- If pulmonary infarction—neutrophilic leukocytosis, high erythrocyte sedimentation rate (ESR), and high LDH.
- Echocardiogram—vigorously contracting the left ventricle and clot in right heart or main pulmonary artery.
- Ventilation and perfusion scan (VQ scan)—reduction of perfusion in major lung area.
- Computed tomography pulmonary angiography (CTPA)—it is sensitive and specific for medium size embolism.
- MRI (if CT is contraindicated)
- Plasma D-dimer—if it is low or undetectable, it excludes pulmonary embolism.
- Pulmonary angiography (may be done in some cases). It is definitive.
- *Other investigations*:
    - Doppler ultrasound of lower limb vessels to see deep venous thrombosis (DVT).
    - Troponins I and T are elevated in 30–50% cases, who have a moderate-to-large pulmonary embolism.
    - Brain natriuretic peptide (BNP)—typically greater in patients with pulmonary embolism compared to patients without pulmonary embolism.

Ques. What are the poor prognostic factors of pulmonary embolism in echocardiogram?

Ans. Only 30–40% patients with pulmonary embolism have echocardiographic abnormalities. Poor prognostic features in echocardiogram are:
- Increased right ventricular size
- Decreased right ventricular function
- Tricuspid regurgitation

Ques. How to treat pulmonary embolism?

Ans. As follows:
- Immediate hospitalization
- High flow oxygen (60–100%)
- Relief of pain by opium (morphine or pethidine)
- Circulatory shock should be treated with intravenous fluid or plasma expander.
- *Anticoagulant:* Low-molecular heparin subcutaneously. Fondaparinux or injection unfractionated heparin 10,000 units IV as a bolus dose, followed by continuous infusion 1,000–2,000 units/hour. Heparin is usually stopped after 5 days.
- *Oral anticoagulant (warfarin):* Started after 48 hours of heparin therapy.
- Warfarin is continued for 6 weeks to 6 months in patients with identifiable reversible risk factor. In recurrent pulmonary embolism or in persistent prothrombotic state, it may be required to continue for lifelong.
- *Fibrinolytic therapy:* Streptokinase (250,000 units by IV infusion over 30 minutes, followed by streptokinase 100,000 units IV hourly for up to 12–72 hours). Or alteplase (60 mg IV over 15 minutes) is used following a major embolism. Heparin should be given subsequently.
- In massive pulmonary embolism with severe hemodynamic compromise, failure of thrombolytic therapy or if it is contraindicated: Surgical embolectomy may be necessary.
- *In case of recurrent pulmonary embolism*: Insertion of a filter in inferior vena cava above the level of renal veins may be done. It is indicated if there is contraindications to anticoagulation, failed anticoagulation, or developed complication due to anticoagulation.

NB: Remember the following points:
- Signs and symptoms of small- and medium-sized pulmonary emboli may be nonspecific, diagnosis is frequently delayed or missed.
- Pulmonary embolism should be considered, if the patient presents with symptoms of unexplained cough, chest pain, hemoptysis, new onset of atrial fibrillation or other tachycardia, or signs of pulmonary hypertension, if no other cause is found.
- Diuretics and β-blocker has no role, also they reduce cardiac output.

DEXTROCARDIA

ECG Criteria of Dextrocardia

- *P wave*: Inverted in L_I (upright in L_{III})
- *R wave*: Tall in V_1, diminishing progressively in V_5 and V_6
- *Right axis*: Deviation

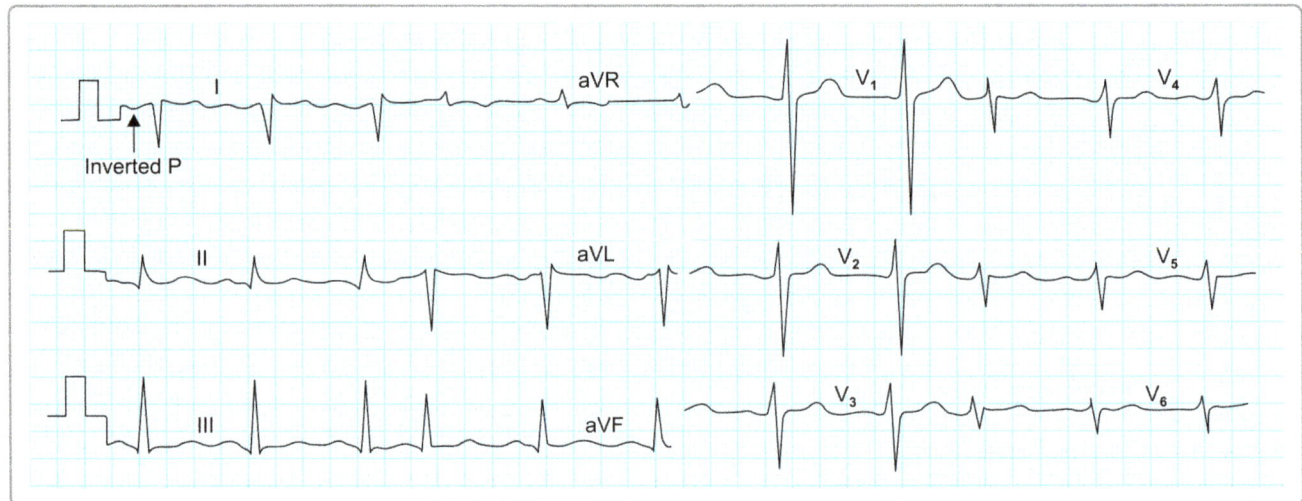

Ques. What is the differential diagnosis of dextrocardia?

Ans. Incorrectly placed or reversed arm electrodes (right one on left and left one on right). It is called technical dextrocardia. In this case, P wave is inverted in L_I, but QRS in chest leads will remain normal (tall R in V_5 and V_6).

Ques. What is dextrocardia?

Ans. It is a congenital disorder in which the heart is located in the right side of chest, but other organs are in their usual positions.

Ques. If the patient has dextrocardia, what else do you want to see?

Ans. I want to see the evidence of Kartagener's syndrome, characterized by:
- Dextrocardia
- Bronchiectasis
- Frontal sinusitis or frontal sinus agenesis

Ques. What other investigations would you suggest?

Ans. As follows:
- CXR (heart on the right side of chest. There may be features of bronchiectasis)
- X-ray of paranasal sinus (PNS)—evidence of frontal sinusitis or frontal sinus agenesis

Ques. What is situs inversus?

Ans. When there is dextrocardia with reversal of the sites of other visceras (stomach on the right side, liver on the left side, right lung is on the left, and left lung is on the right).

Ques. What is levocardia?

Ans. When the heart is on the left side of chest, but there is reversal of the sites of other visceras, it is called levocardia (stomach on the right side, liver on the left side, right lung is on the left, and left lung is on the right).

Chapter 2: ECG Changes in Different Diseases

Ques. What is mesocardia?

Ans. When the cardiac apex is in the midline, it is called mesocardia.

NB: Remember the following points:
- If dextrocardia is associated with situs inversus, the heart is usually otherwise normal.
- In case of isolated dextrocardia or levocardia, there may also be multiple cardiac anomalies.

Ques. What is the clinical importance of situs inversus?

Ans. As follows:
- Diagnosis of acute appendicitis may be missed, as appendix is on the left side.
- As the liver is on the left side, during liver biopsy, care should be taken, so that the biopsy needle is not mistakenly given on the right side.

Ques. What is the prognosis of situs inversus or dextrocardia?

Ans. Normal life span.

HYPOTHERMIA

ECG Criteria of Hypothermia (ECG Findings are Nonspecific)

- J wave (at the junction of distal limb of QRS)
- *Other findings*:
  - Sinus bradycardia
  - First- and second-degree heart block
  - Prolongation of QT interval
  - Ectopics
  - Atrial fibrillation (if temperature <29°C)
  - May be ventricular tachycardia and ventricular fibrillation (if temperature <30°C)
  - Tracing may be low voltage

Ques. What is hypothermia?

Ans. The core temperature <35°C is called hypothermia. Causes are:
- Exposure to cold or immersion in cold water
- *Drugs*: Excess of antipyretics, hypnotics, and alcohol
- Hypothyroidism
- Adrenal insufficiency
- *Others*: Hypovolemic shock, hepatic failure, and stroke

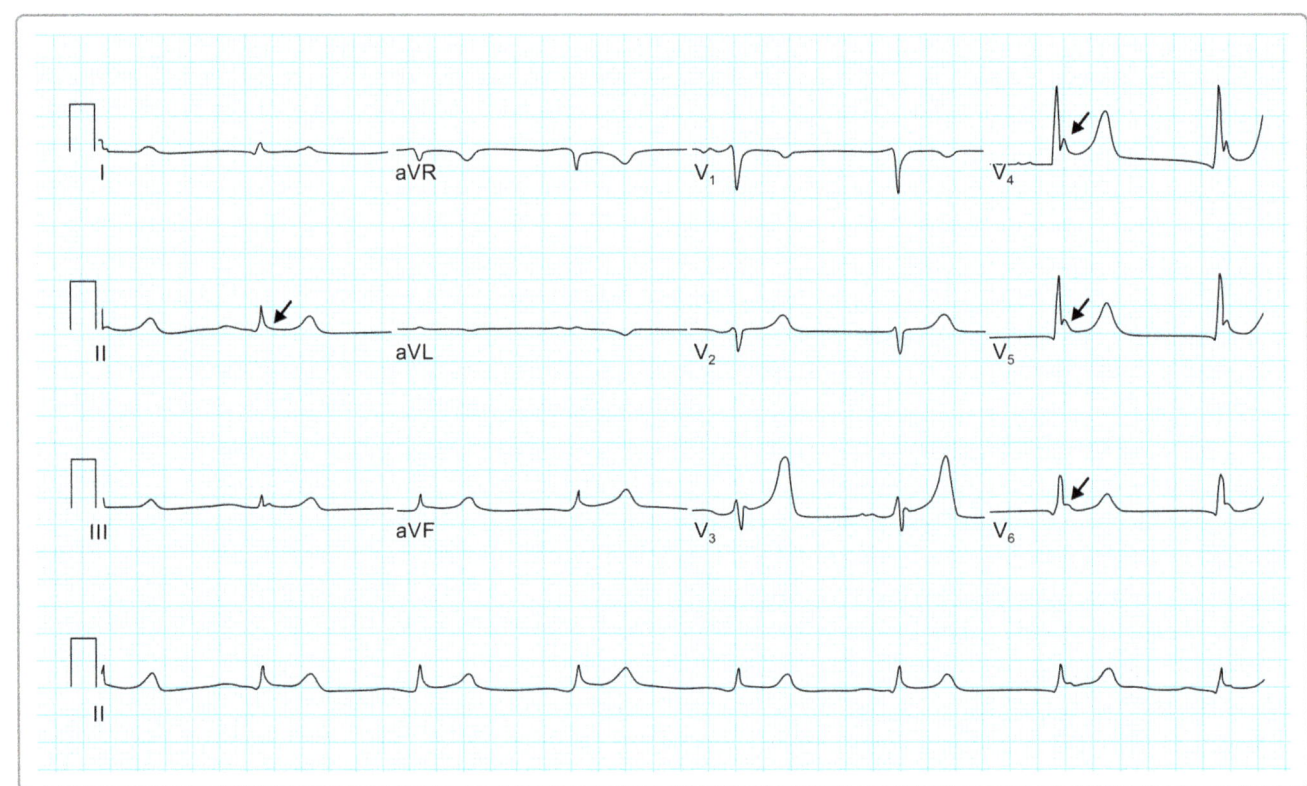

CHRONIC OBSTRUCTIVE PULMONARY DISEASE

Following ECG changes may occur:
- Low-voltage tracing
- P pulmonale (RAH)
- Tall R in V_1 (RVH)
- RAD
- Poor R wave progression (V_1 to V_6)
- Occasionally, MAT

NB: In COPD, RAH (P pulmonale) with RVH (tall R in V1) indicates presence of cor pulmonale.

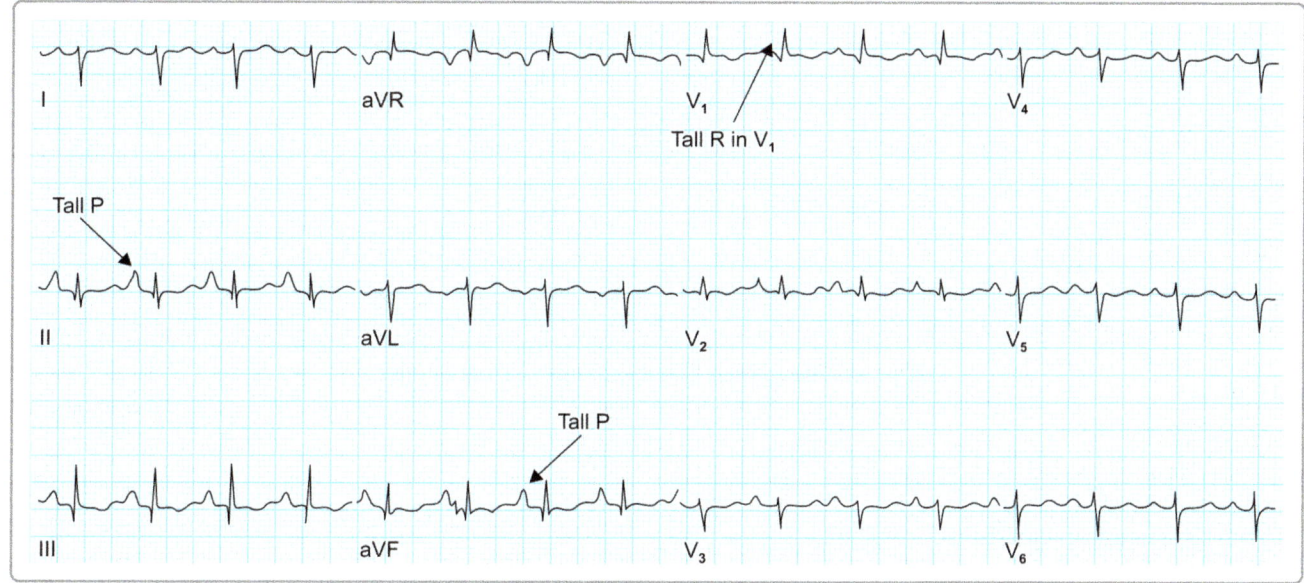

Ques. What is COPD?

Ans. Chronic obstructive pulmonary disease is a preventable and treatable disease characterised by persistent air flow limitation that is usually progressive associated with enhance chronic inflammatory response in the air ways and the lung to noxious particles or gases.

Ques. How to diagnose COPD?

Ans. It can be diagnosed by spirometry and reversibility test.

ATRIAL SEPTAL DEFECT

There are two types of ASDs: (1) Ostium primum (10%) and (2) ostium secundum (90%).

ECG Criteria in Ostium Primum Defect

- Incomplete or complete RBBB
- LAD

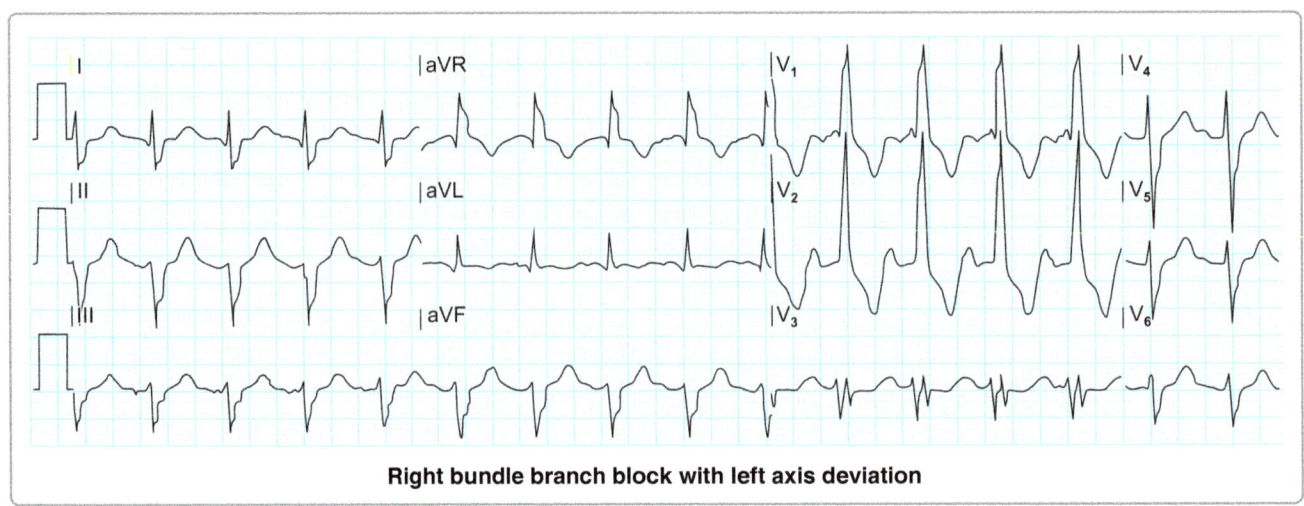

Right bundle branch block with left axis deviation

ECG Criteria in Ostium Secundum Defect

- Incomplete or complete RBBB
- RAD

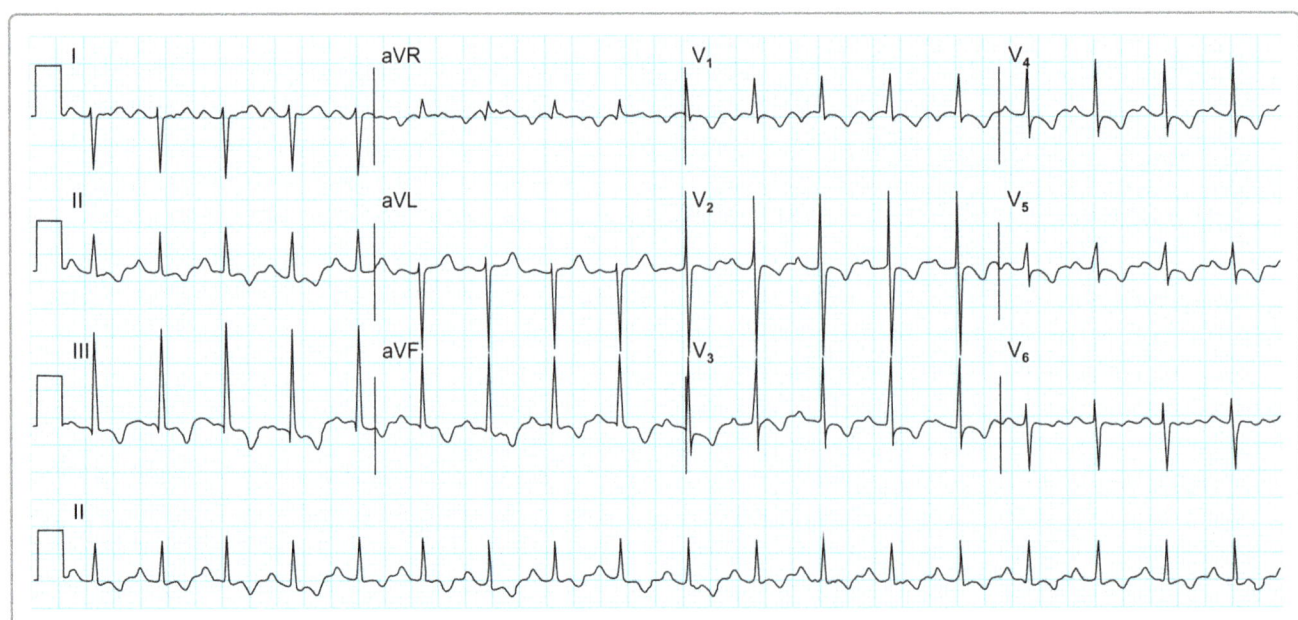

Ques. How to diagnose clinically?

Ans. As follows:
- Wide and fixed splitting of second heart sound
- Ejection systolic murmur (ESM) in left second and third intercostal space

Ques. What investigations should be done?

Ans. As follows:
- CXR PA view
- Color Doppler echocardiography
- Cardiac catheterization in some cases

Ques. What are the complications of ASD?

Ans. As follows:
- Pulmonary hypertension with reversal of shunt (Eisenmenger's syndrome)
- Arrhythmia (AF commonest)
- Embolism (pulmonary and systemic)
- Brain abscess
- Infective endocarditis
- Recurrent pulmonary infection

Ques. How to treat ASD?

Ans. As follows:
- Small ASD: no surgery needed. Follow up should be done (patient can live normal life)
- Moderate to large ASD: surgical closure is needed
- During the catheterization, closure may be done with transcatheter clamshell device.
- In Eisenmenger's syndrome develop, surgical closure is contraindicated. Then medical treatment is given such as-
  - Diuretics,
  - Digoxin in some case
  - Venesection (if polycythaemia)
  - Heart-lung transplantation may be considered

HYPOTHYROIDISM

ECG Criteria of Hypothyroidism

- Low-voltage tracing
- Sinus bradycardia
- T inversion

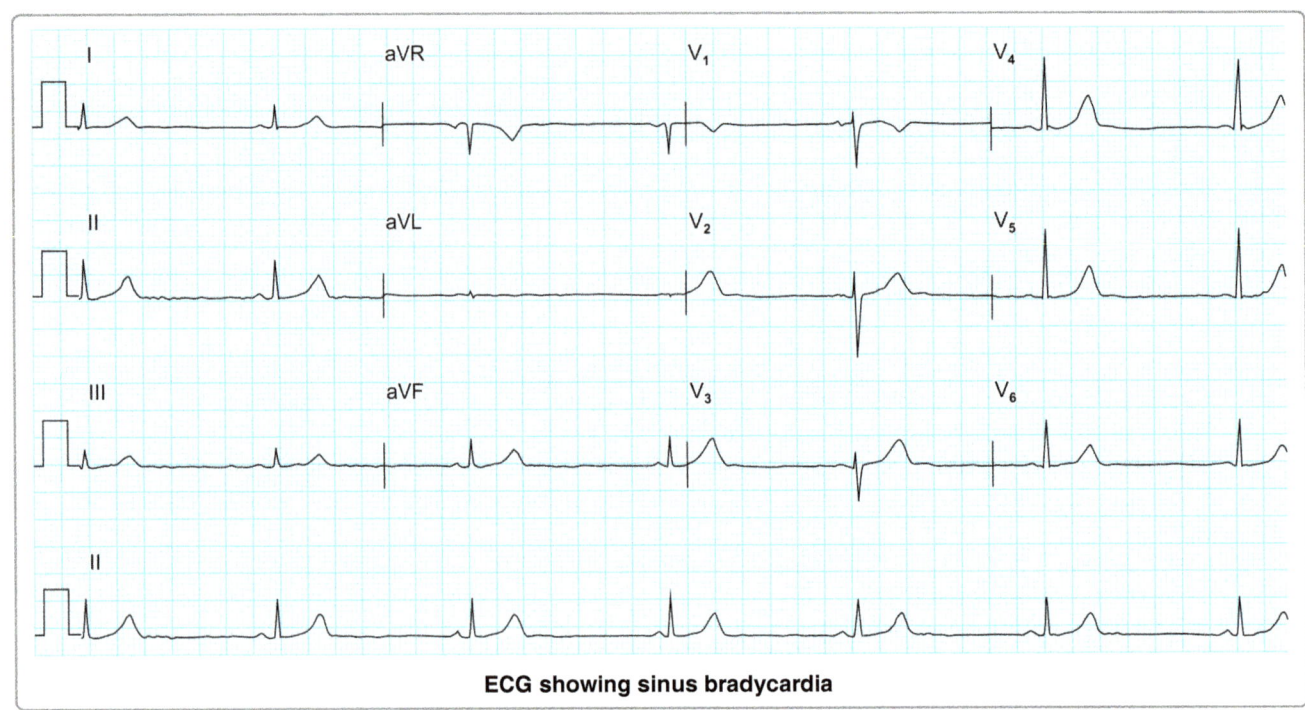

ECG showing sinus bradycardia

Ques. What are the cardiac complication of hypothyroidism?

Ans. As follows:
- Pericardial effusion
- Congestive cardiac failure
- Ischemic heart disease
- Sinus bradycardia
- Atherosclerosis

HYPERTHYROIDISM

ECG Criteria of Hyperthyroidism

- Sinus tachycardia (common)
- Arrhythmia—atrial fibrillation and ectopic beat

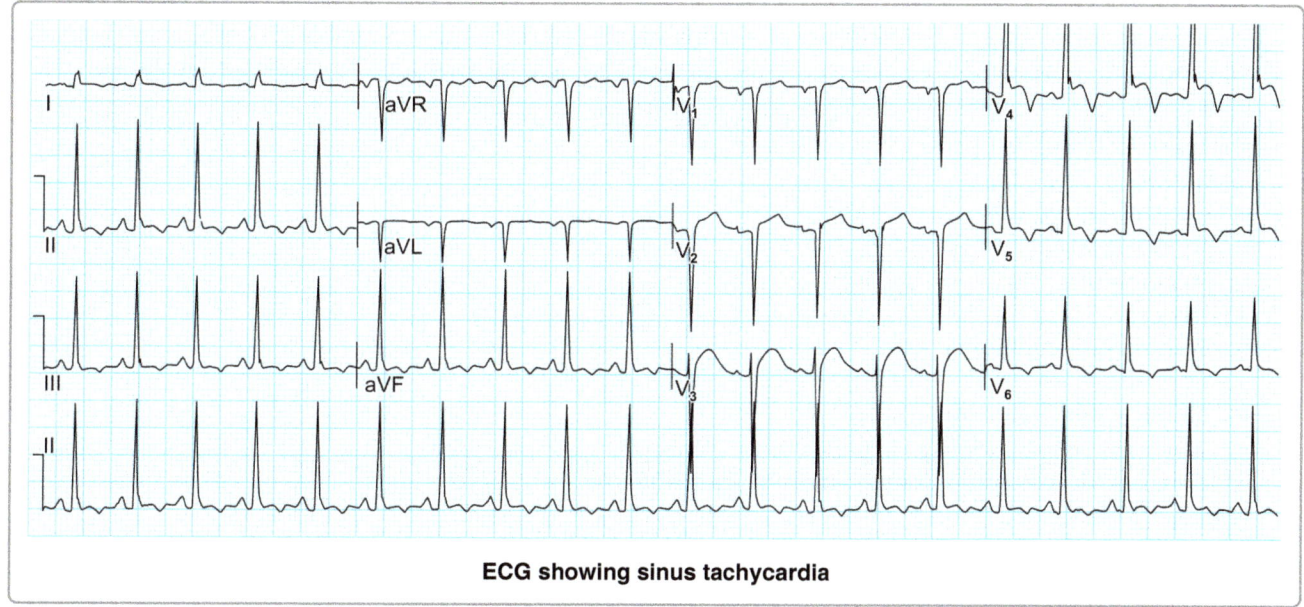

ECG showing sinus tachycardia

Ques. What are the cardiac complication of hyperthyroidism?

Ans. As follows:
- Sinus tachycardia
- High output cardiac failure
- Atrial fibrillation
- Hypertension (systolic)

PULSELESS ELECTRICAL ACTIVITY OR ELECTROMECHANICAL DISSOCIATION

ECG Criteria of Electromechanical Dissociation (EMD)

- P, QRS, and T—all are normal
- Evidence of the cause

Ques. What is pulseless electrical activity (PEA)?

Ans. It is a clinical condition, in which the heart continues to work electrically, but unable to contract. So, there will be no cardiac output, no pulse, no blood pressure, and the patient is unconscious. PEA has previously been referred to as EMD.

Ques. What are the causes of PEA?

Ans. As follows:
- Cardiac tamponade
- Hypovolemia
- Hypothermia
- Hypoxia
- Tension pneumothorax
- Cardiac rupture
- Massive pulmonary embolism
- Electrolyte imbalance (e.g., hypokalemia)
- Drug overdose—cardio-depressant drug, e.g., β-blocker

Ques. How to treat PEA?

Ans. Treatment depends on underlying causes.
- Intubate and IV access
- Injection adrenaline (1 mg IV)
- CPR
- *Other therapy*: Pressor agents, calcium, etc.
- Specific treatment of underlying cause

NB: Remember the following points:

- EMD is frequently a late event in cardiac arrest and indicates a poor prognosis.
- When EMD is the presenting feature, it suggests the possibility of underlying ventricular rupture and it is unlikely that the patient will be resuscitated.
- However, potentially treated causes should not be overlooked.

RAISED INTRACRANIAL PRESSURE

ECG Criteria of Raised ICP

- Widespread giant T-wave inversions ("cerebral T waves")
- QT prolongation
- Bradycardia (Cushing reflex—indicates imminent brainstem herniation)

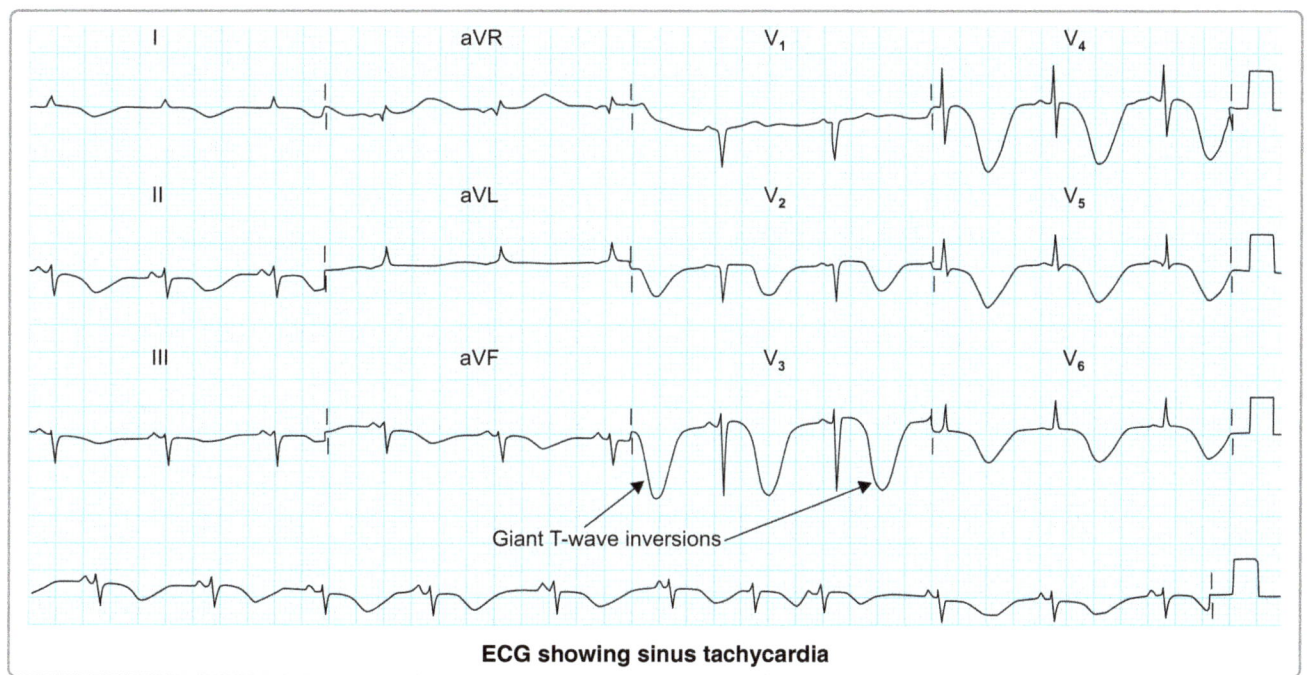

ECG showing sinus tachycardia

CHAPTER 3

151 Tracings of ECG

"Most of the doctors can competently interpret ECG without getting submerged in its complexities"

Remember *"there is no need for the ECG to be daunting: Just as most people drive car without knowing much about the engines and the gardeners do not necessarily need to be a botanist"*

151 ECG tracings are included here.
The reader should interpret by himself and then
compare the findings given in the last pages.
In this way, it will offer a good
self-learning and exercise in ECG.

ECG in Medical Practice

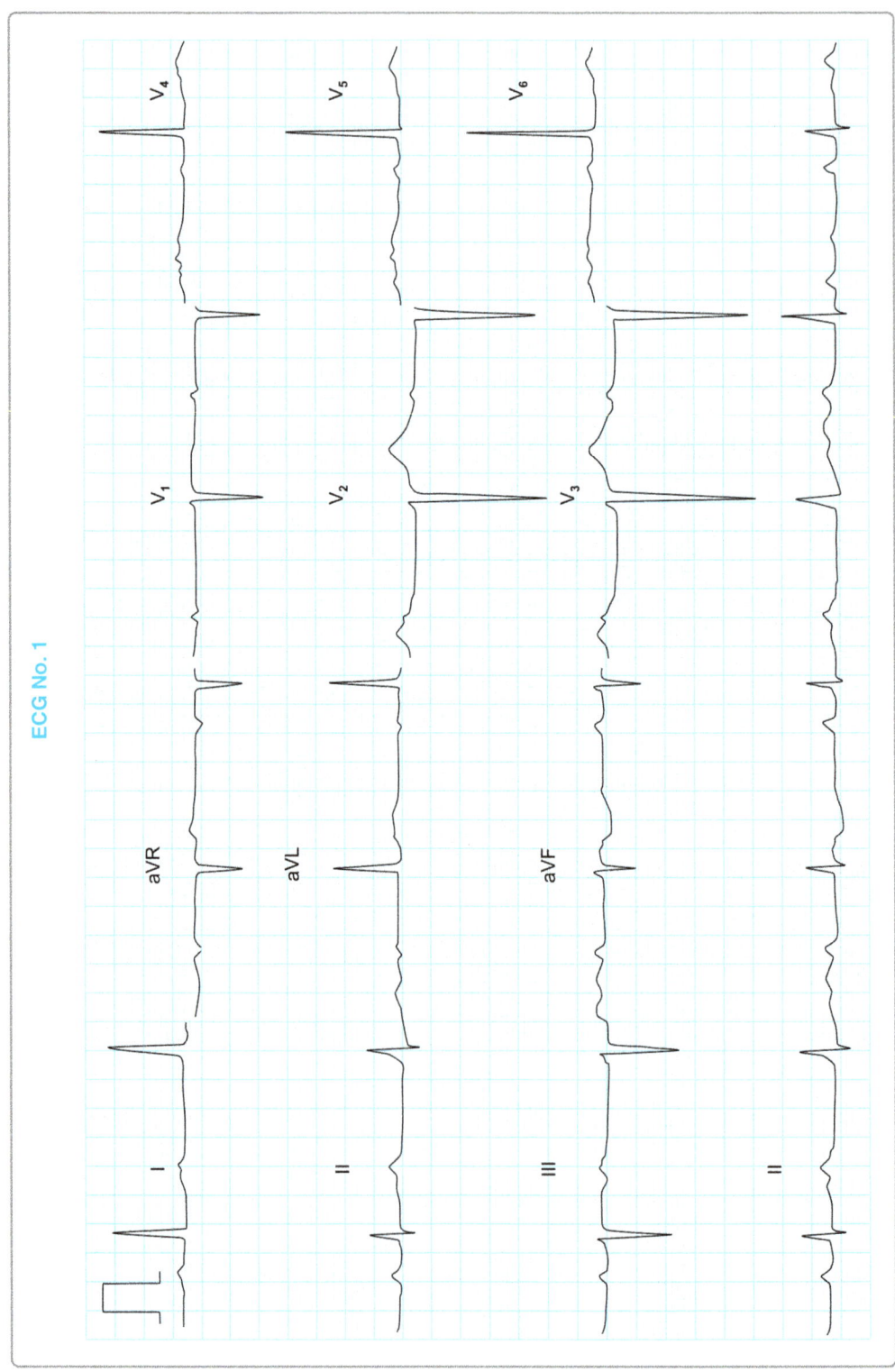

ECG No. 1

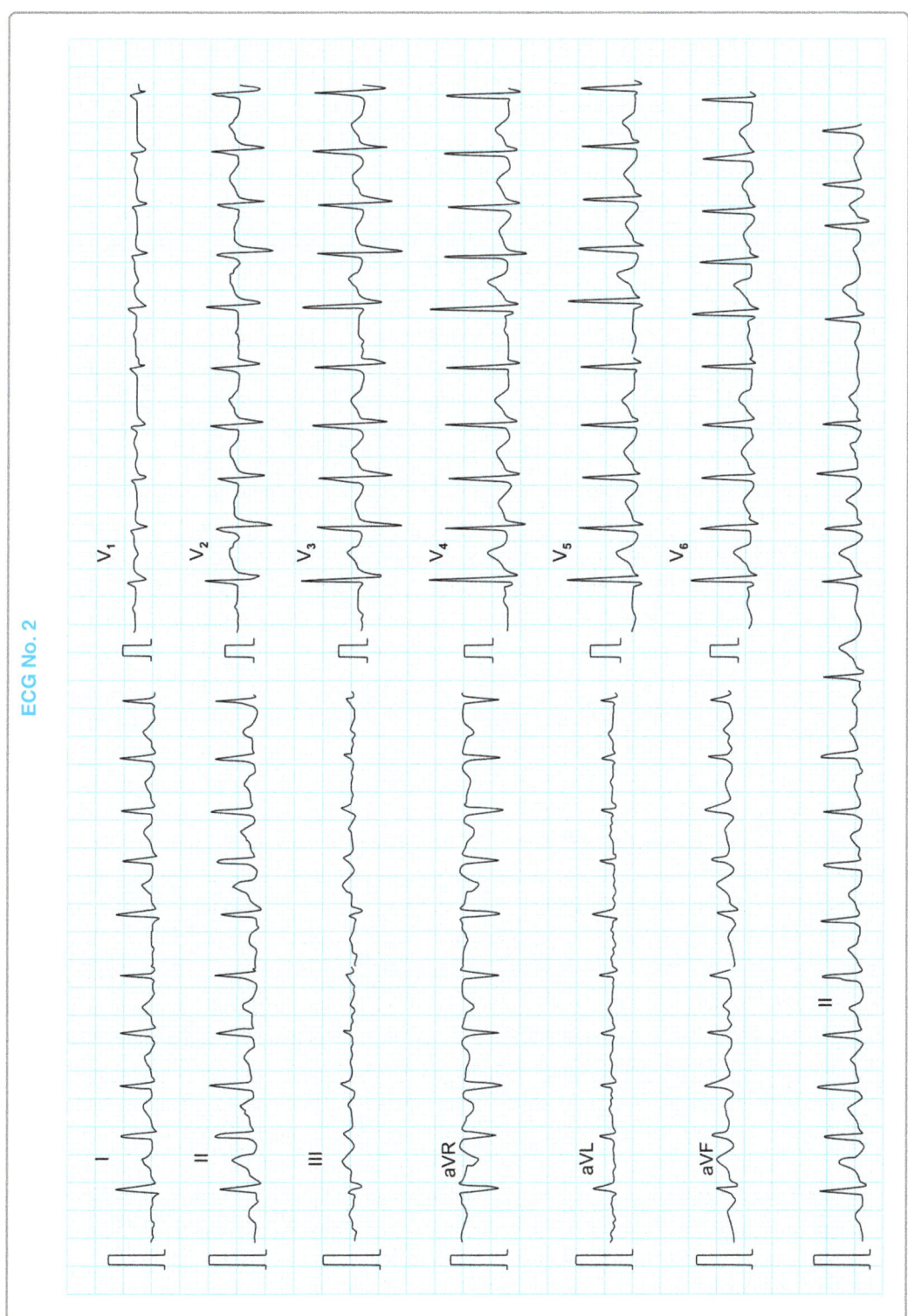

ECG in Medical Practice

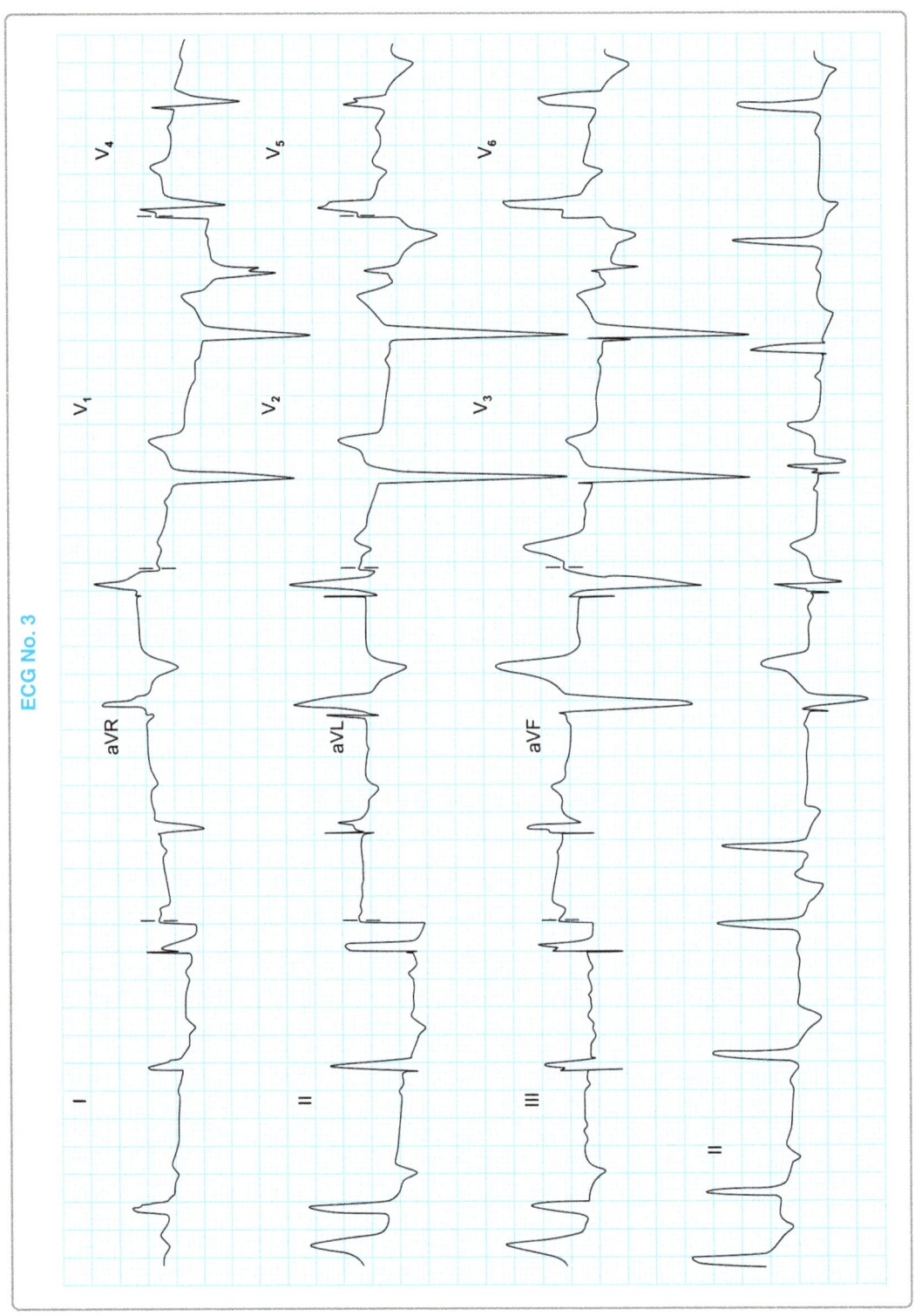

ECG No. 3

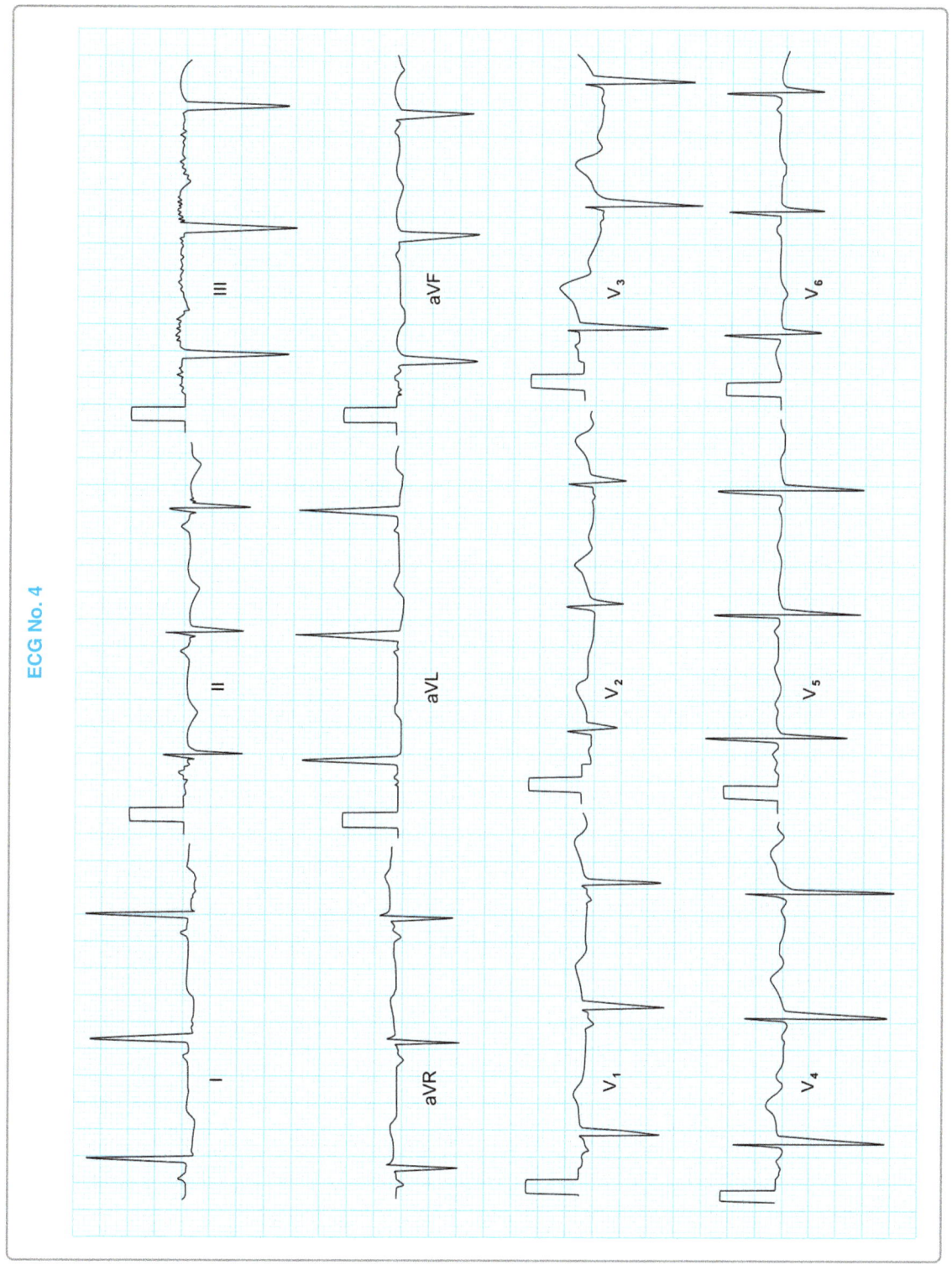

ECG No. 4

ECG in Medical Practice

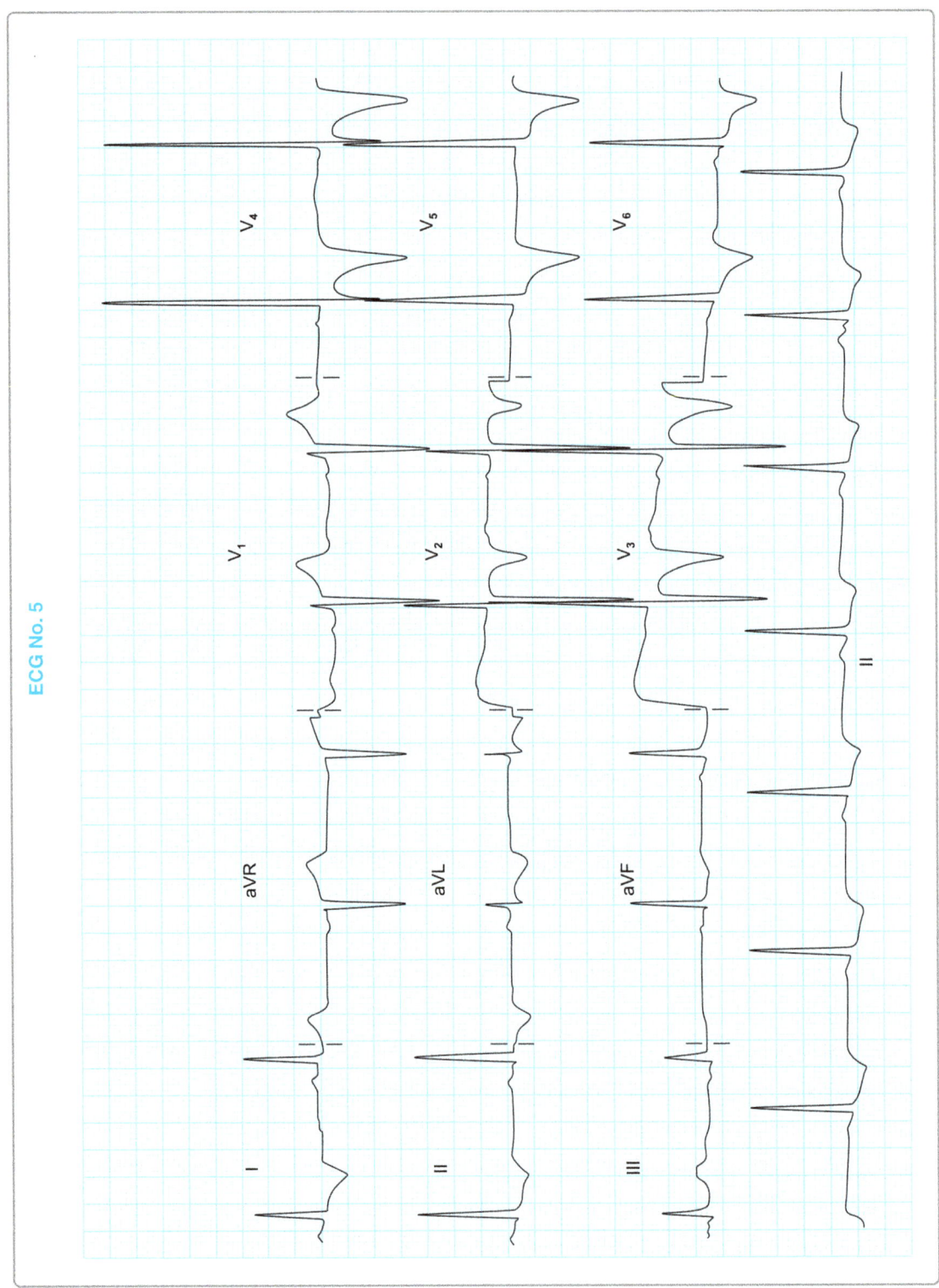

ECG No. 5

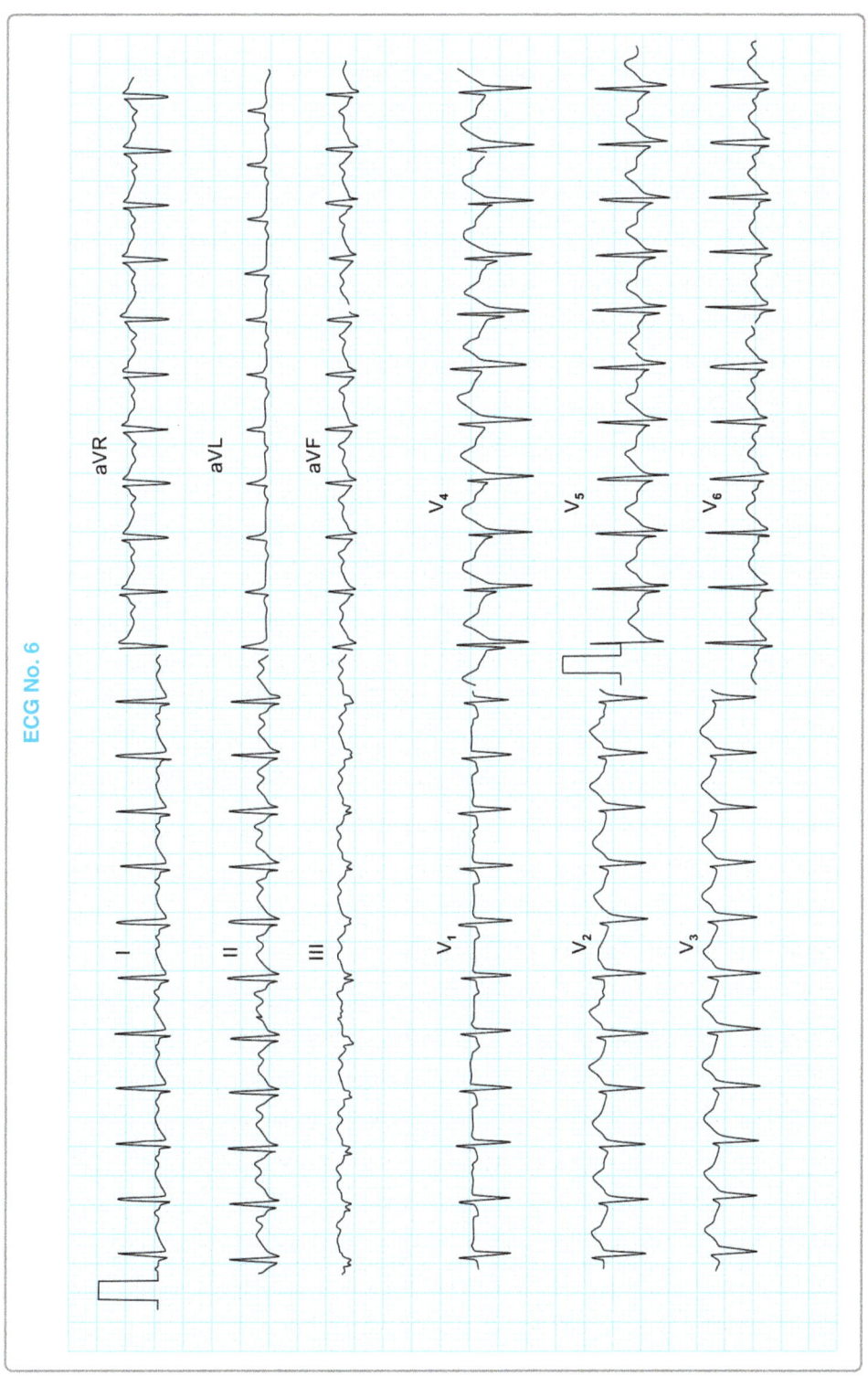

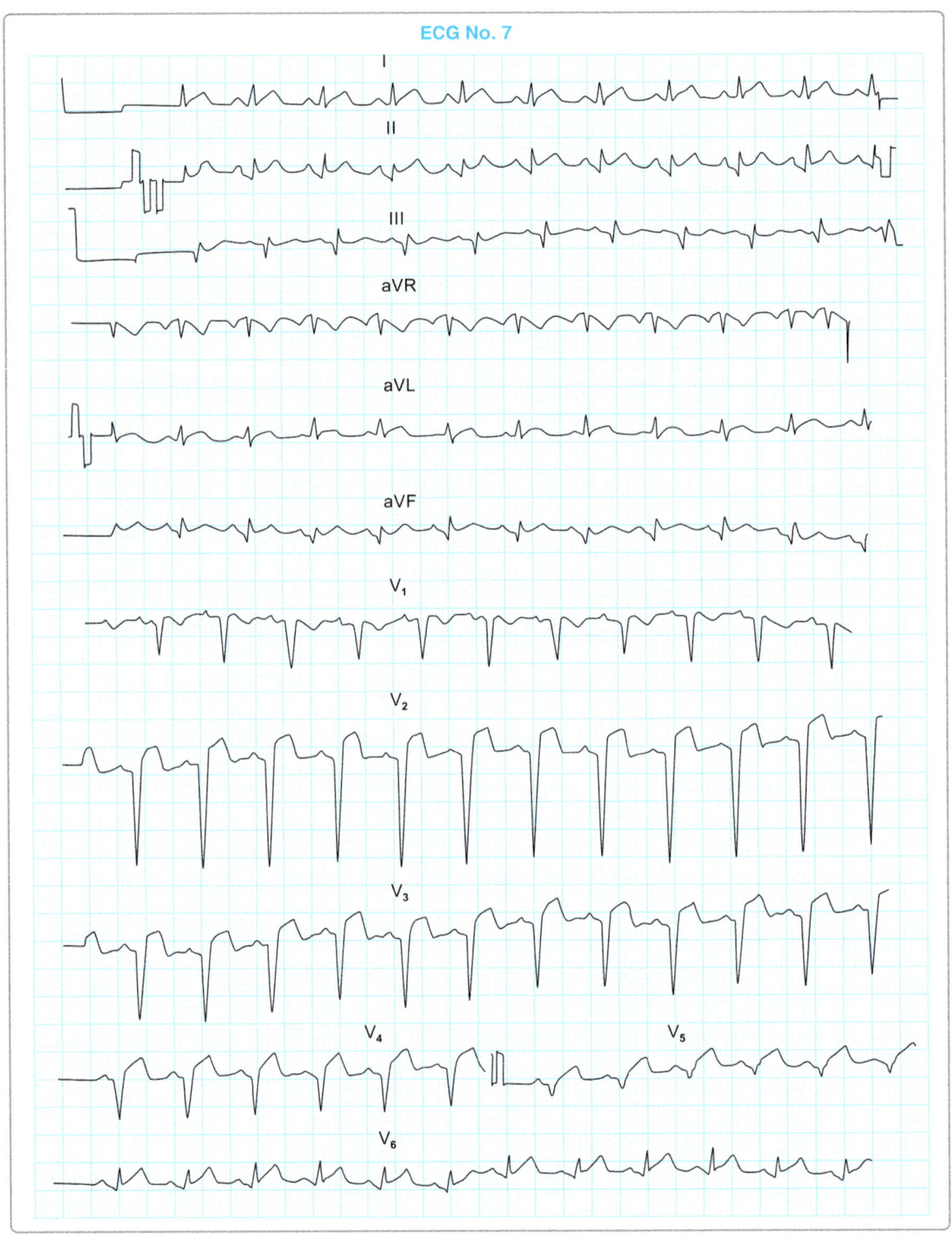

ECG No. 8

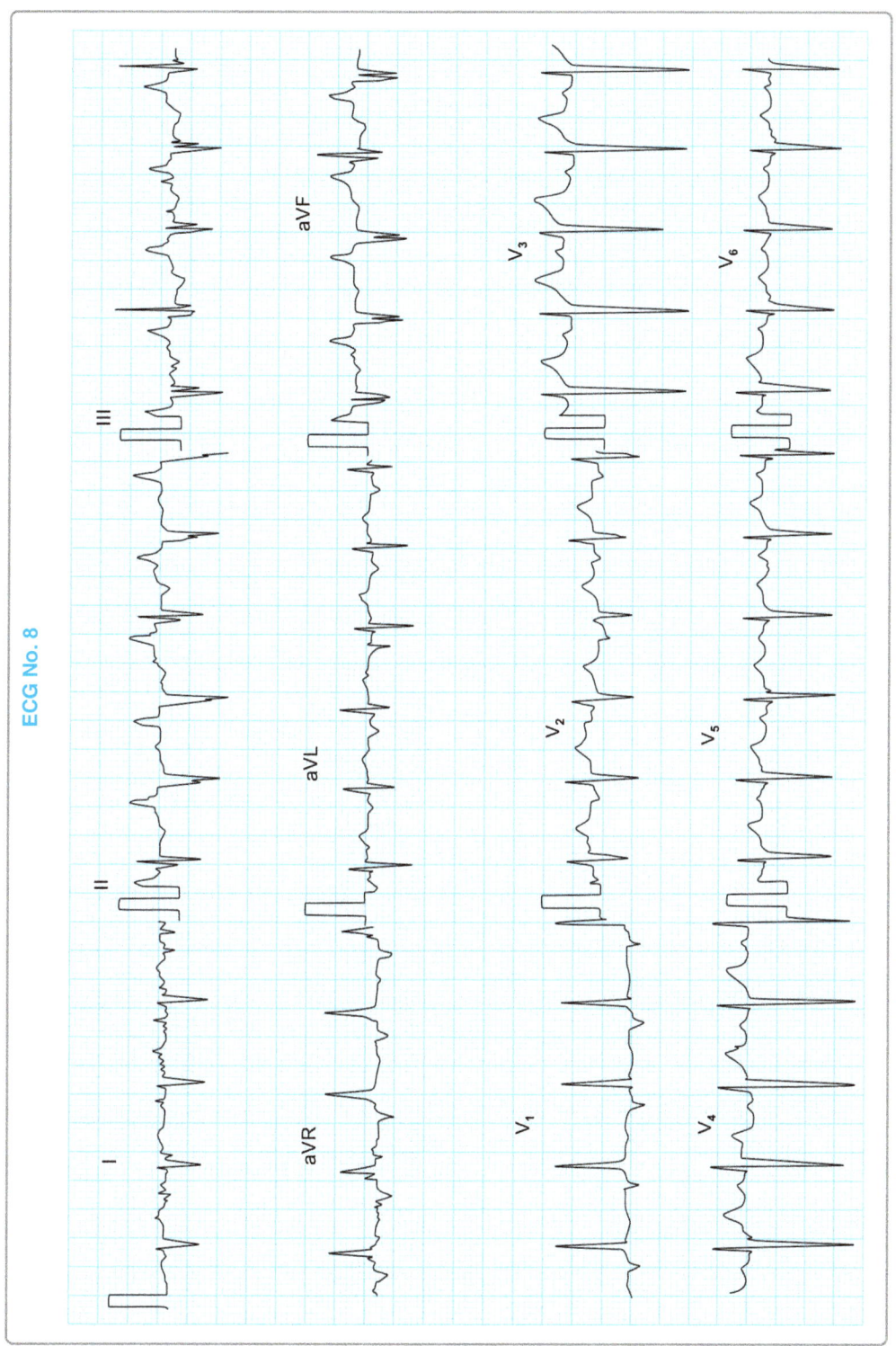

ECG in Medical Practice

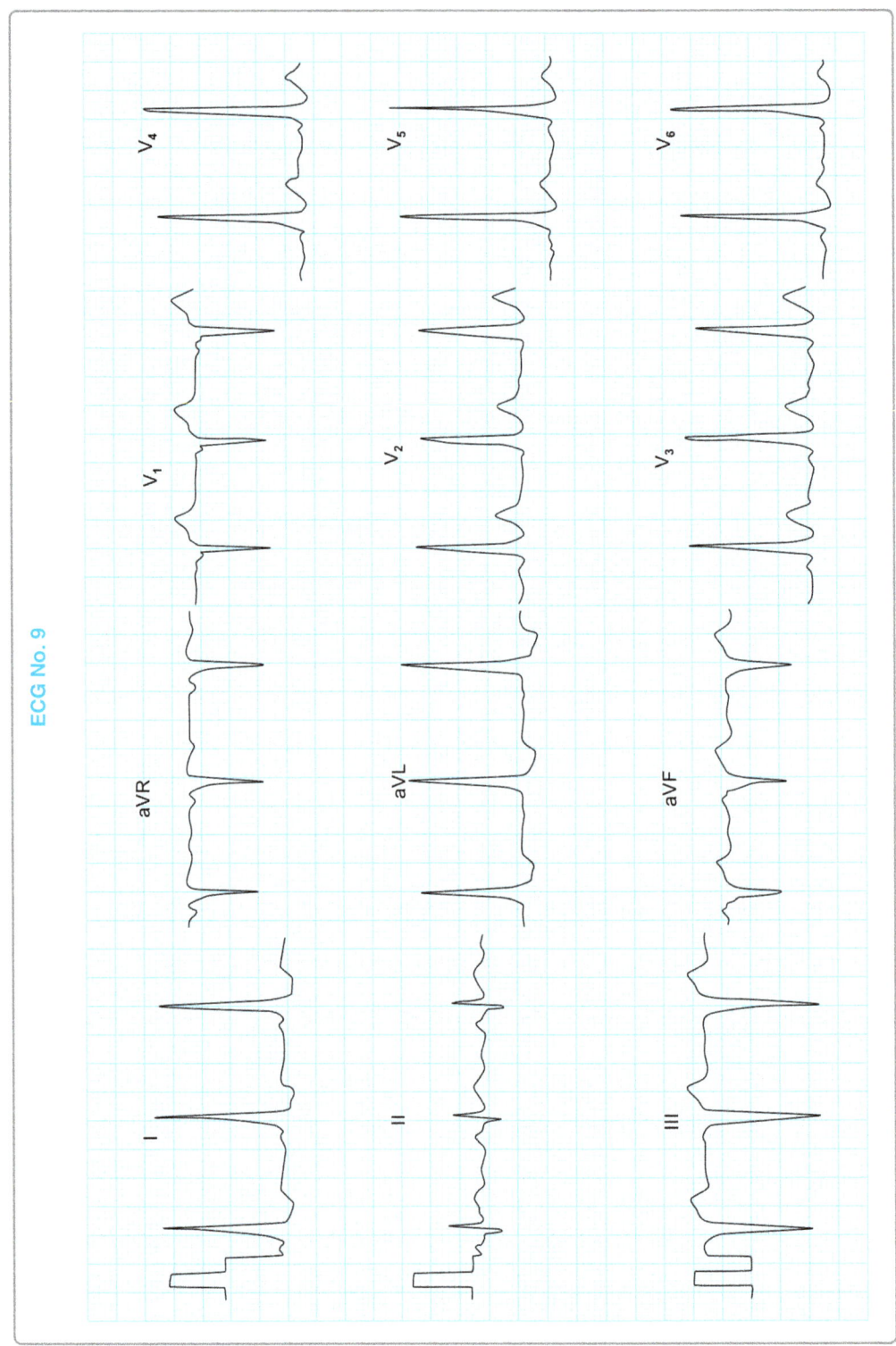

ECG No. 9

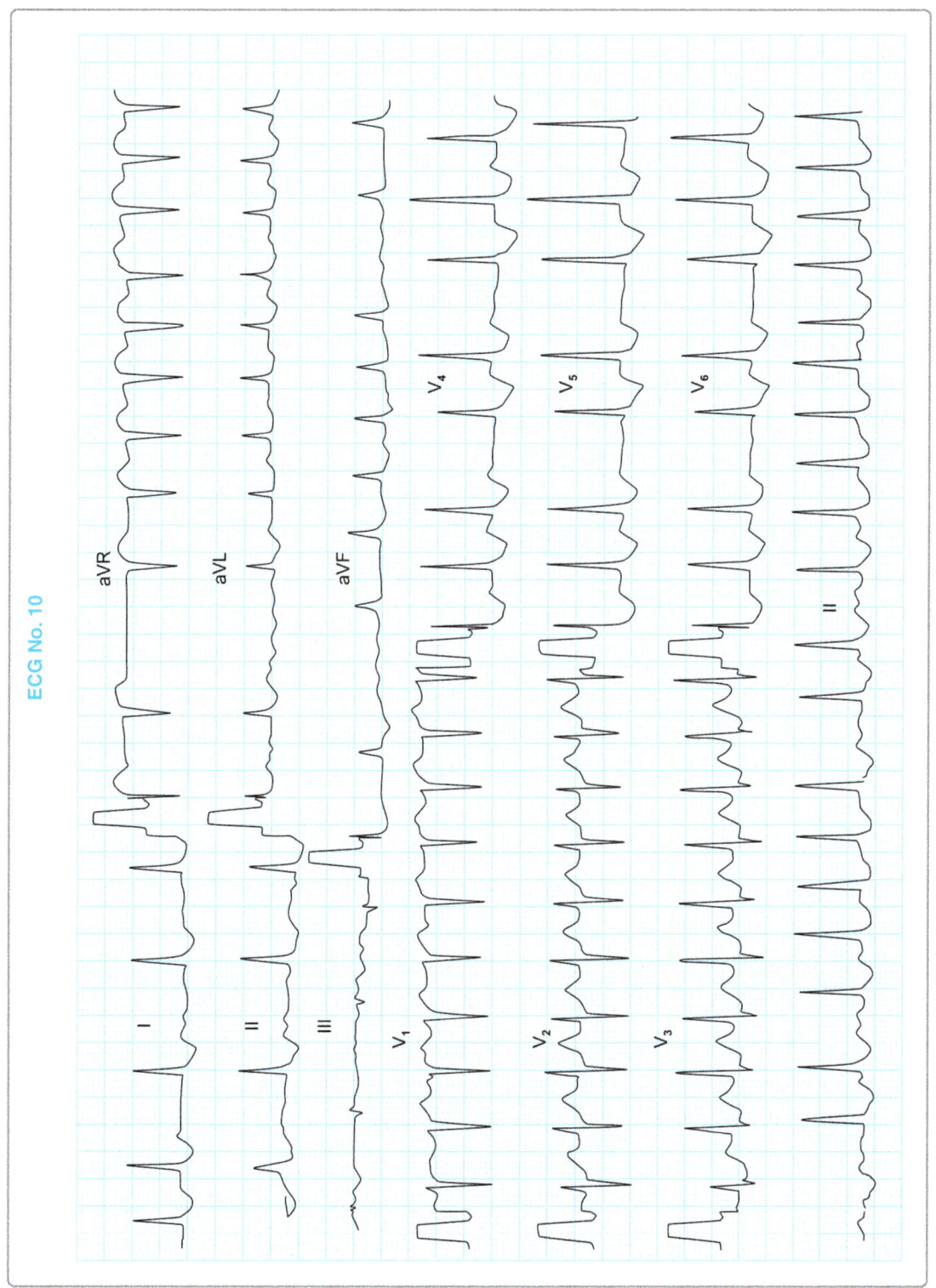

ECG No. 10

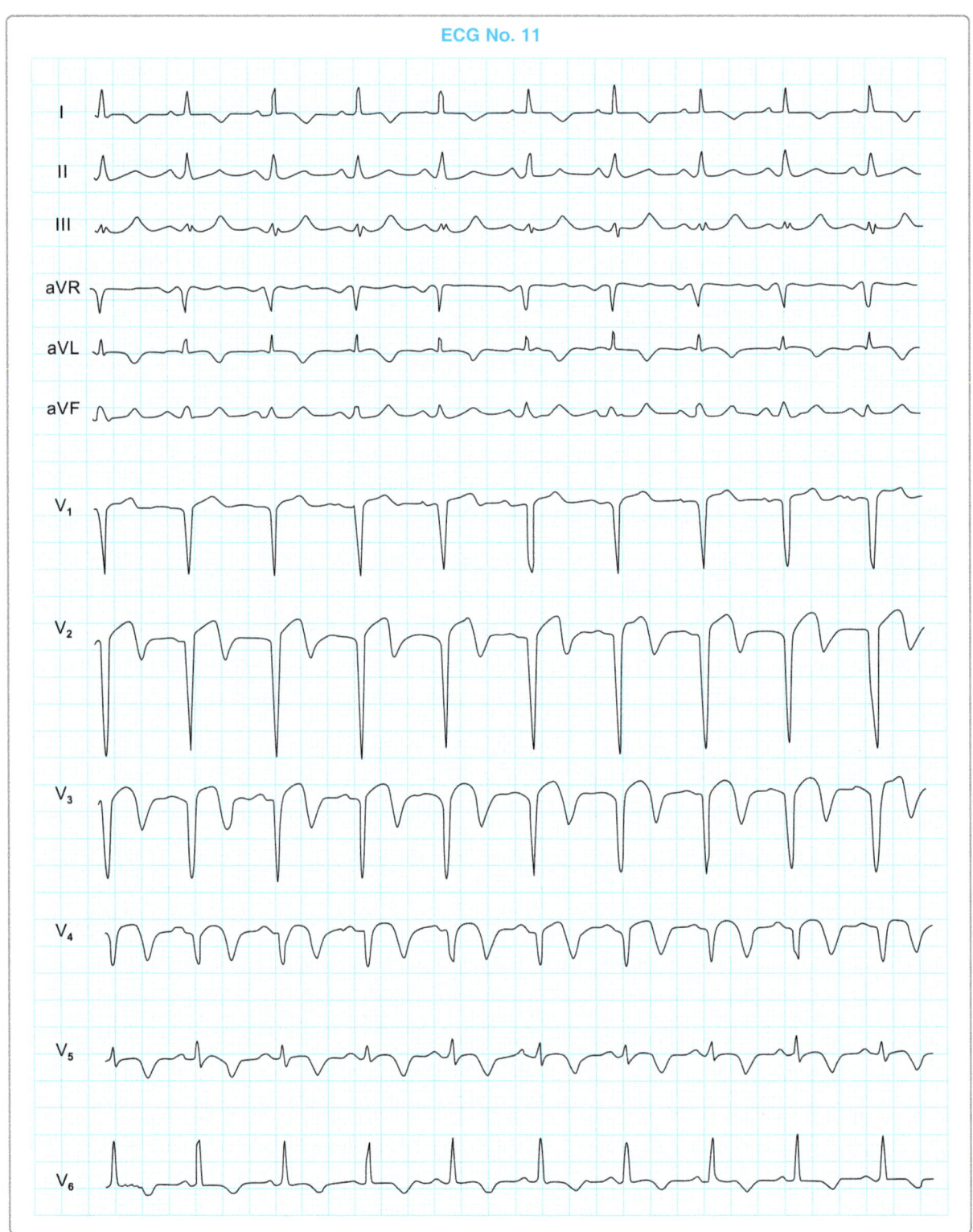

Chapter 3: 151 Tracings of ECG

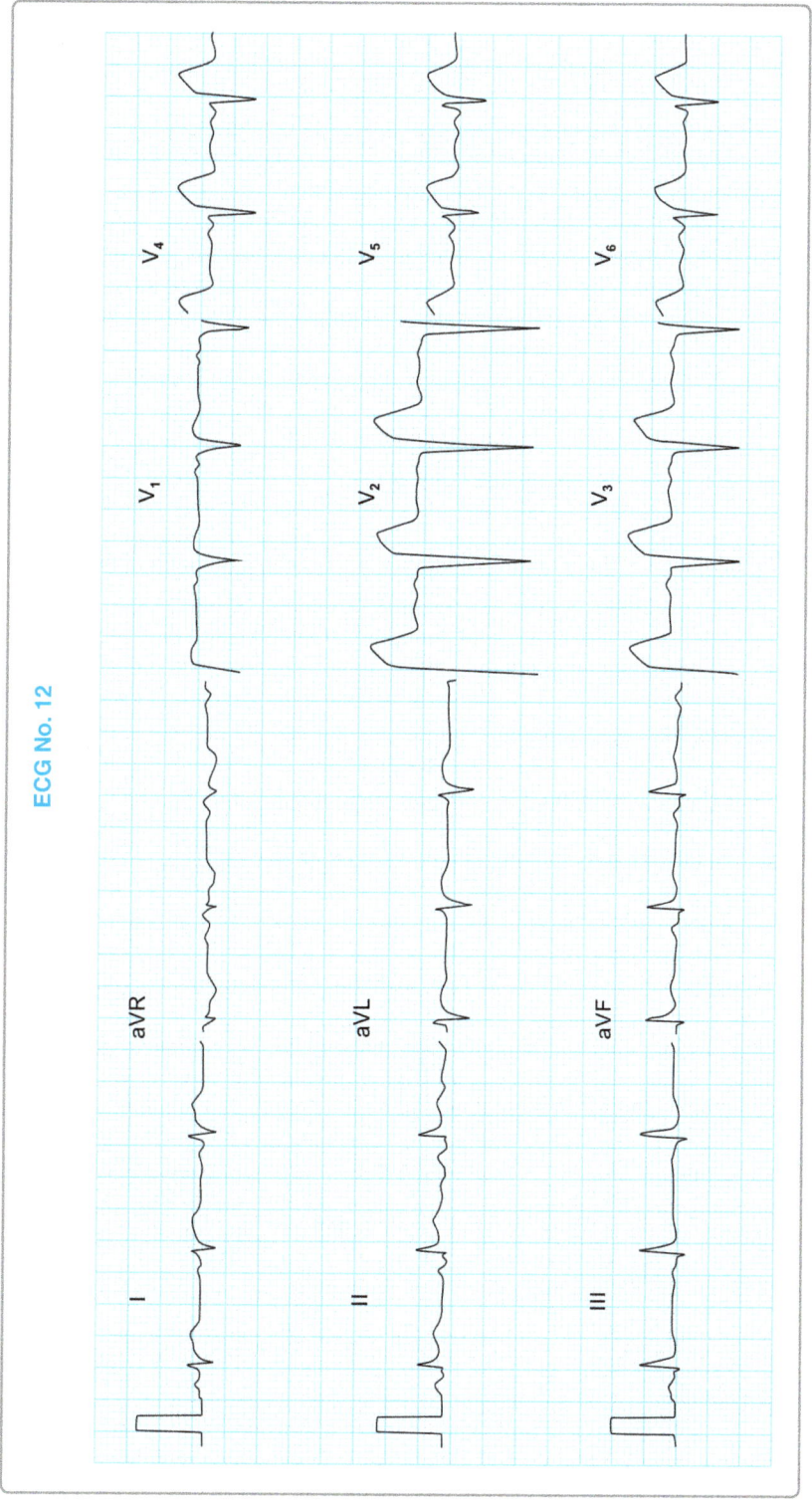

ECG No. 12

ECG in Medical Practice

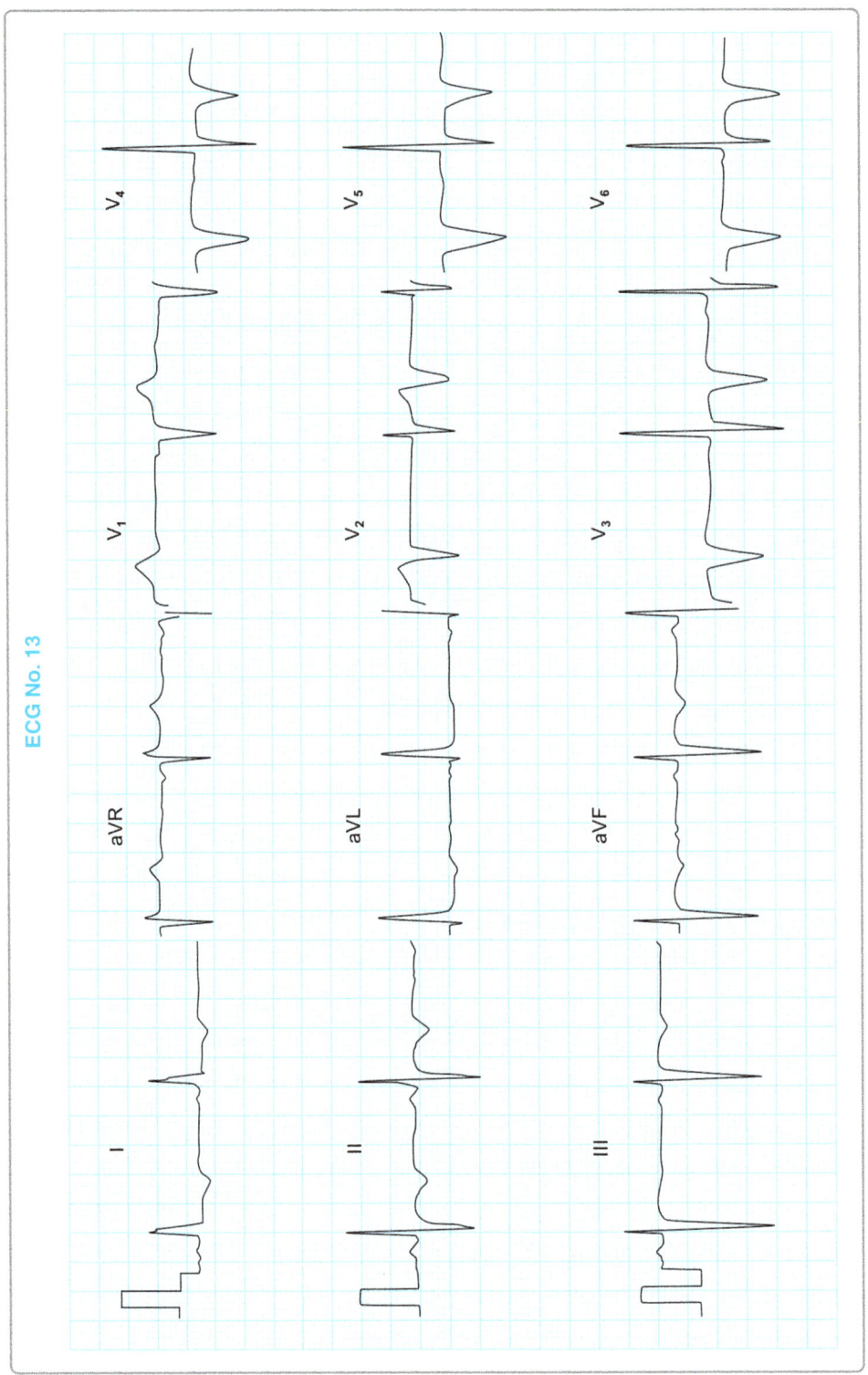

ECG No. 13

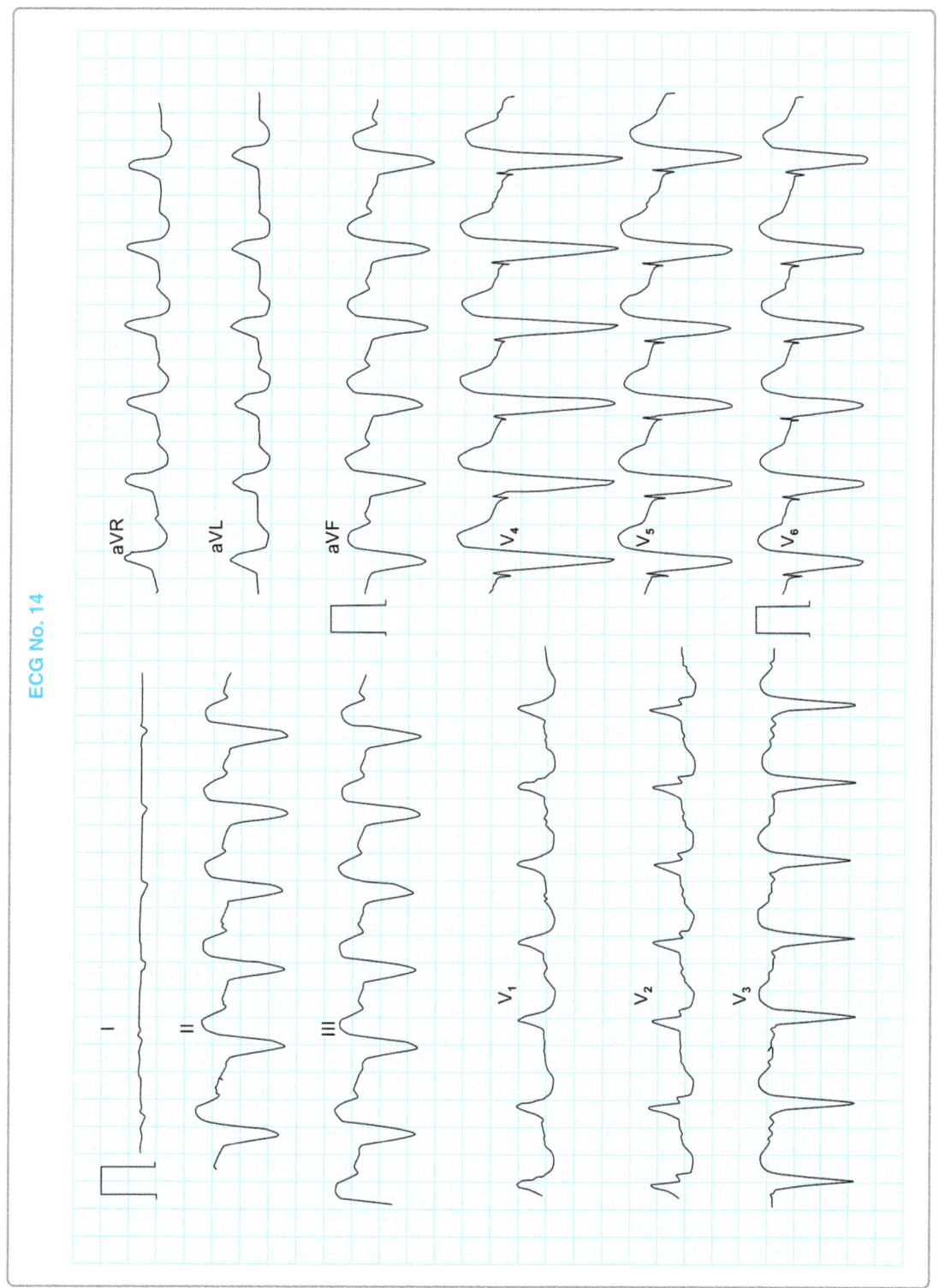

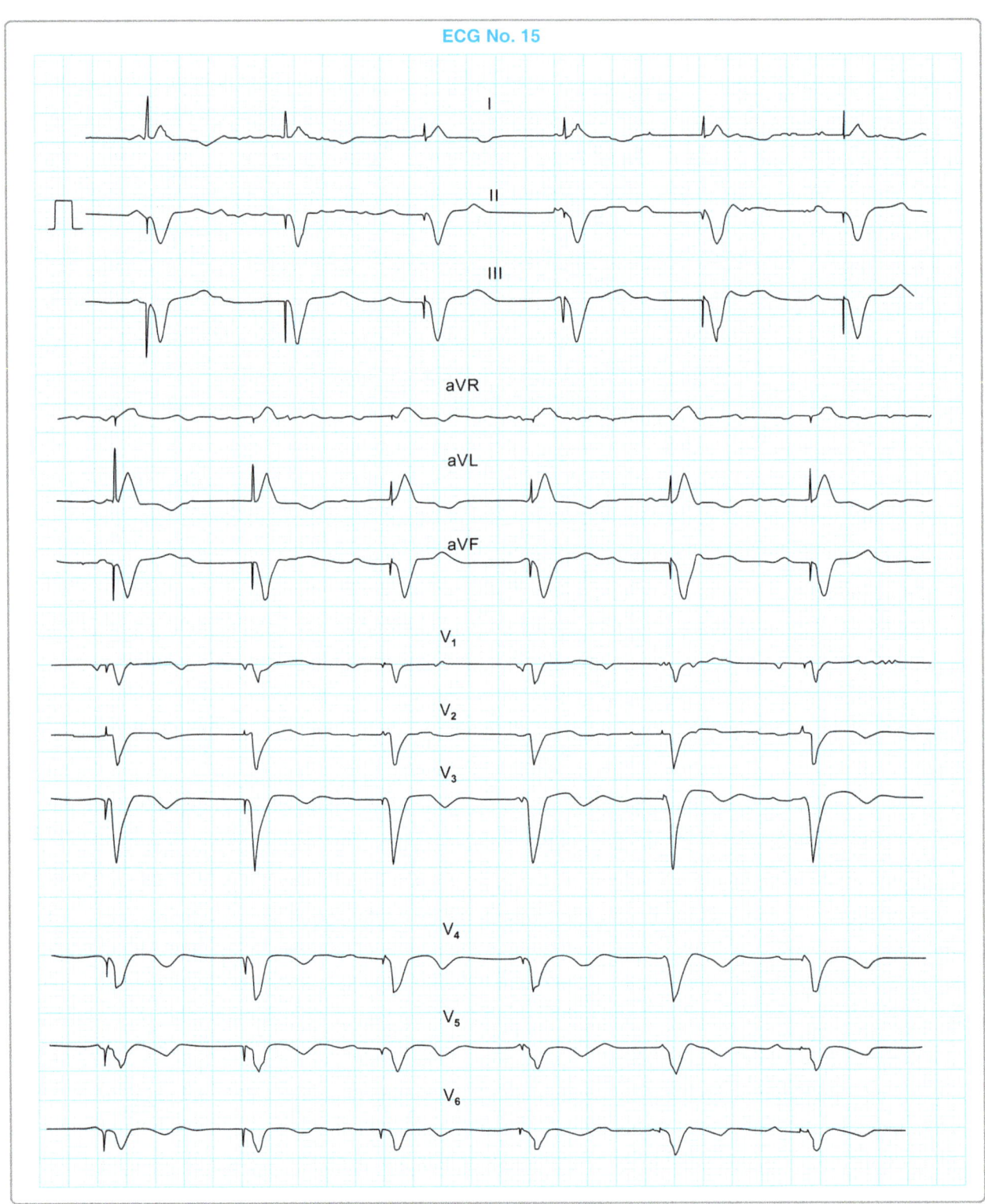

ECG No. 15

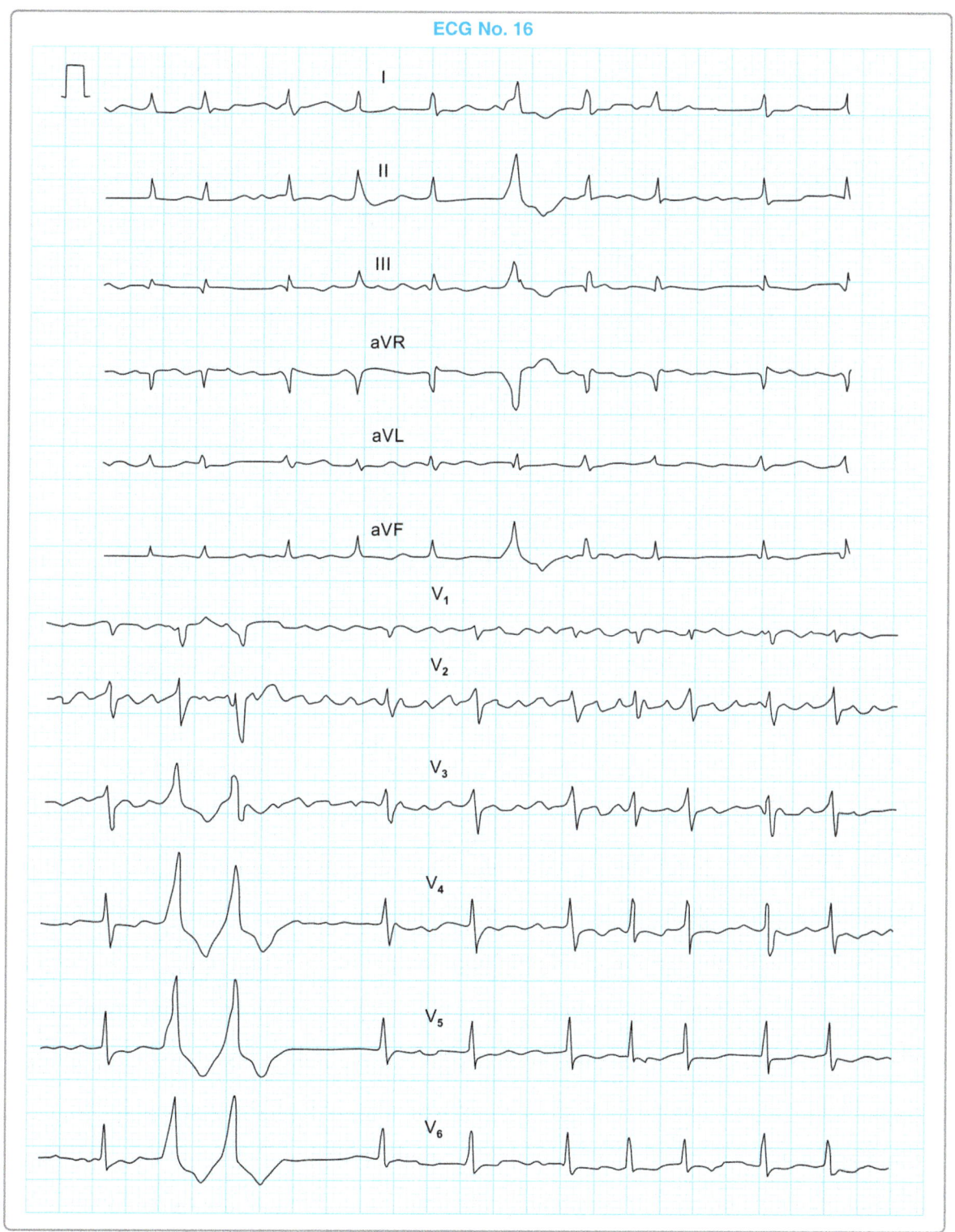

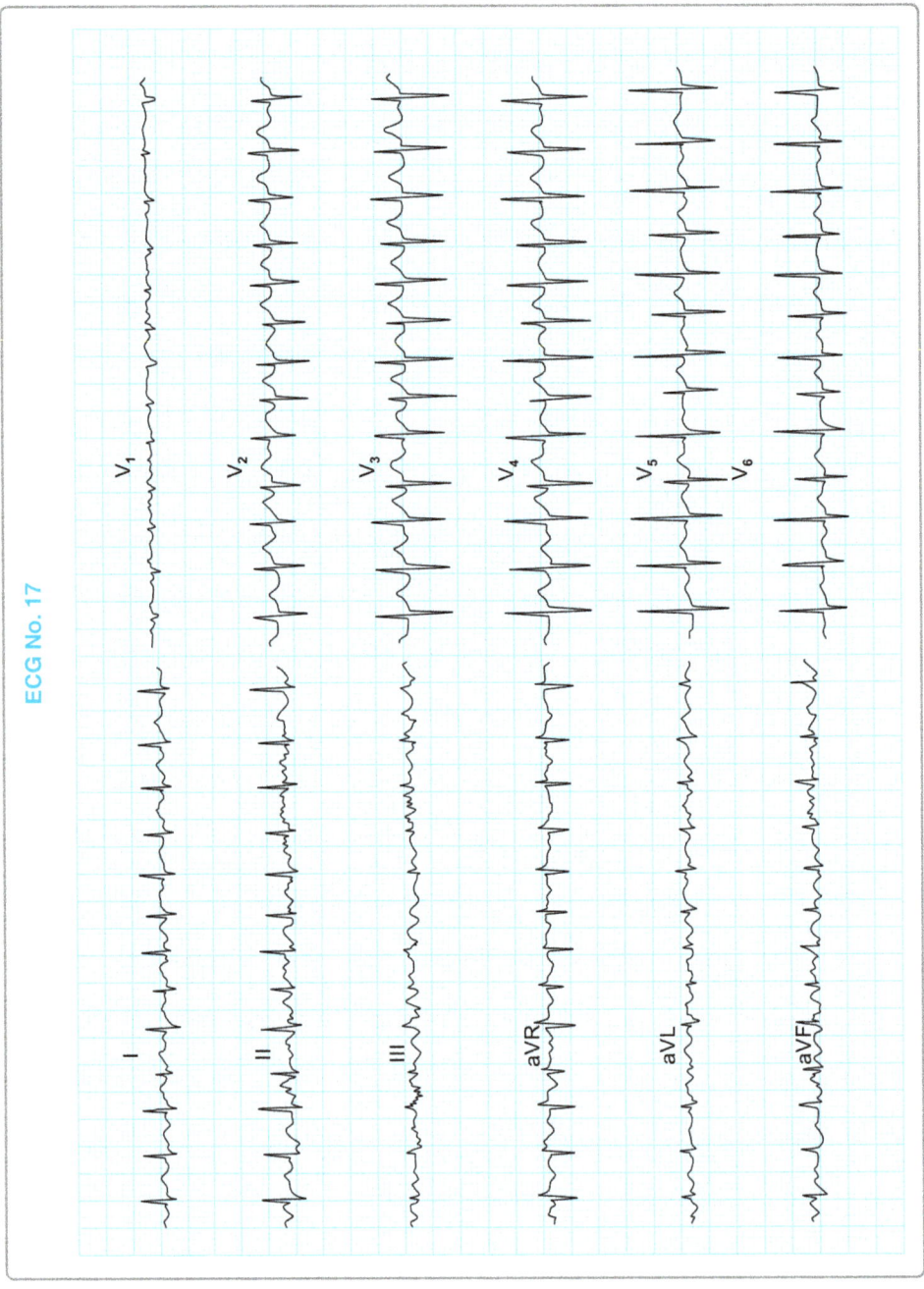

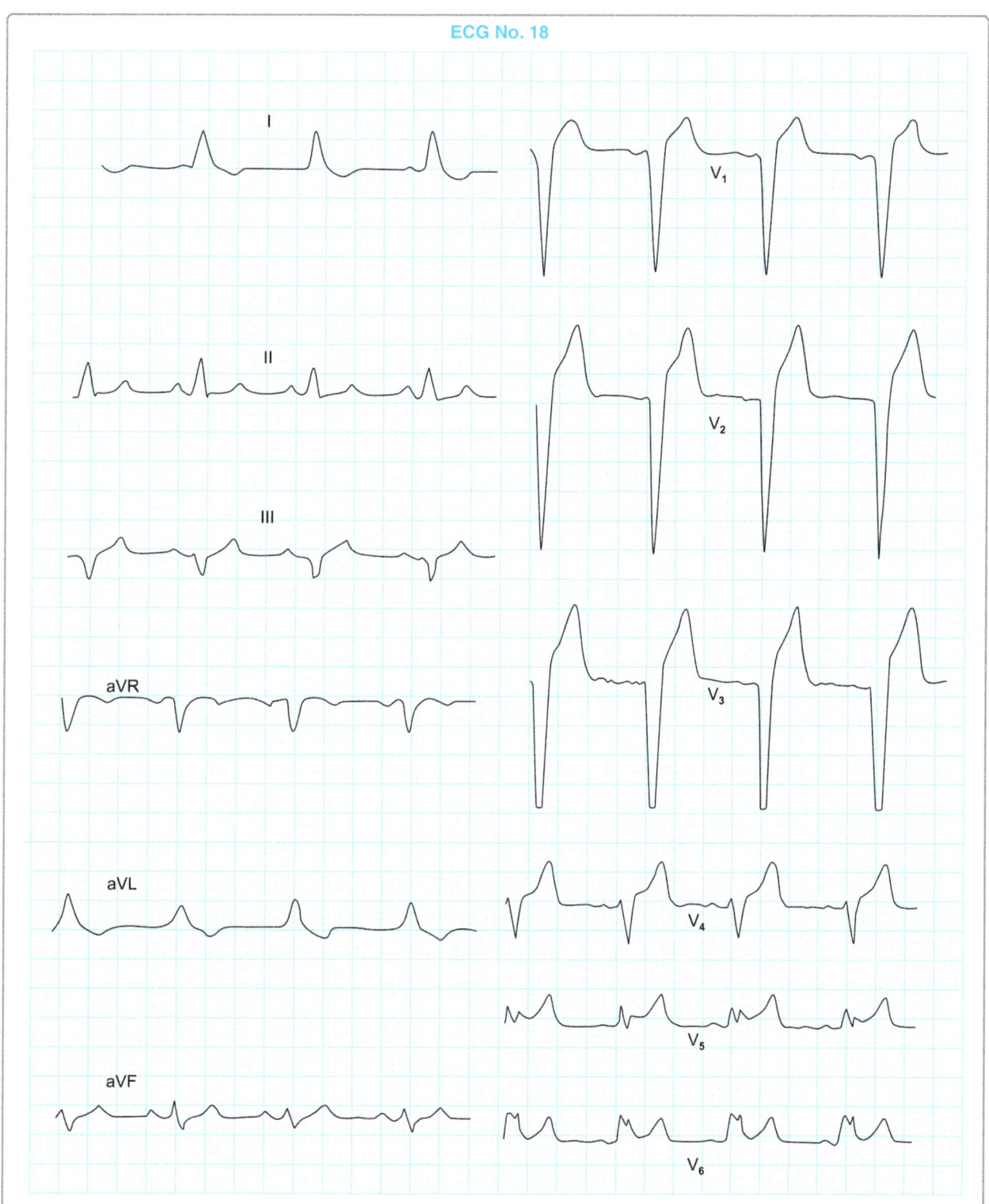

ECG in Medical Practice

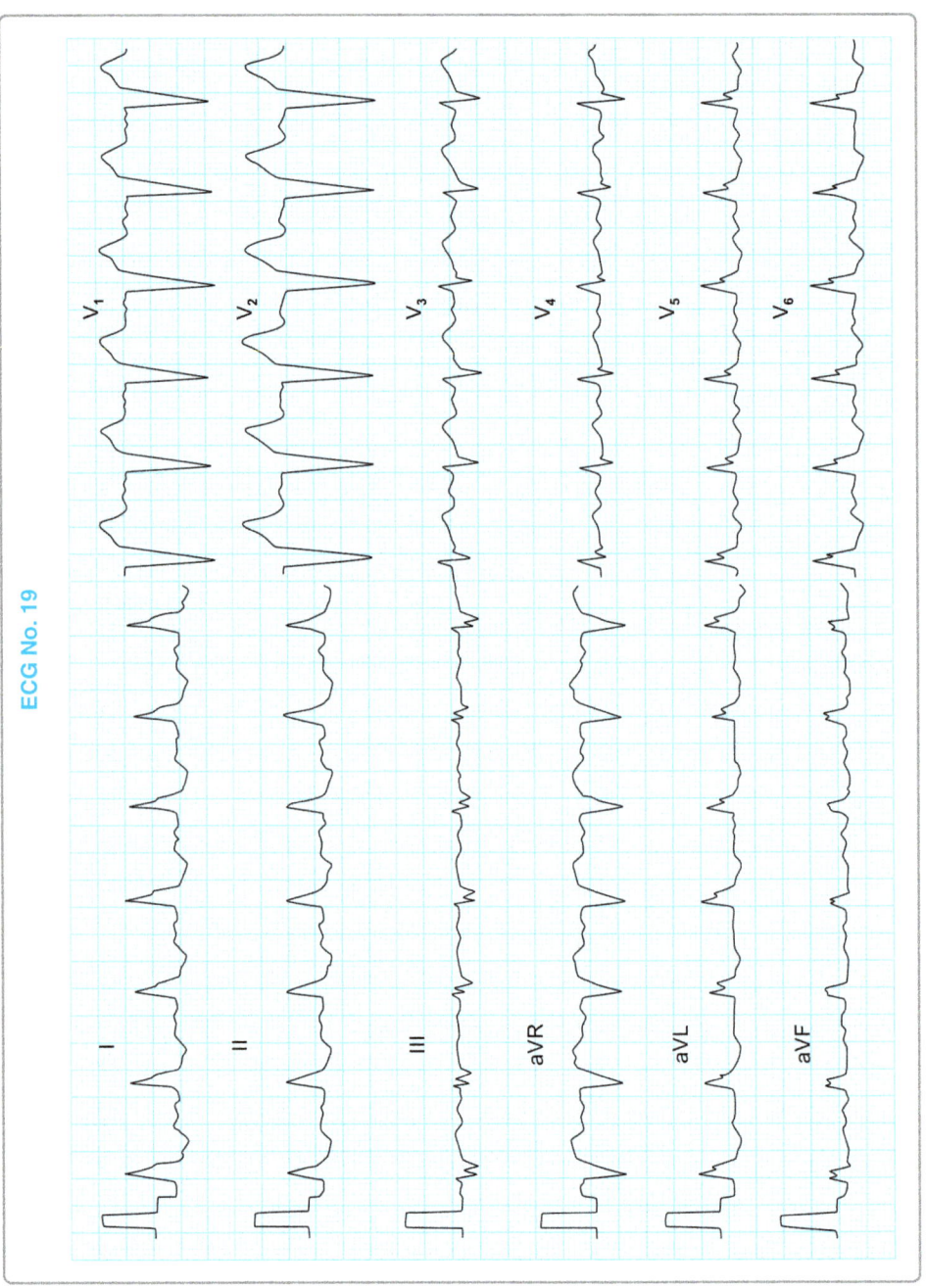

ECG No. 19

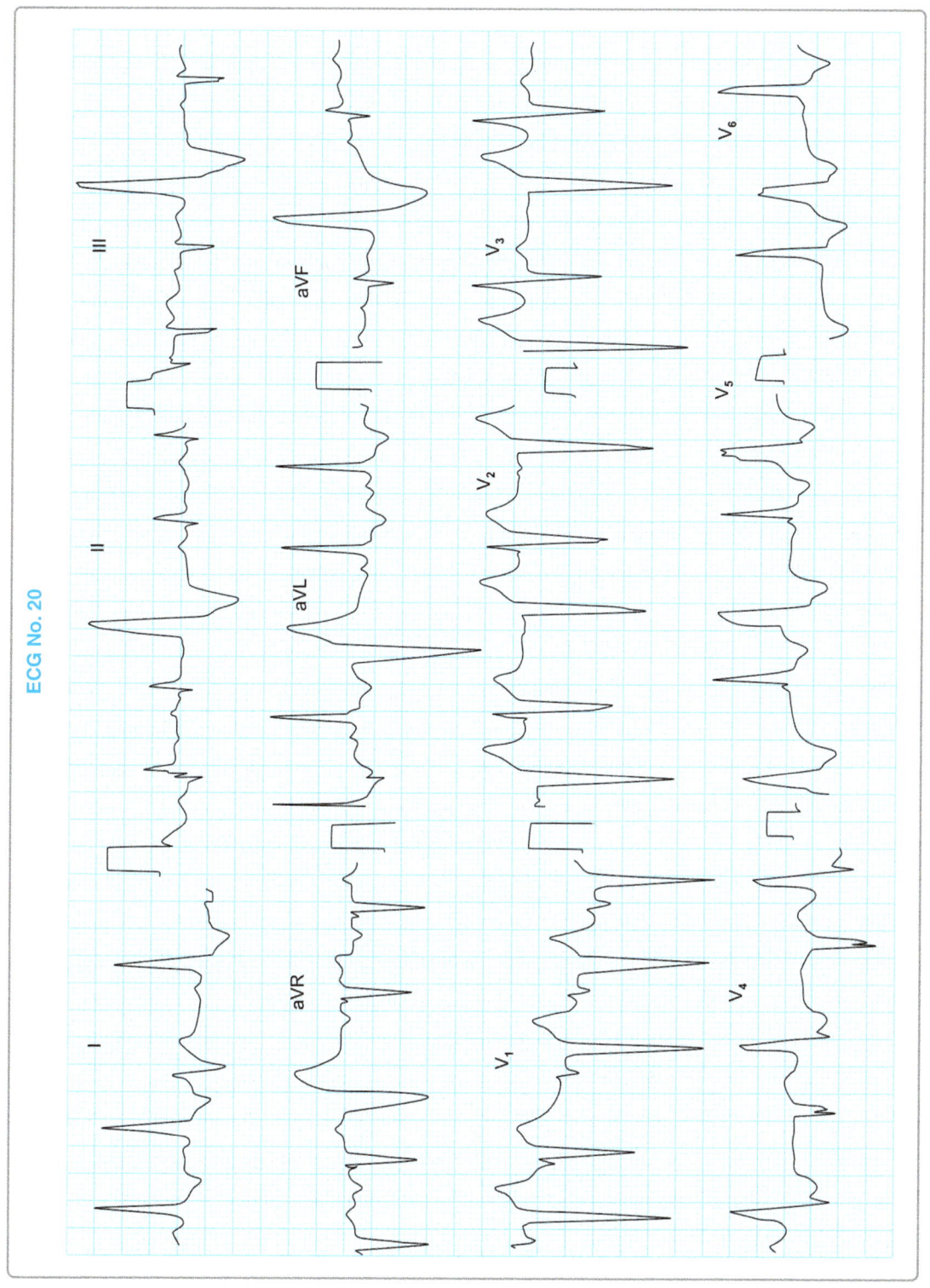

ECG No. 20

ECG in Medical Practice

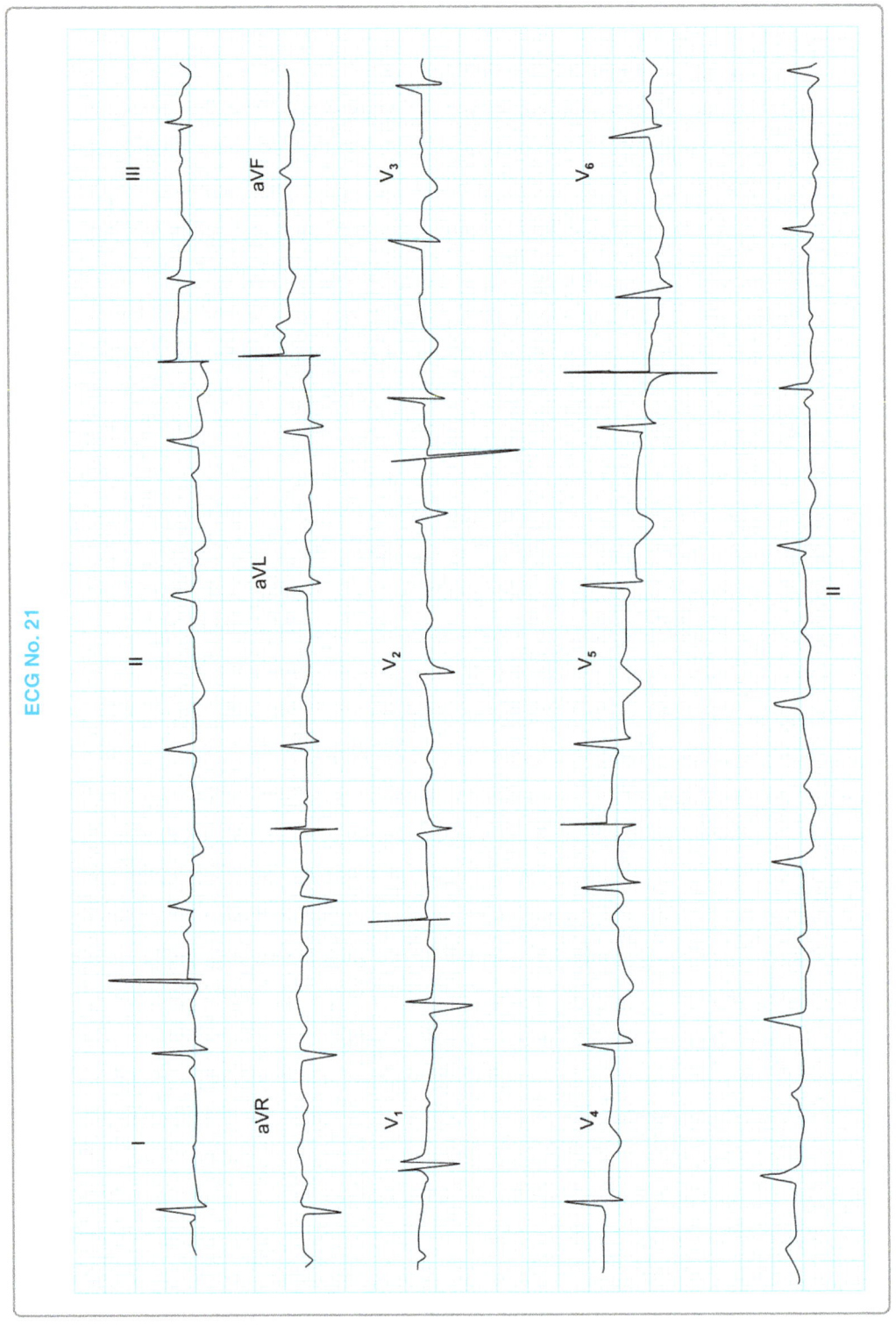

ECG No. 21

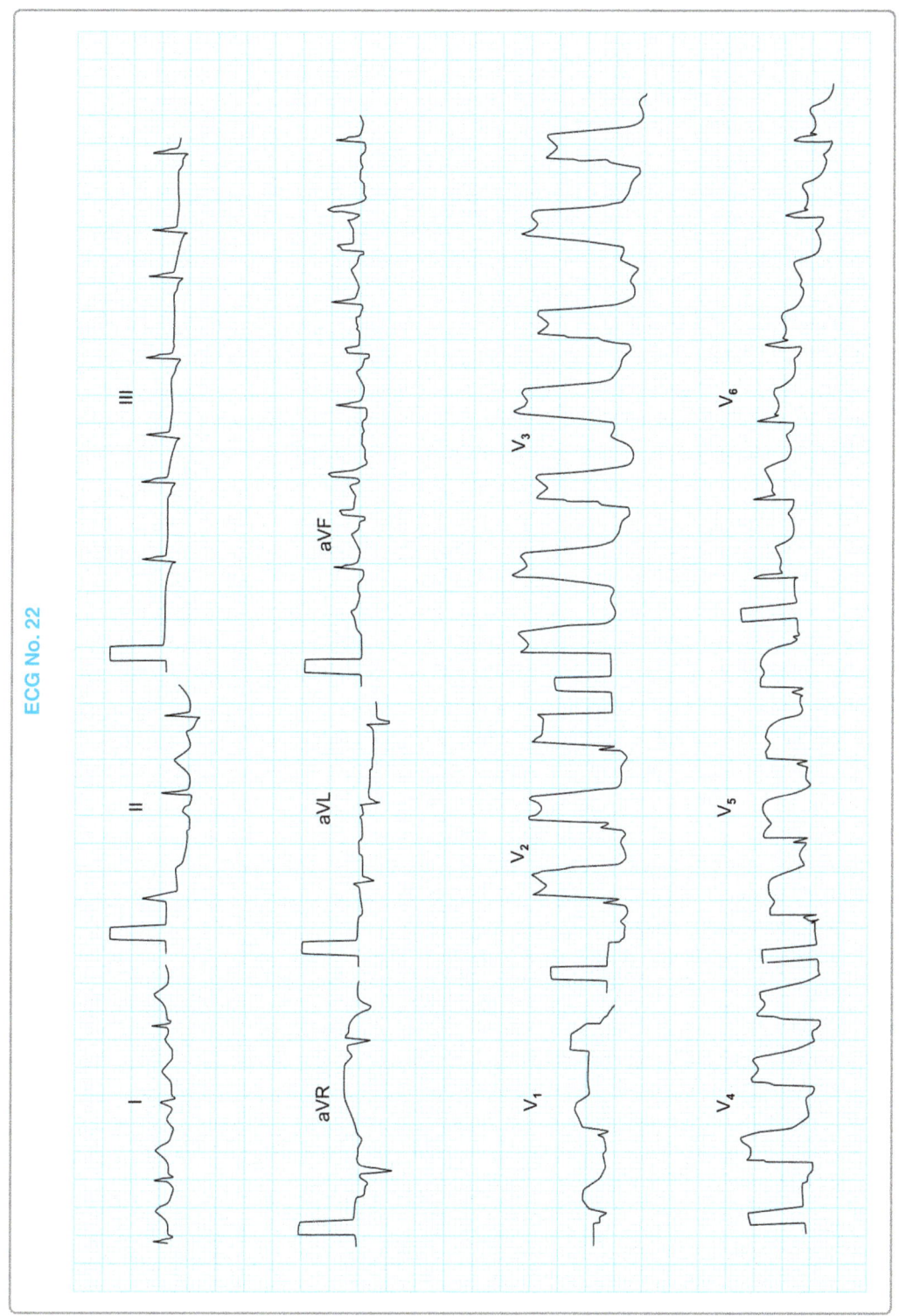

ECG No. 22

ECG in Medical Practice

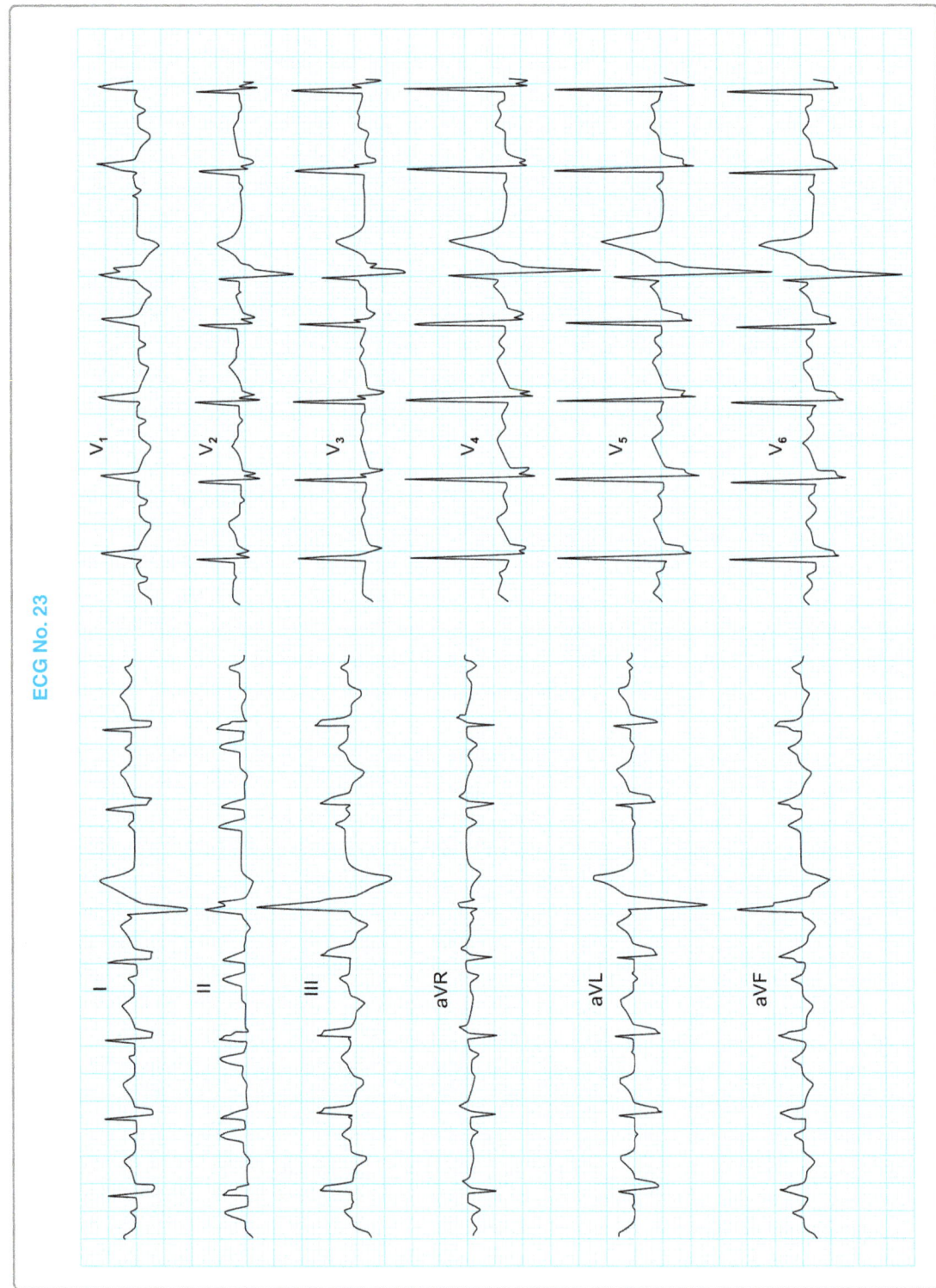

ECG No. 23

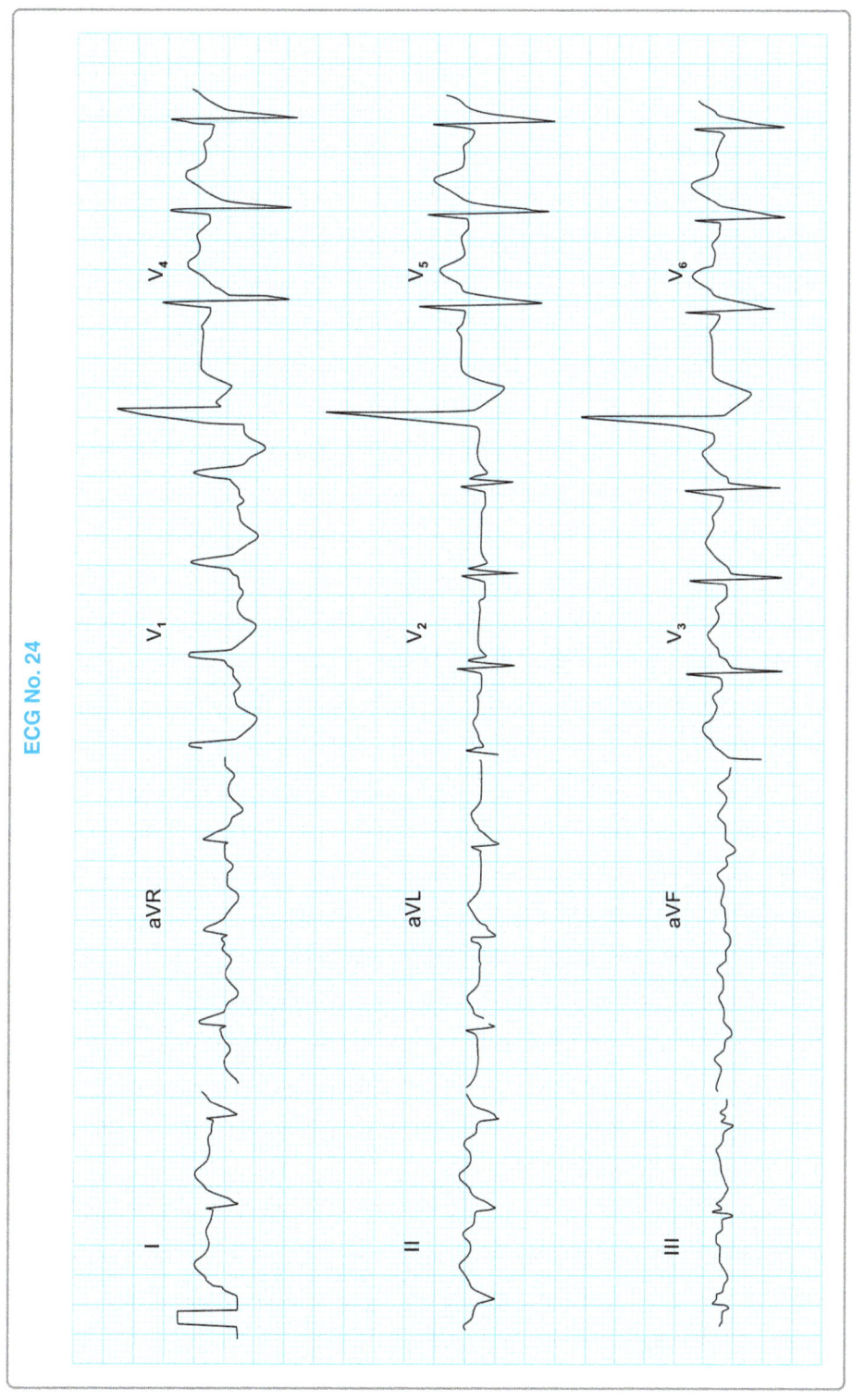

ECG in Medical Practice

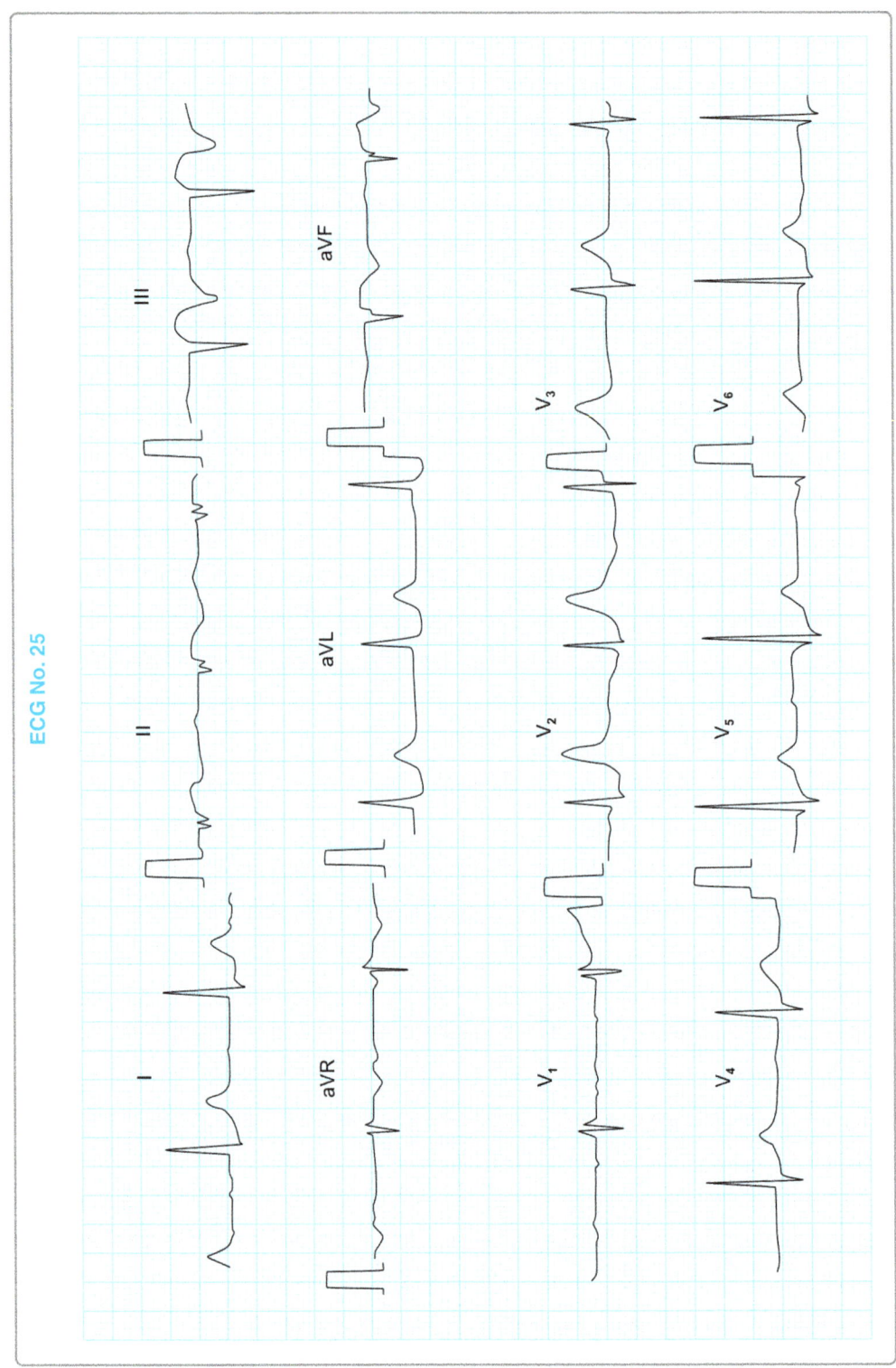

ECG No. 25

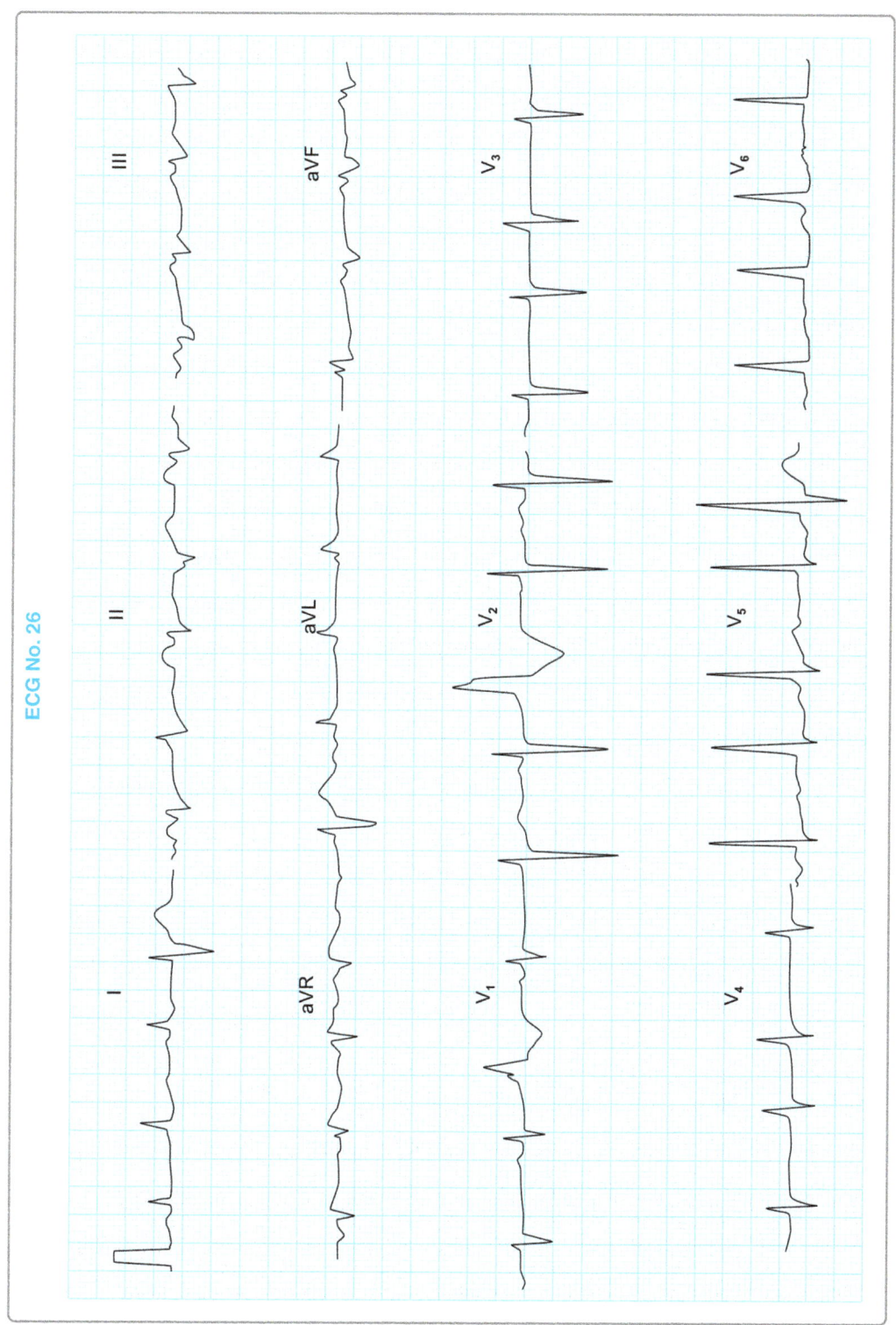

ECG in Medical Practice

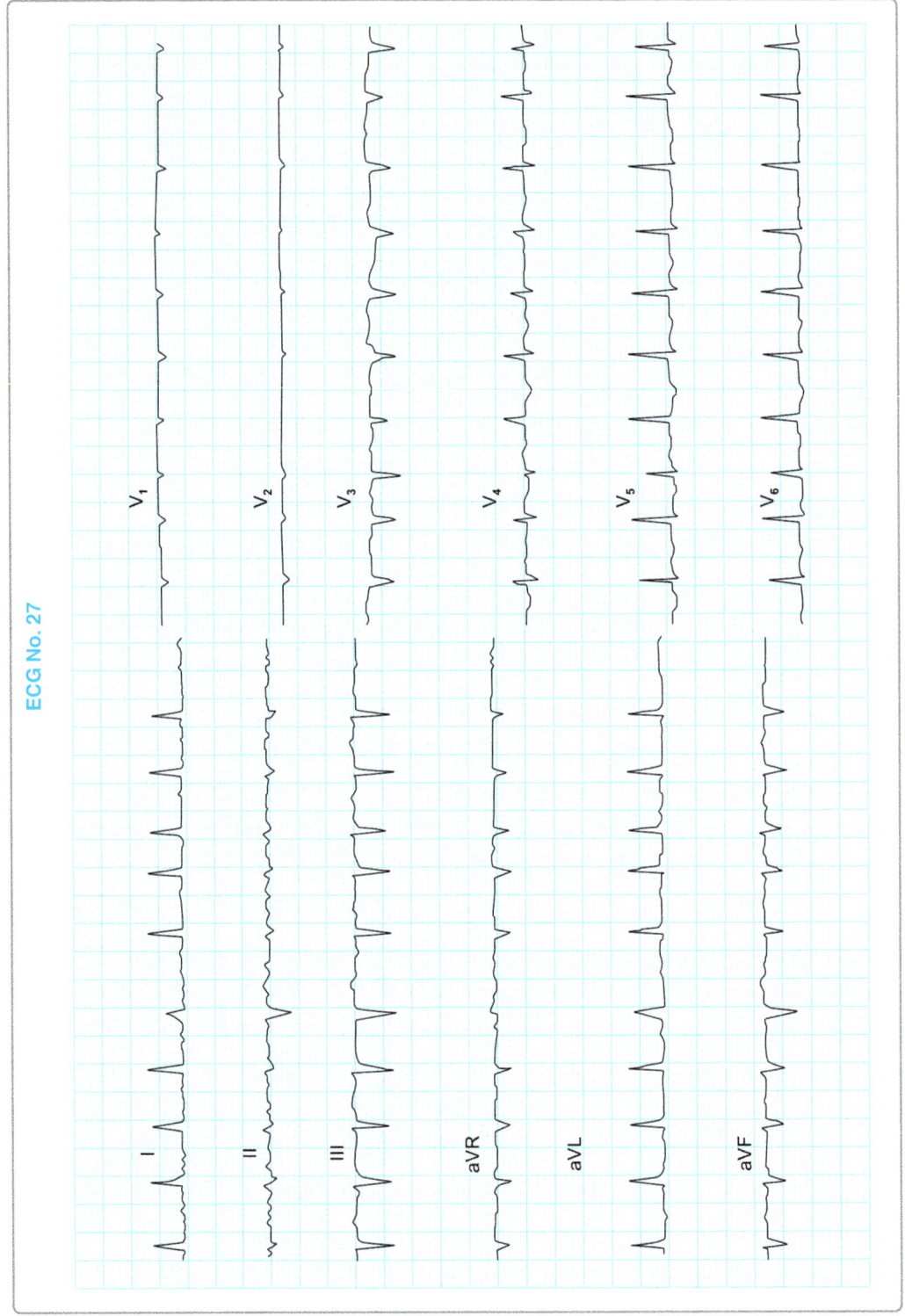

ECG No. 27

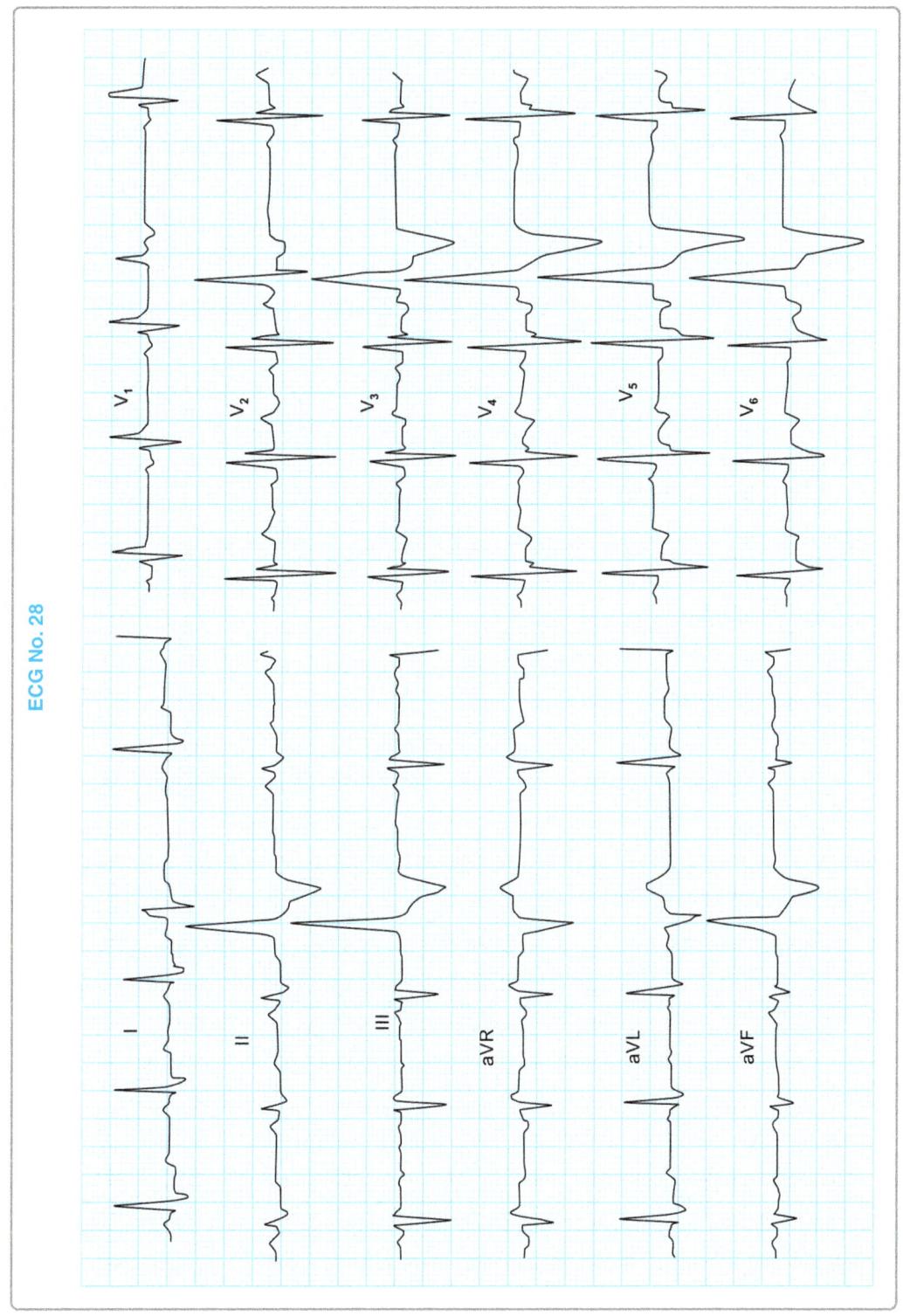

ECG in Medical Practice

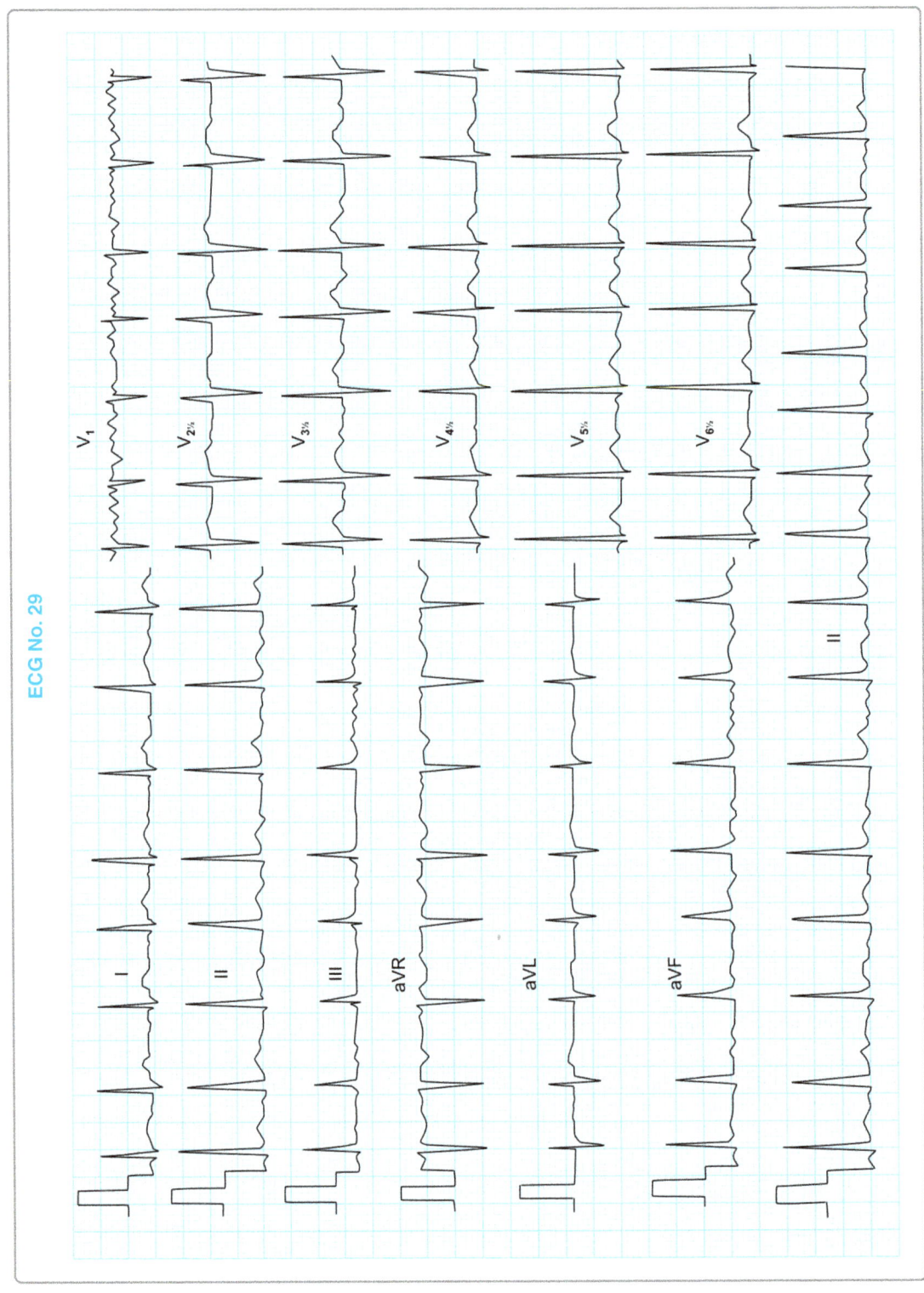

ECG No. 29

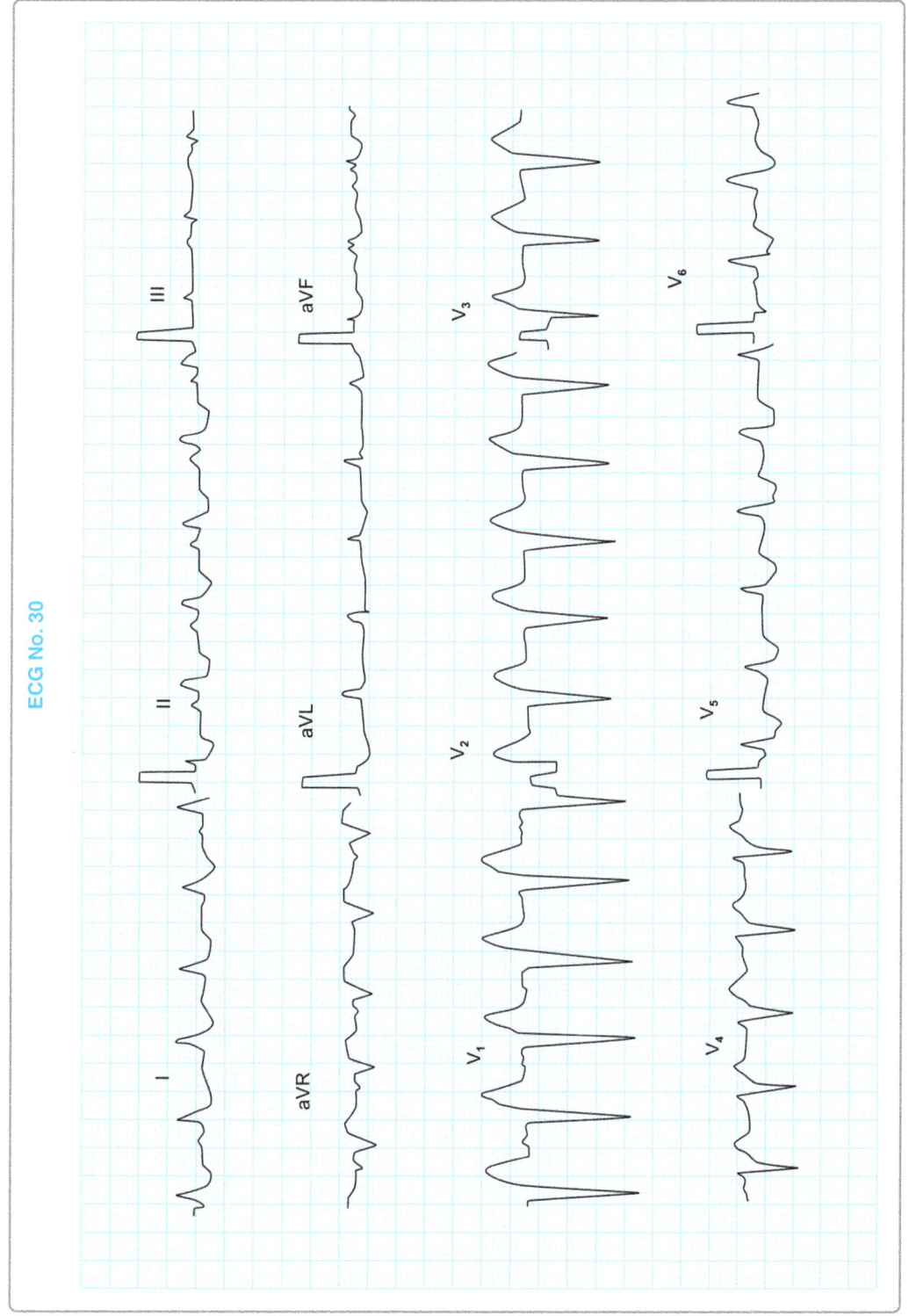

ECG No. 31

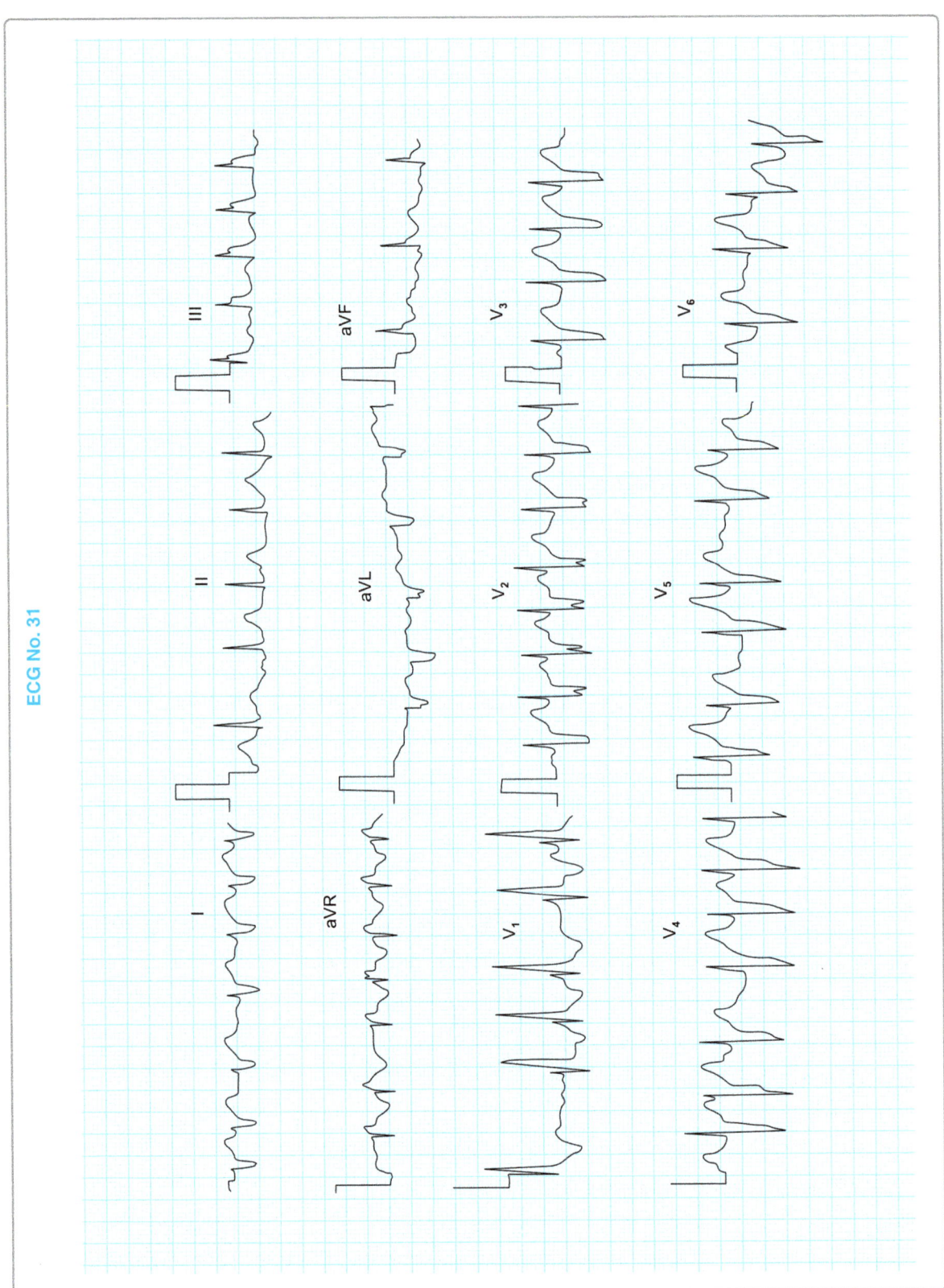

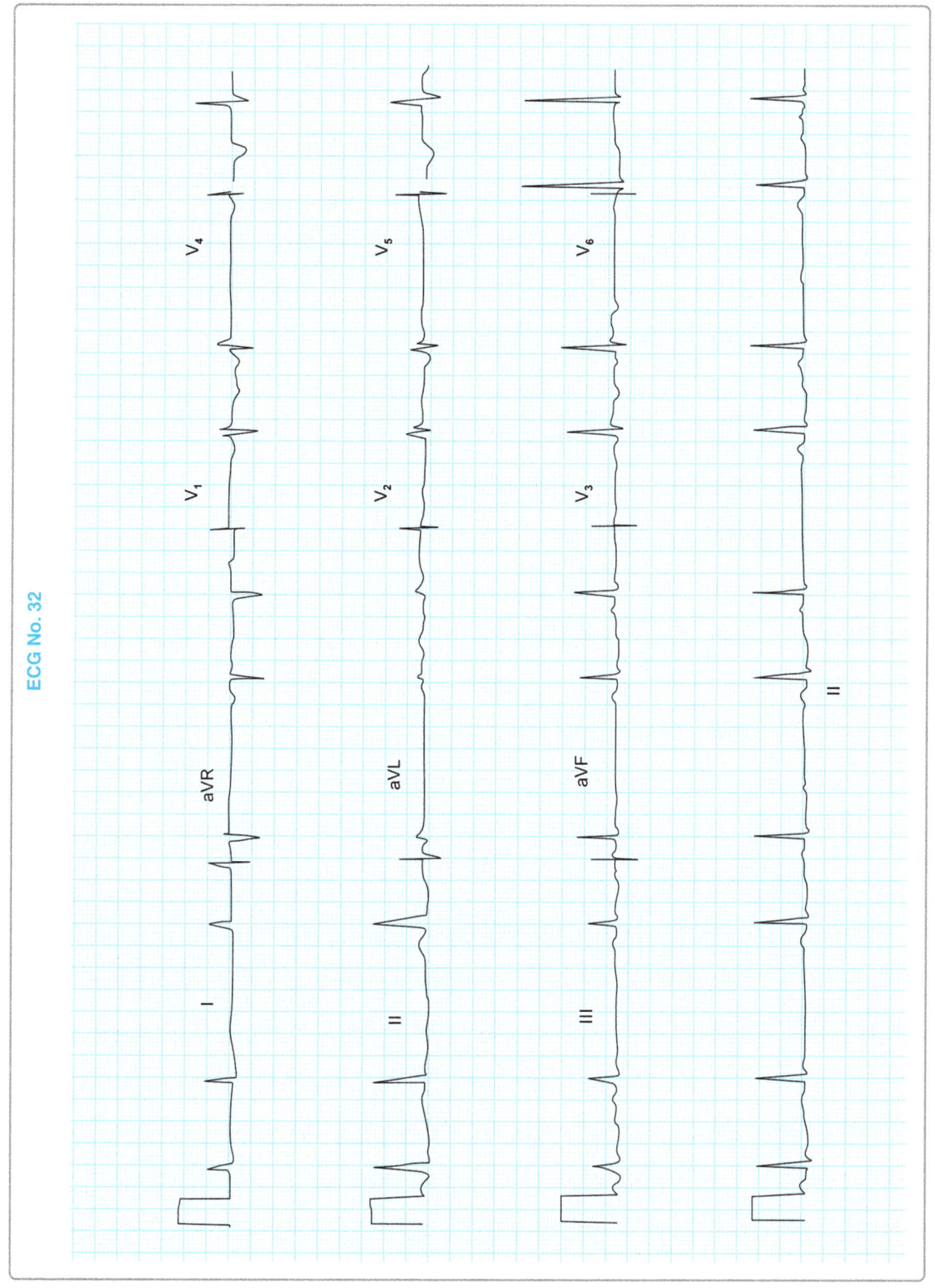

ECG No. 32

ECG in Medical Practice

ECG No. 33

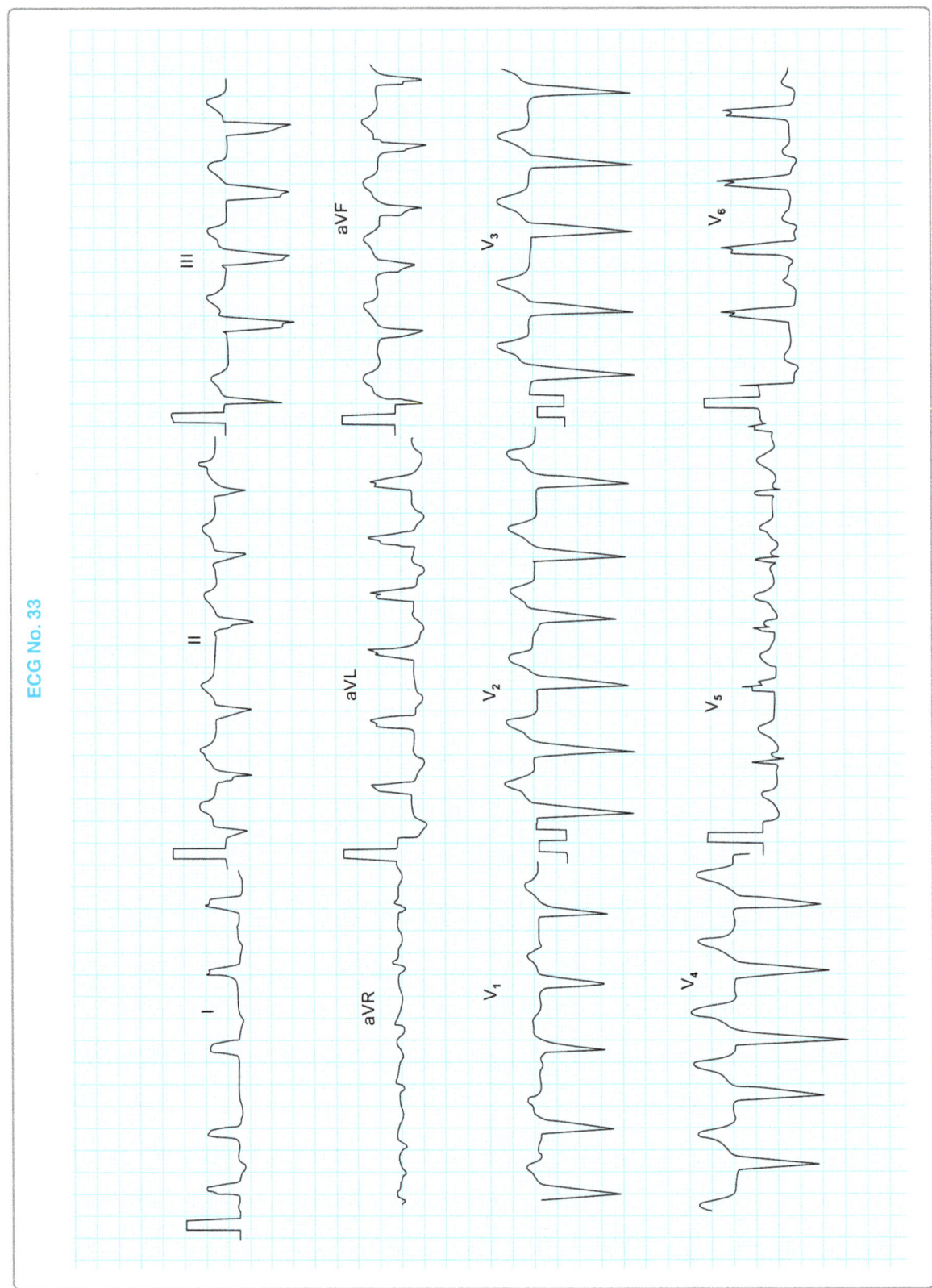

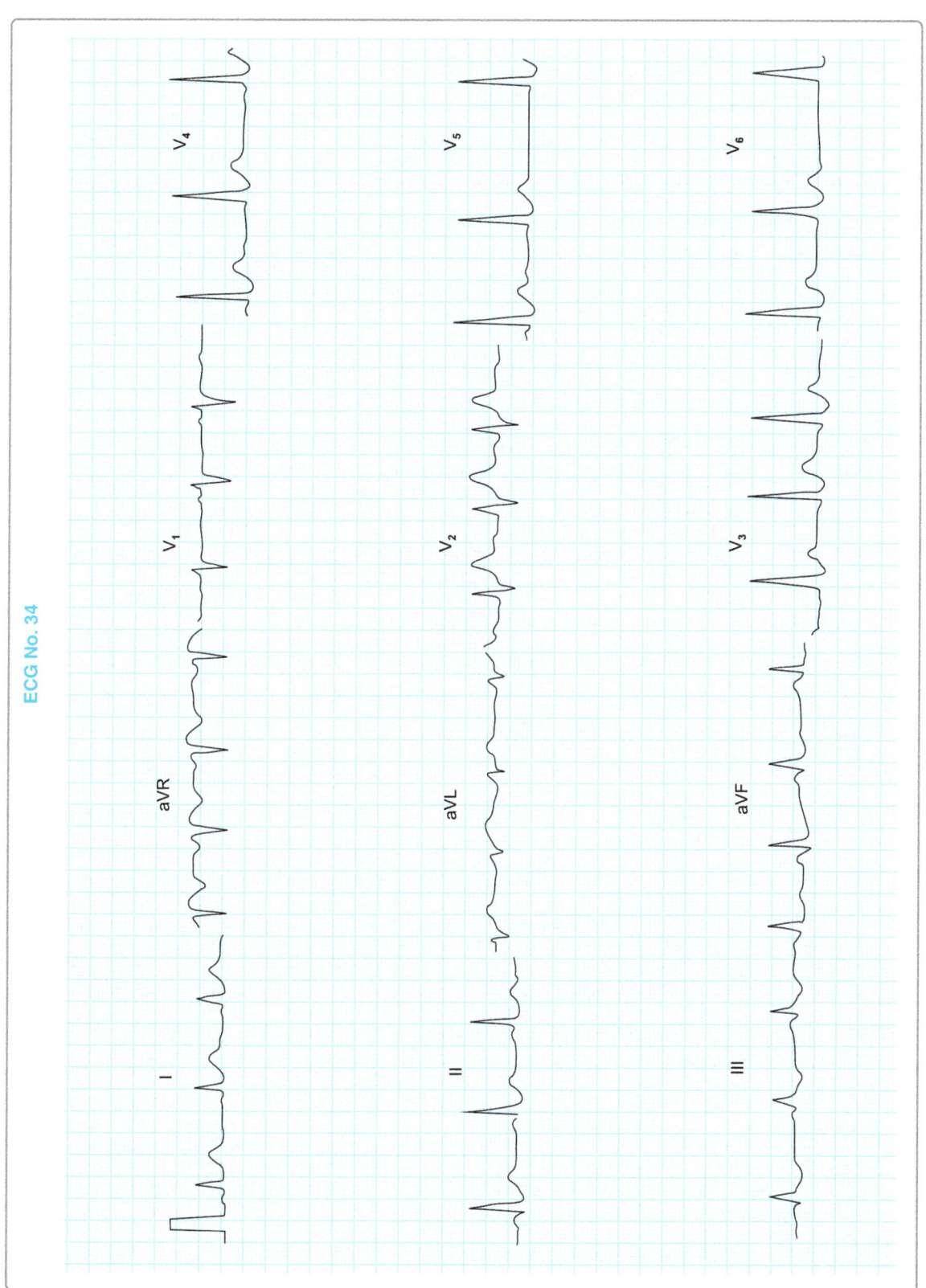

ECG No. 34

ECG in Medical Practice

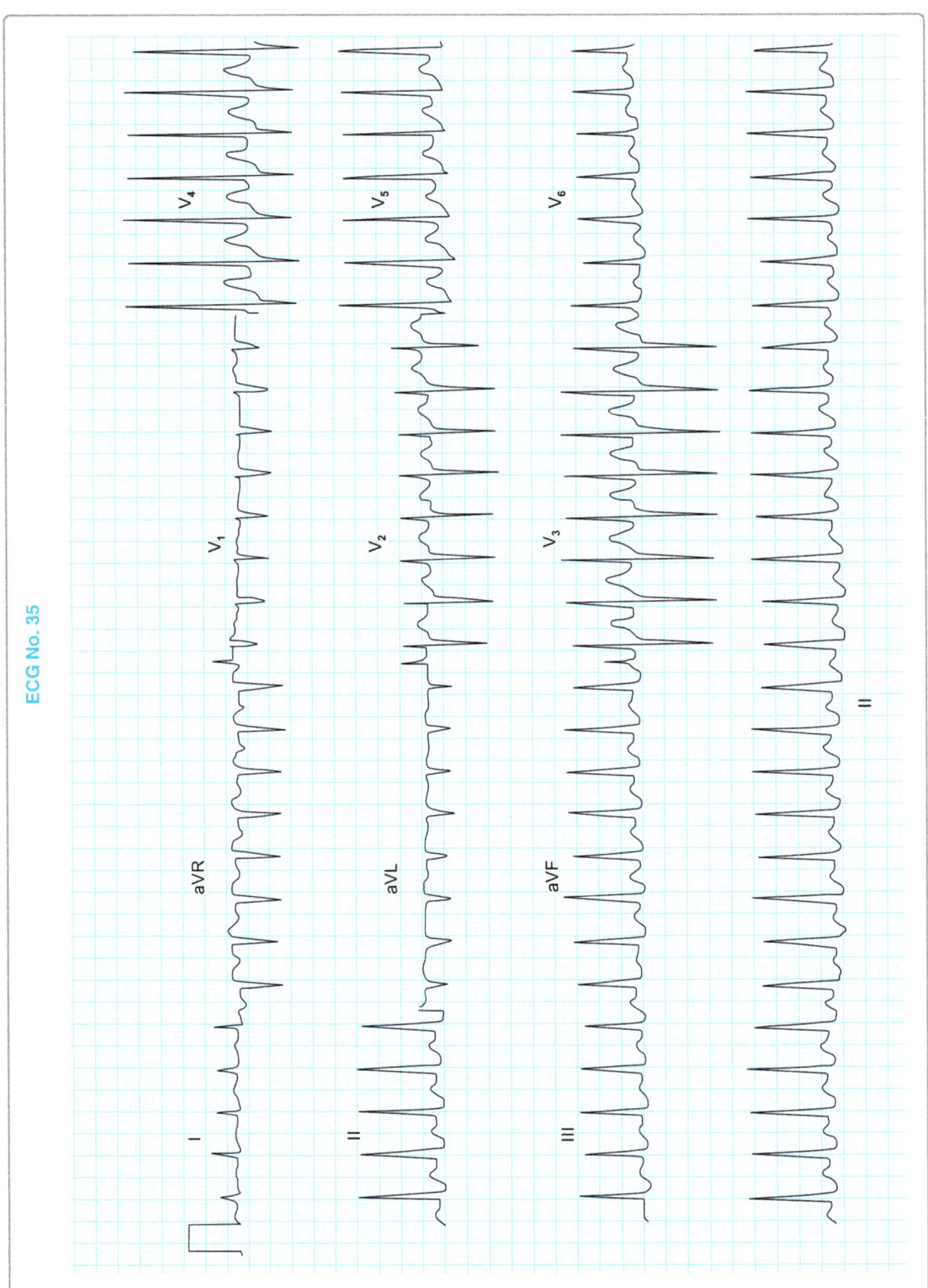

ECG No. 35

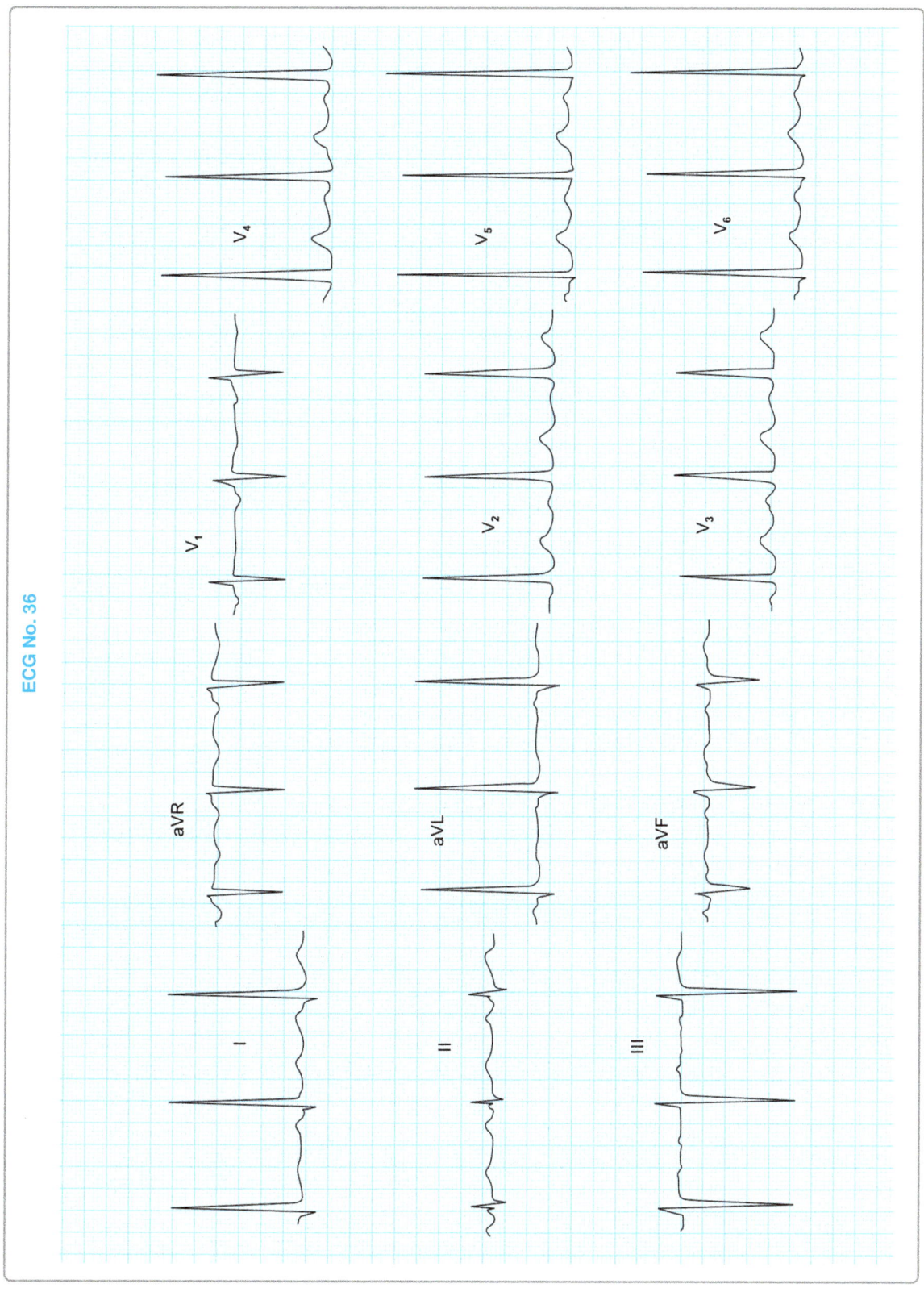

ECG No. 36

ECG in Medical Practice

ECG No. 37

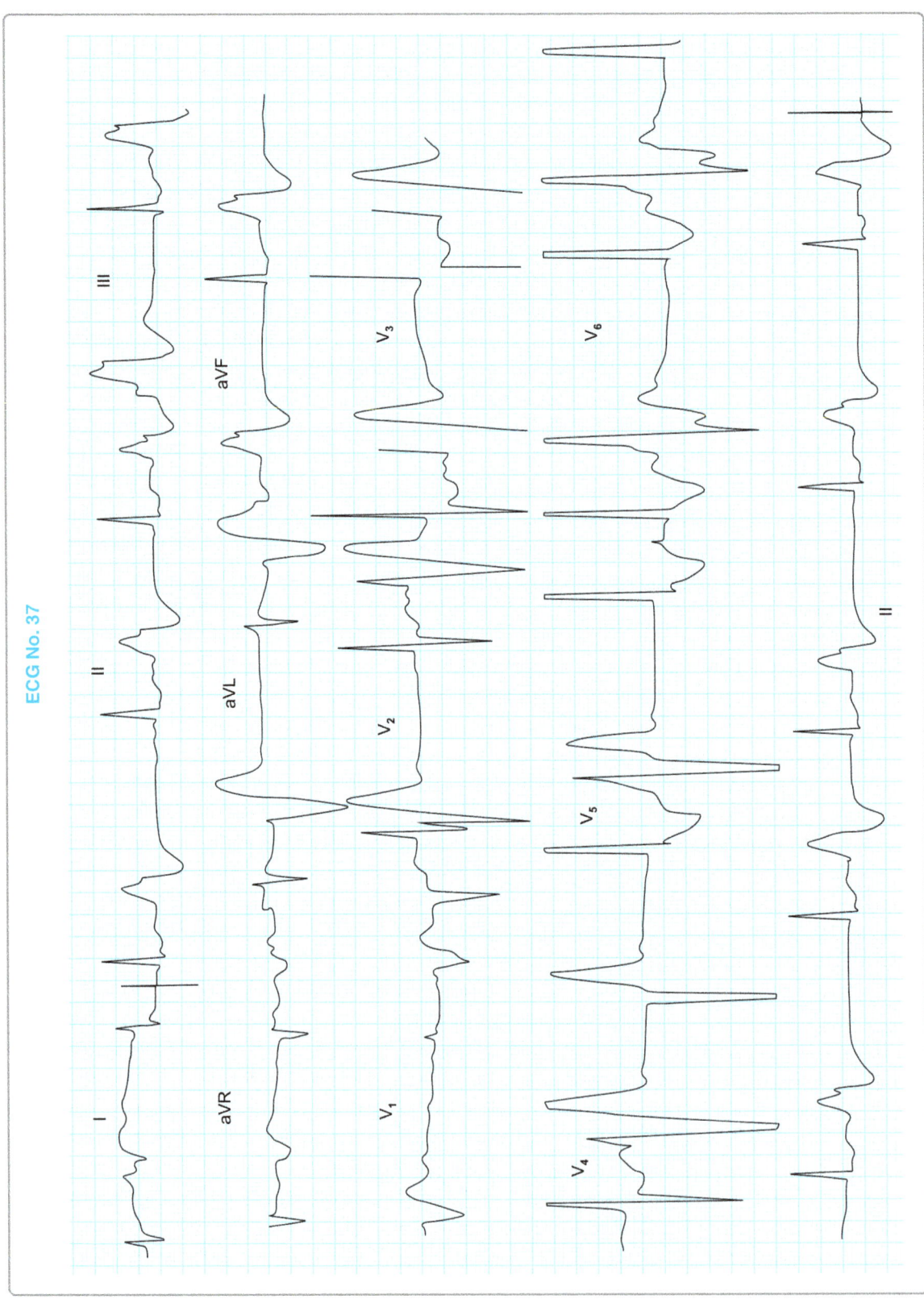

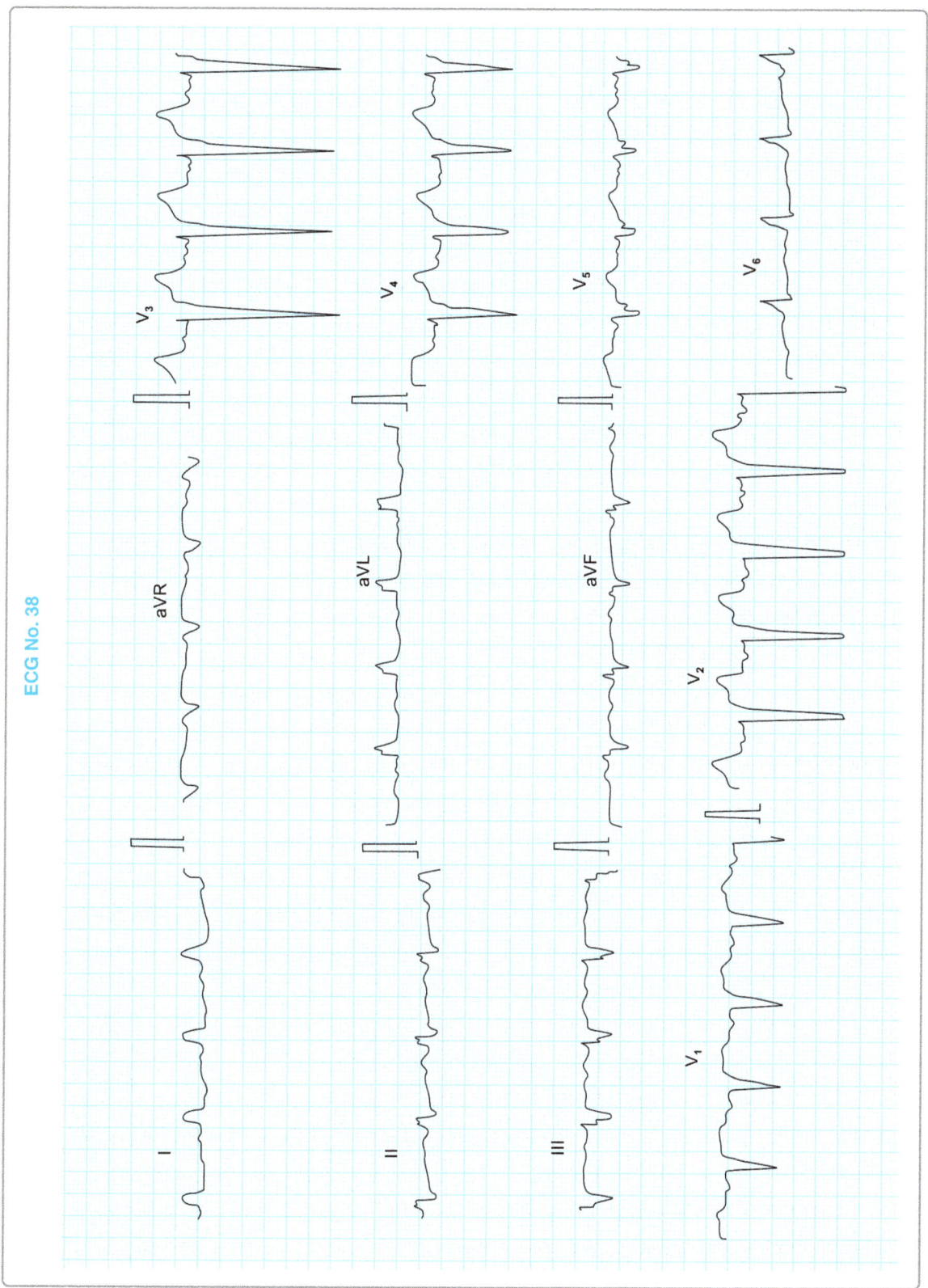

ECG No. 38

ECG in Medical Practice

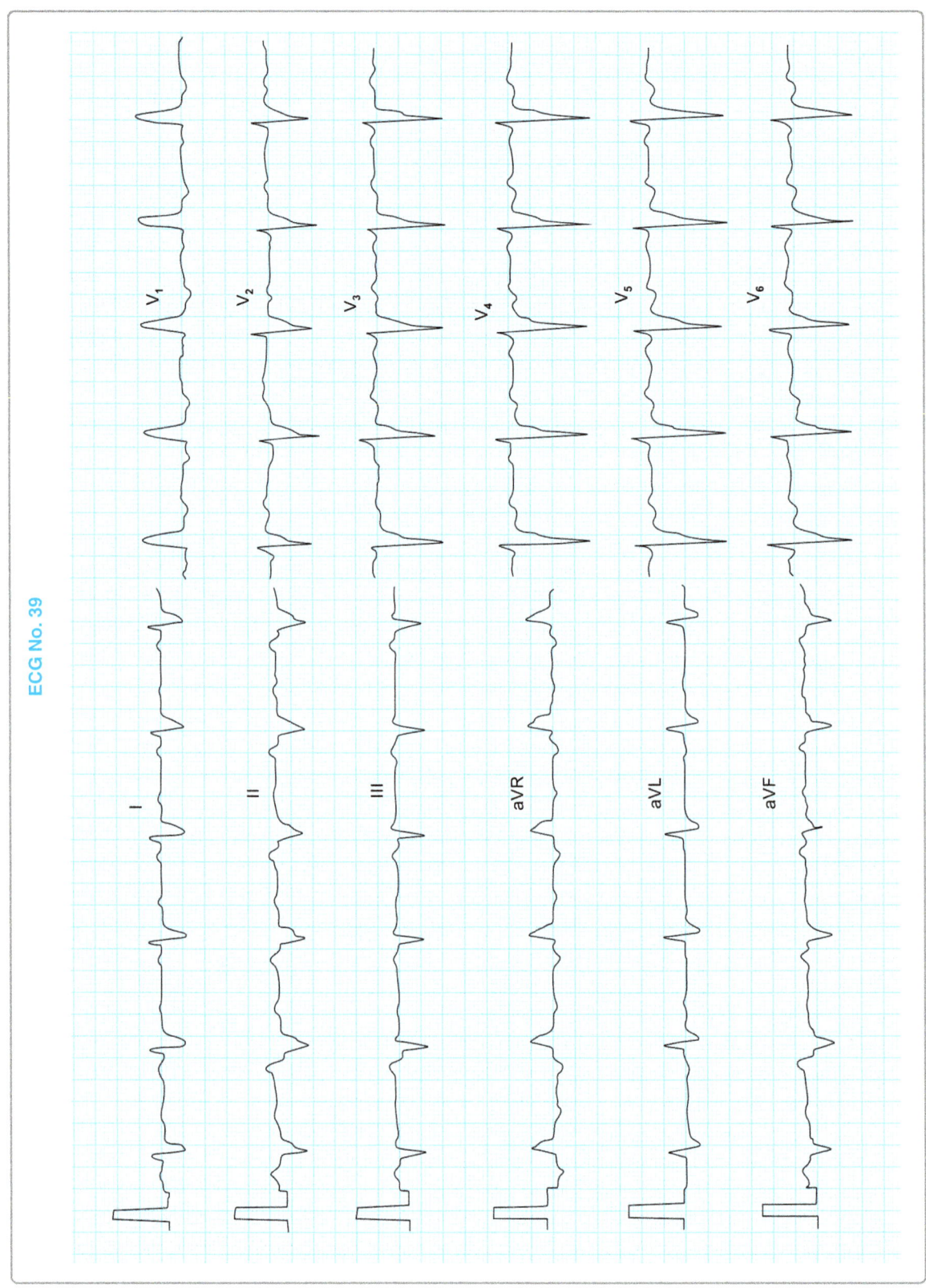

ECG No. 39

Chapter 3: 151 Tracings of ECG

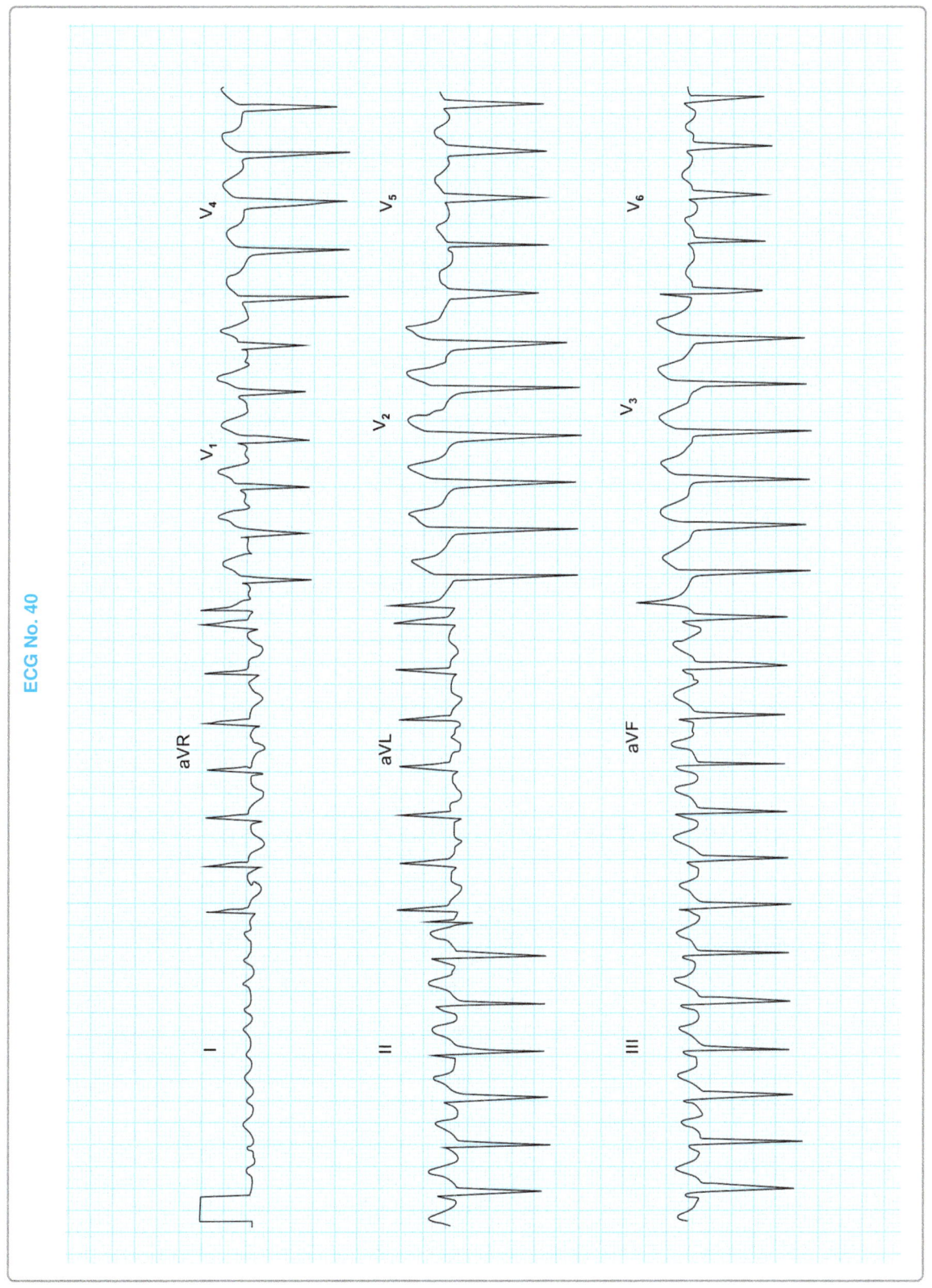

ECG No. 40

ECG in Medical Practice

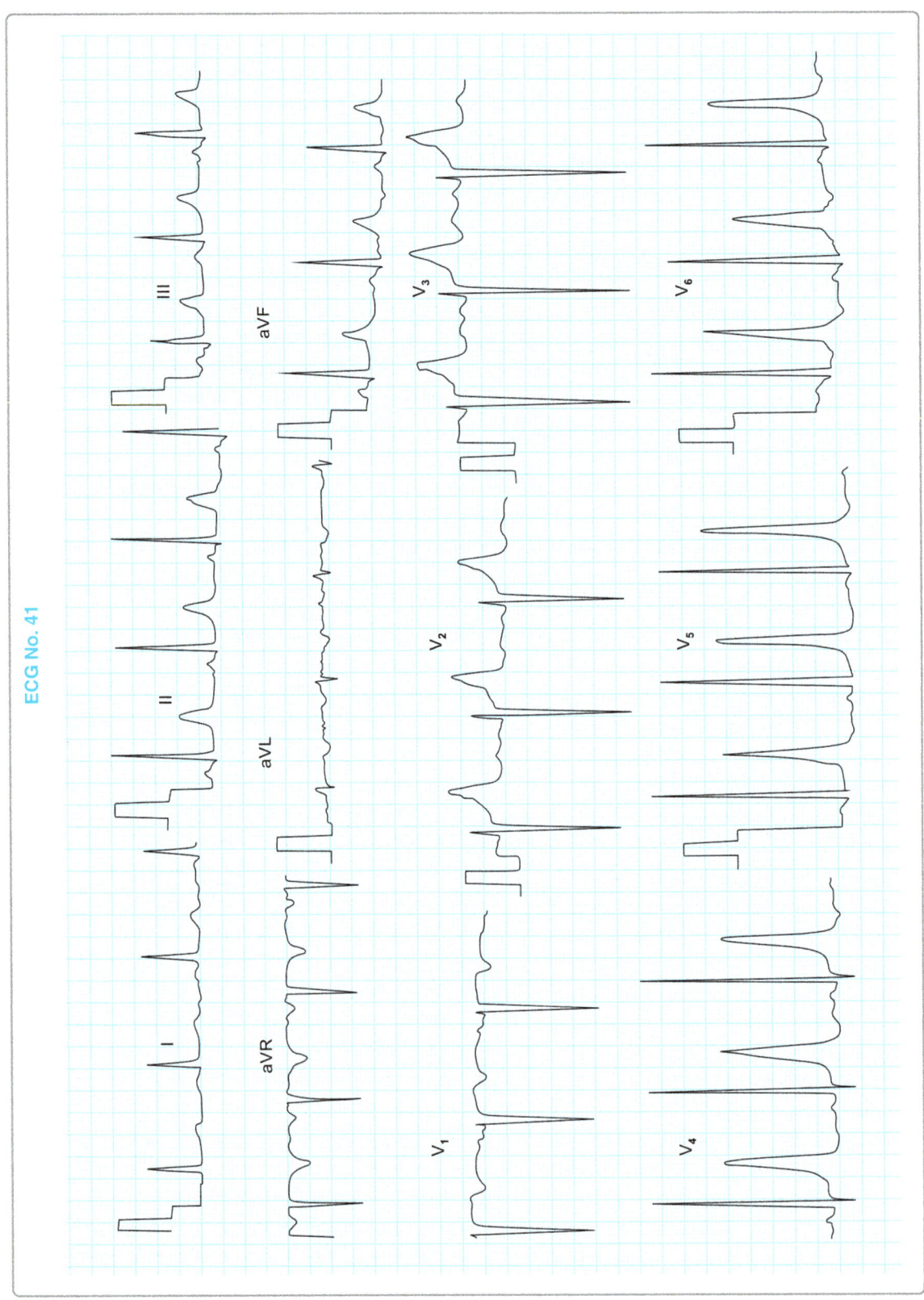

ECG No. 41

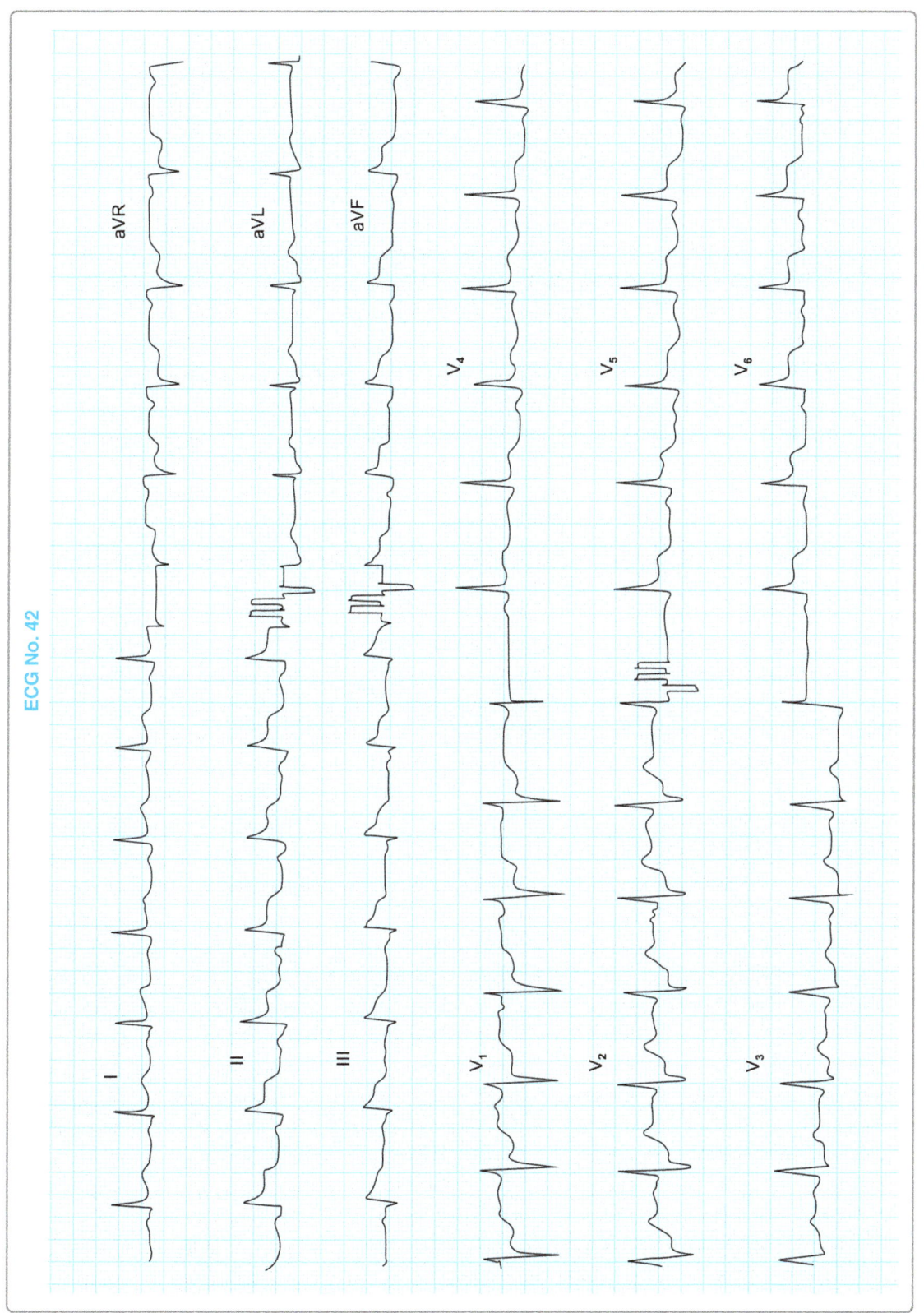

ECG in Medical Practice

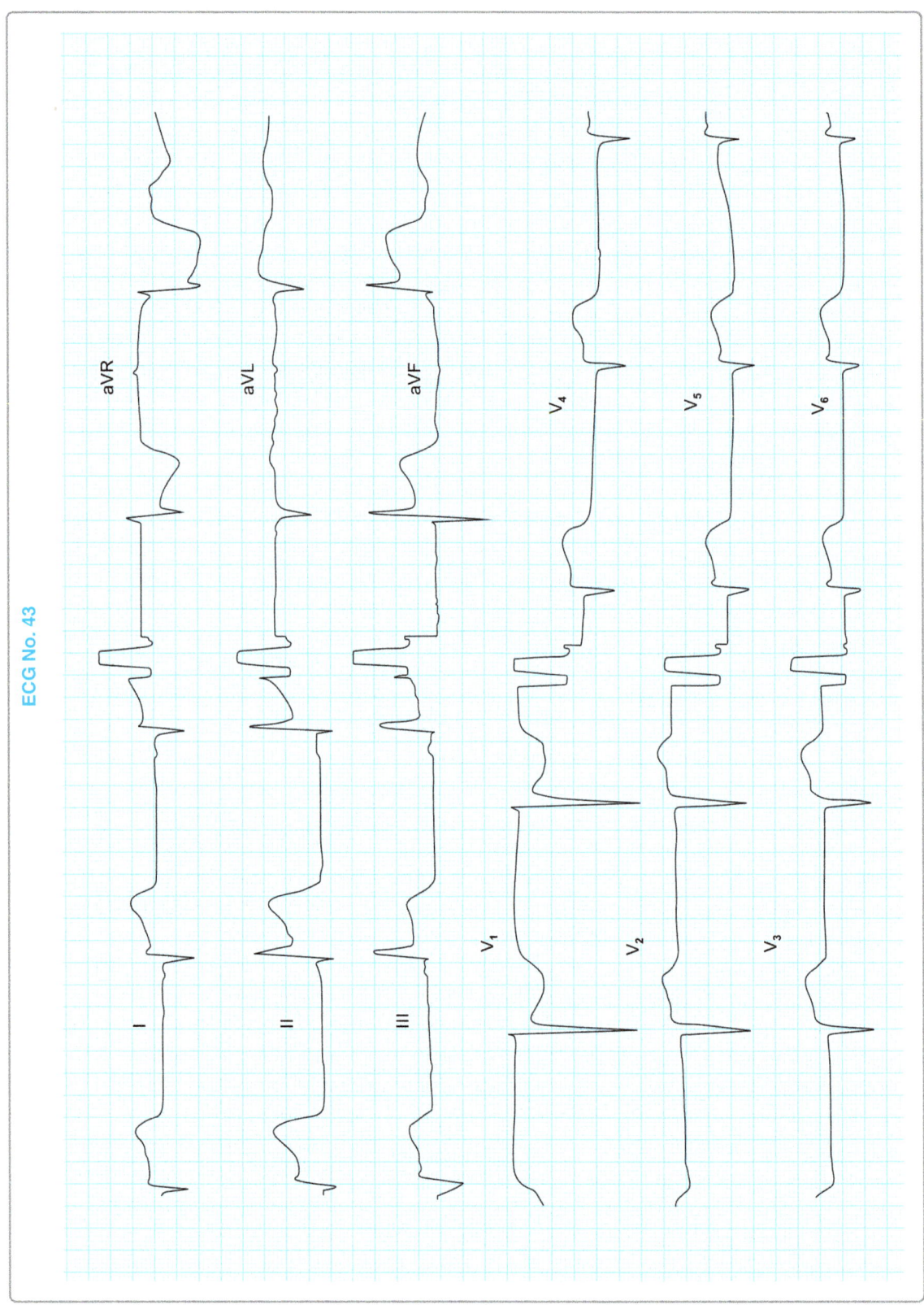

ECG No. 43

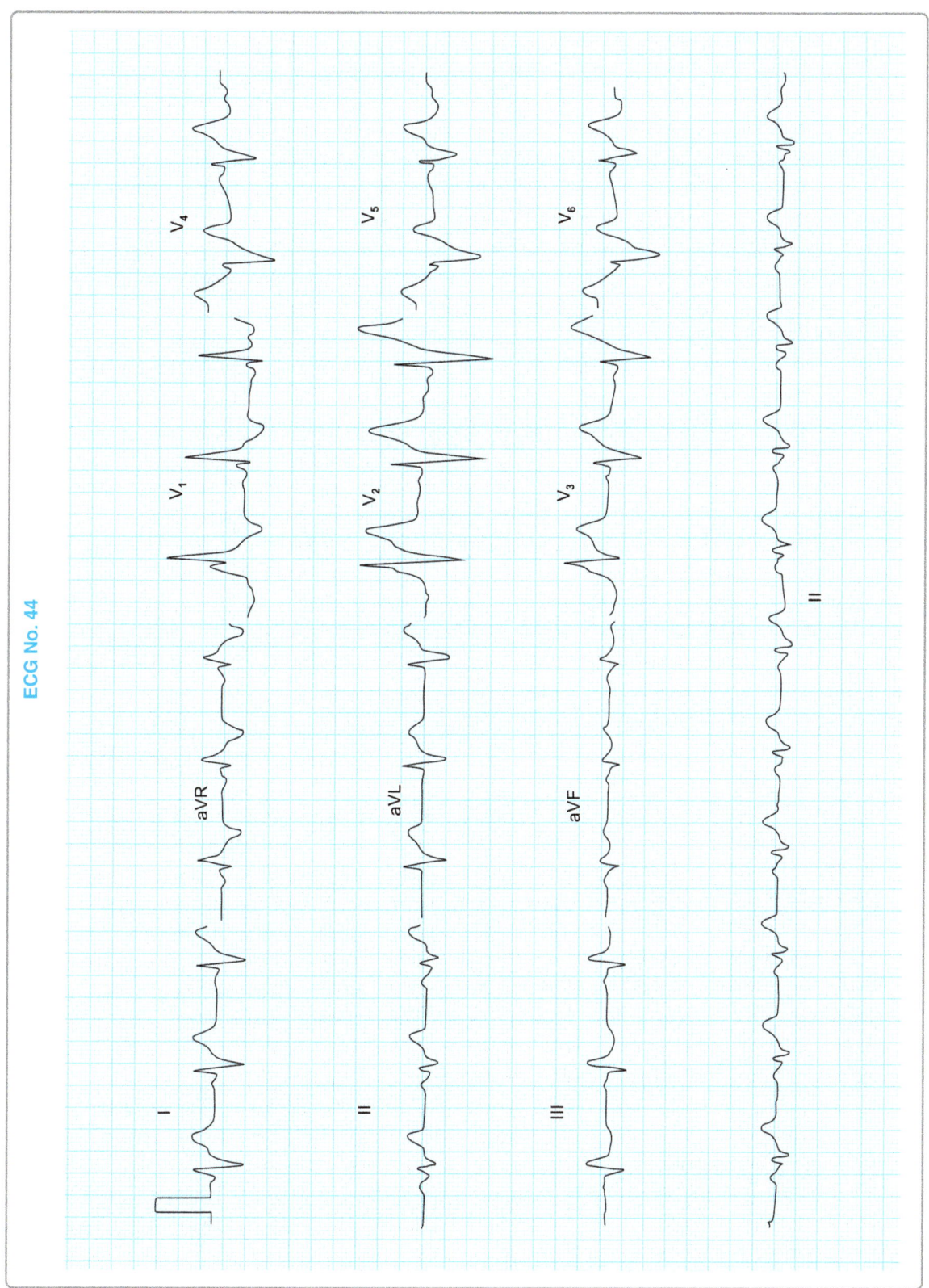

ECG in Medical Practice

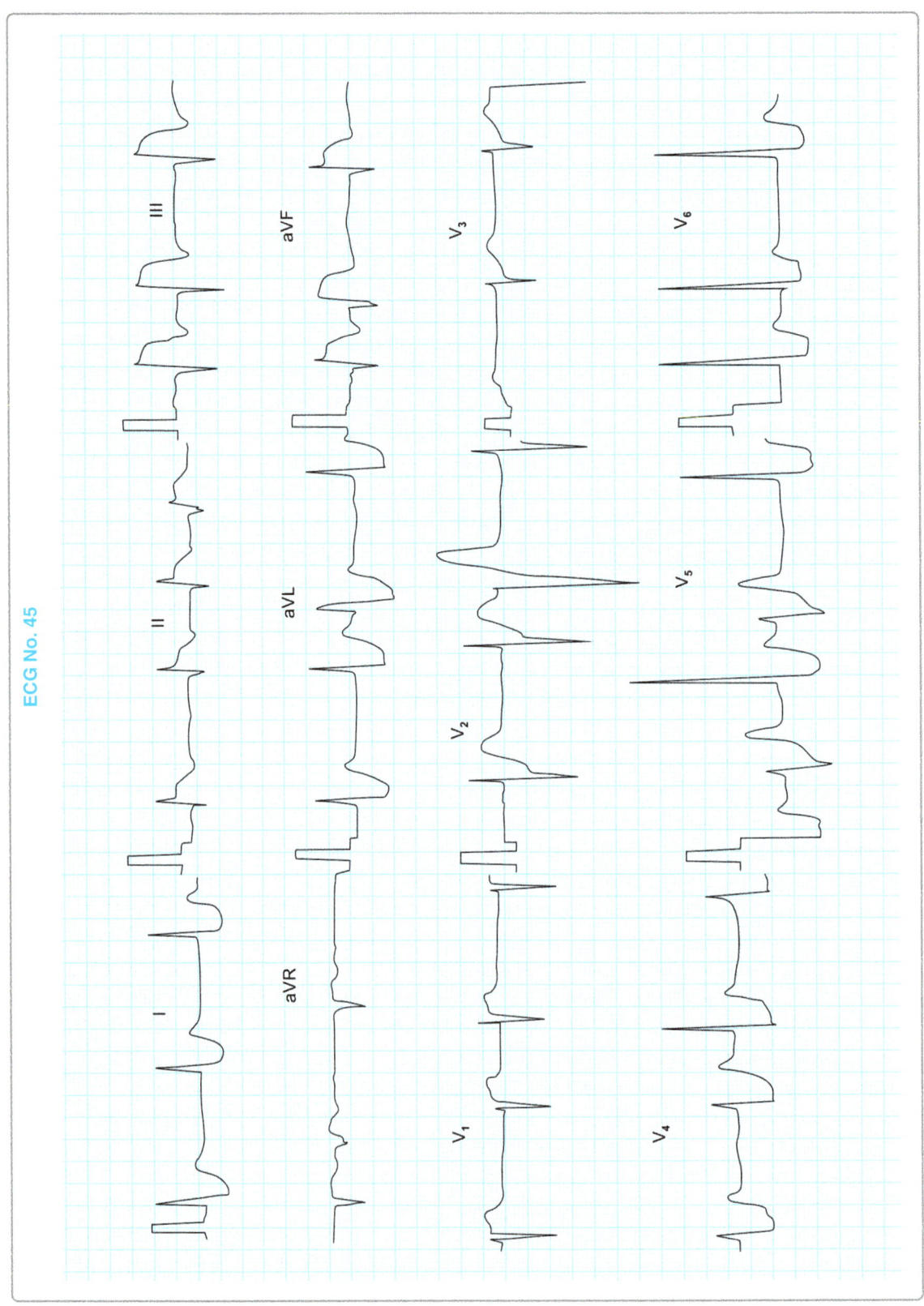

ECG No. 45

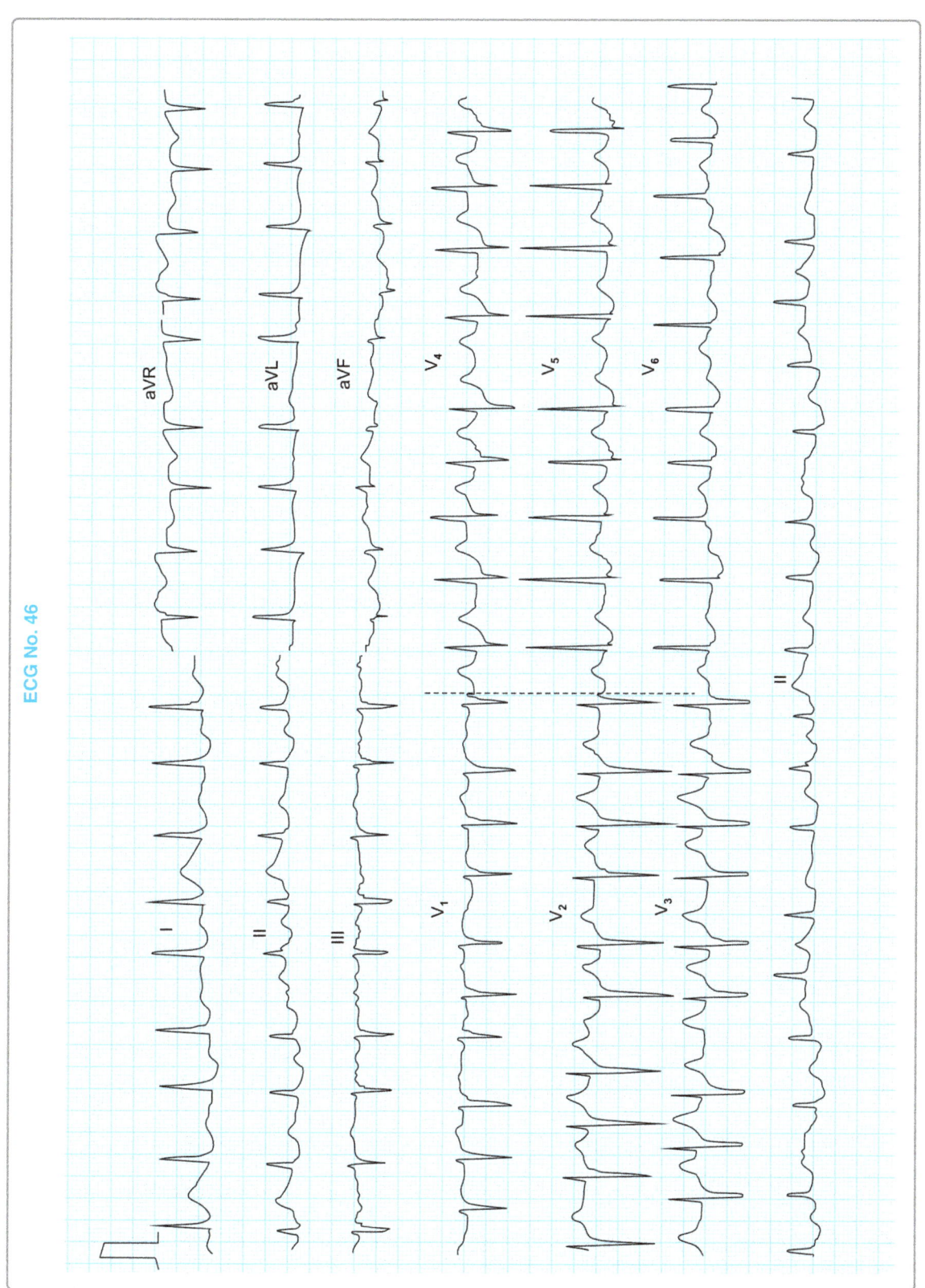

ECG No. 46

ECG in Medical Practice

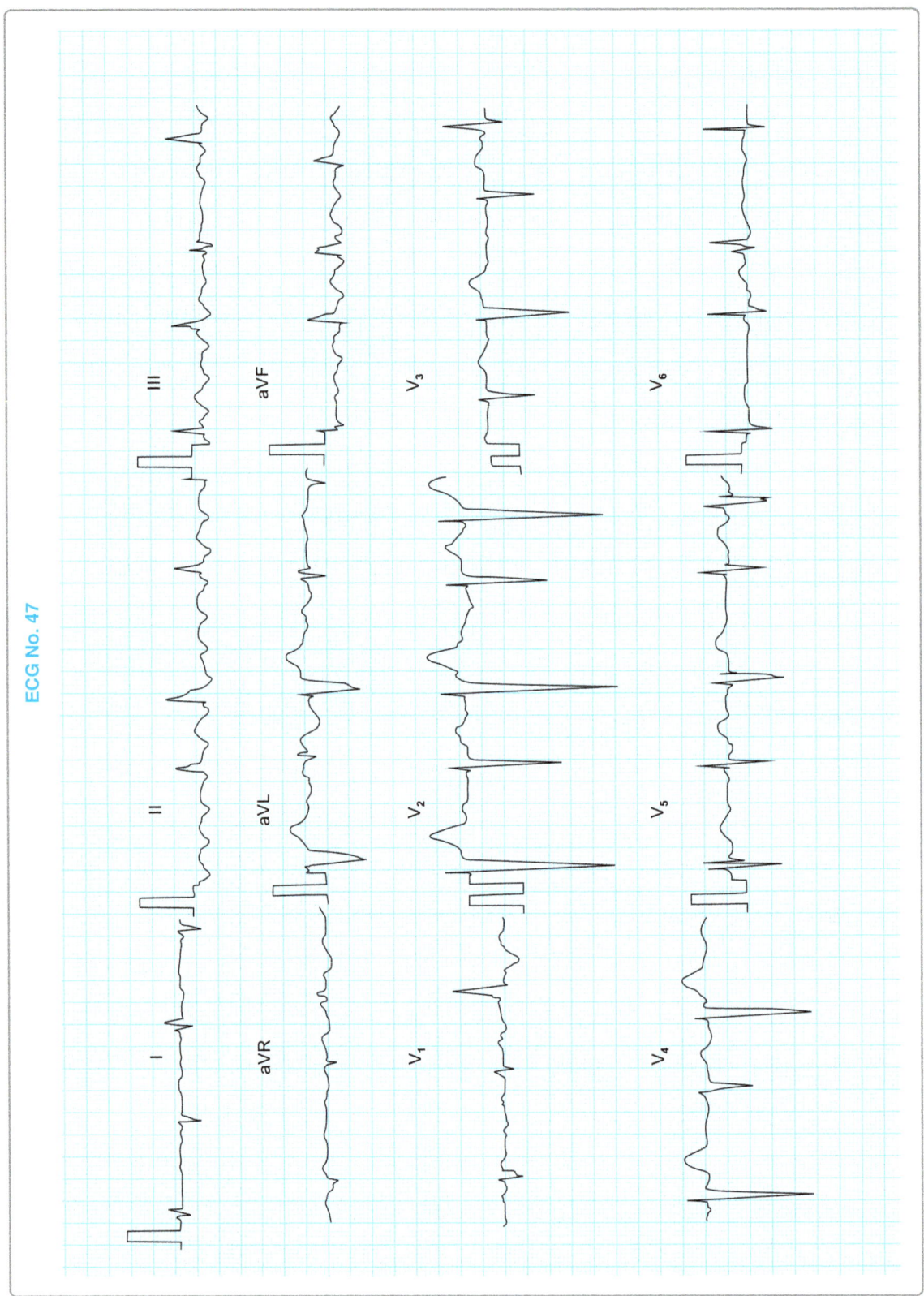

ECG No. 47

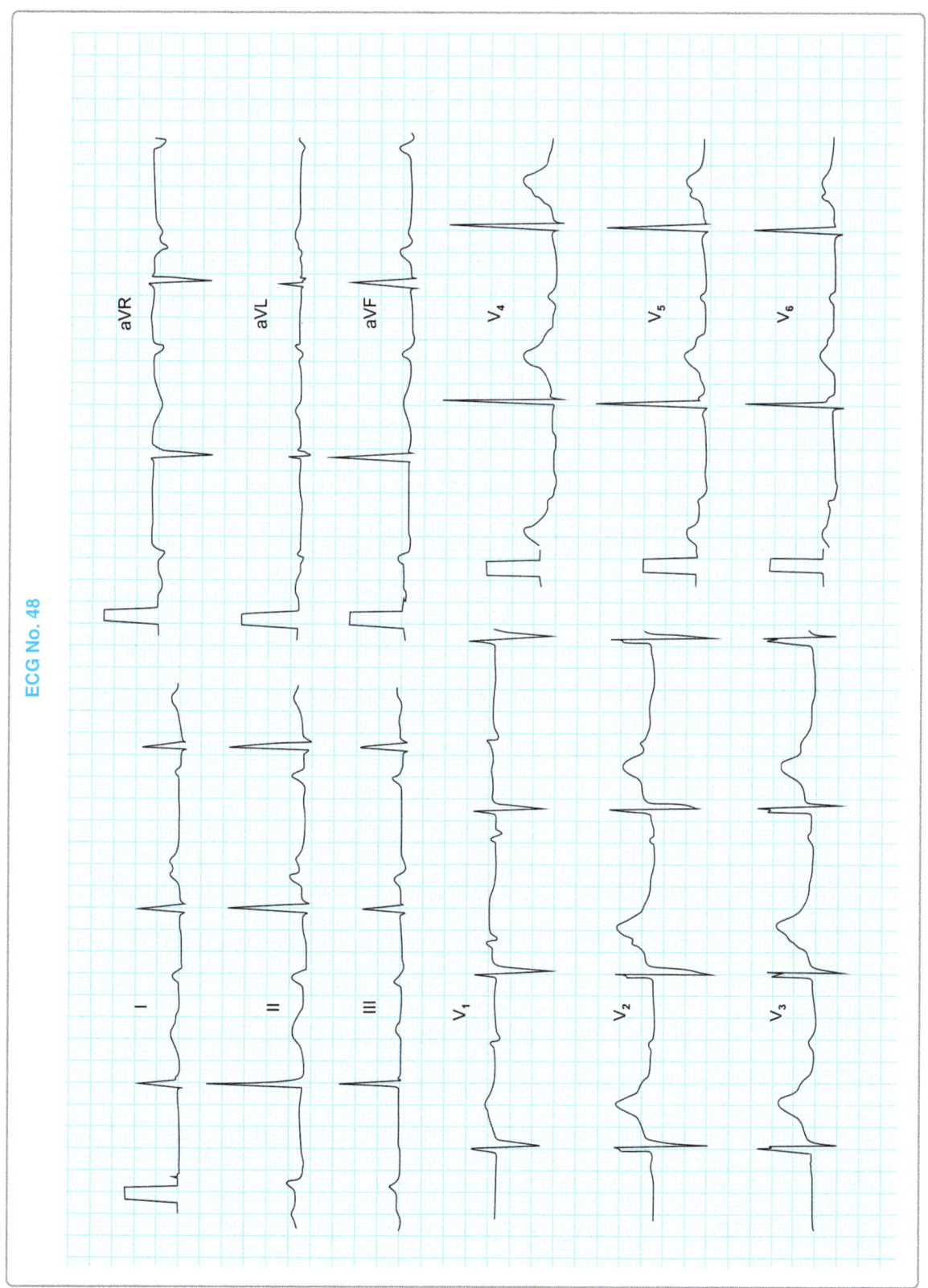

ECG No. 48

ECG in Medical Practice

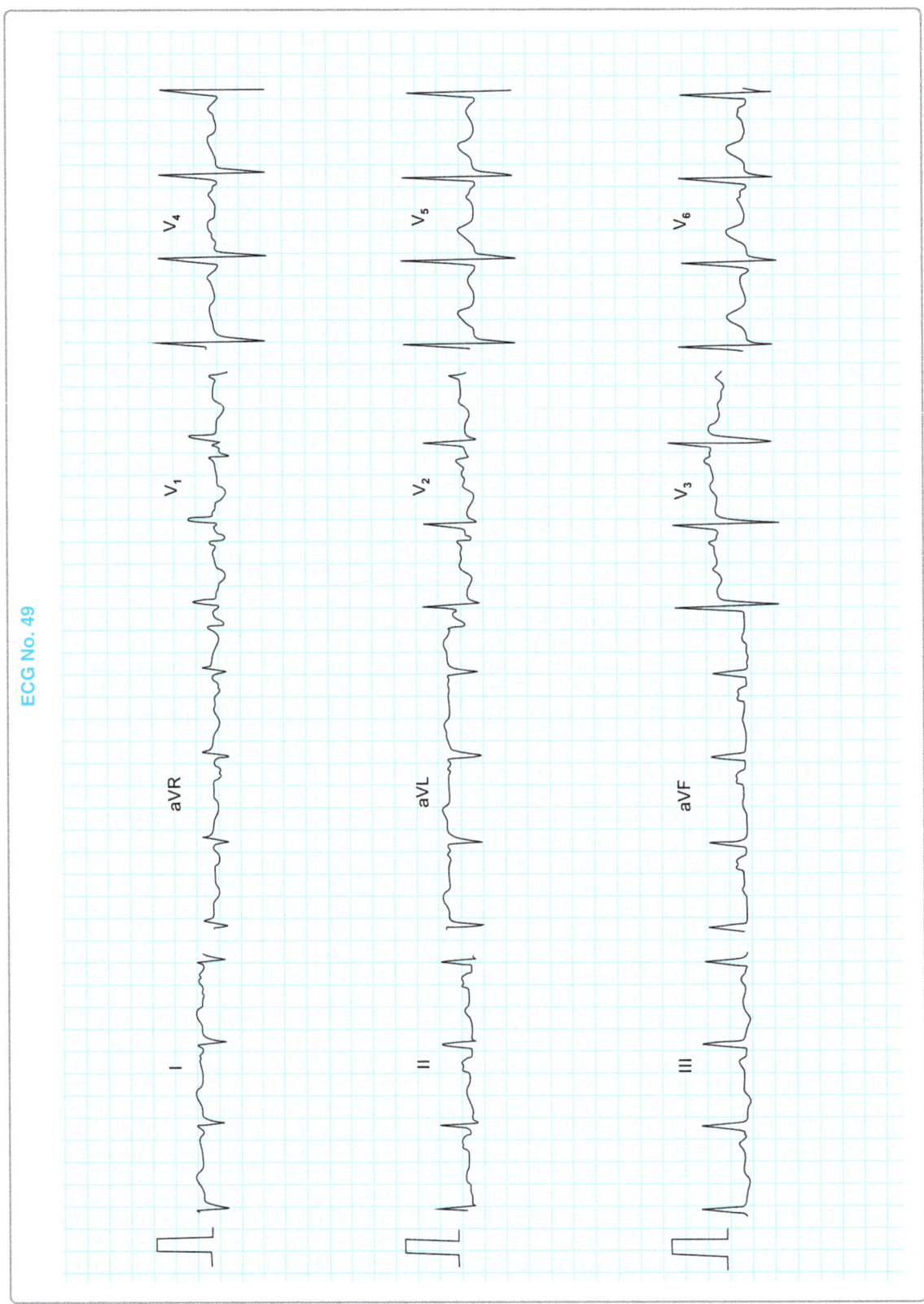

ECG No. 49

224

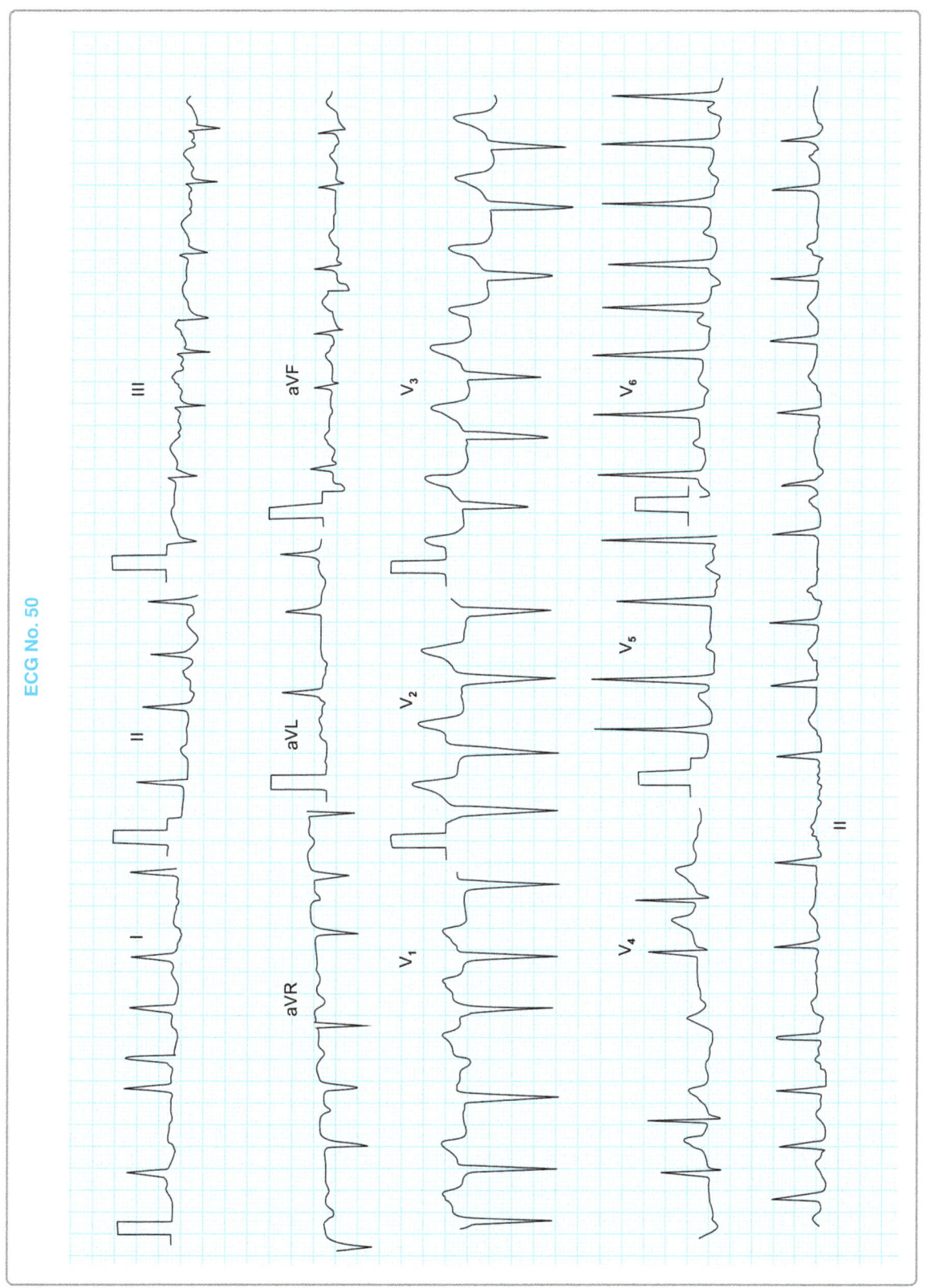

ECG in Medical Practice

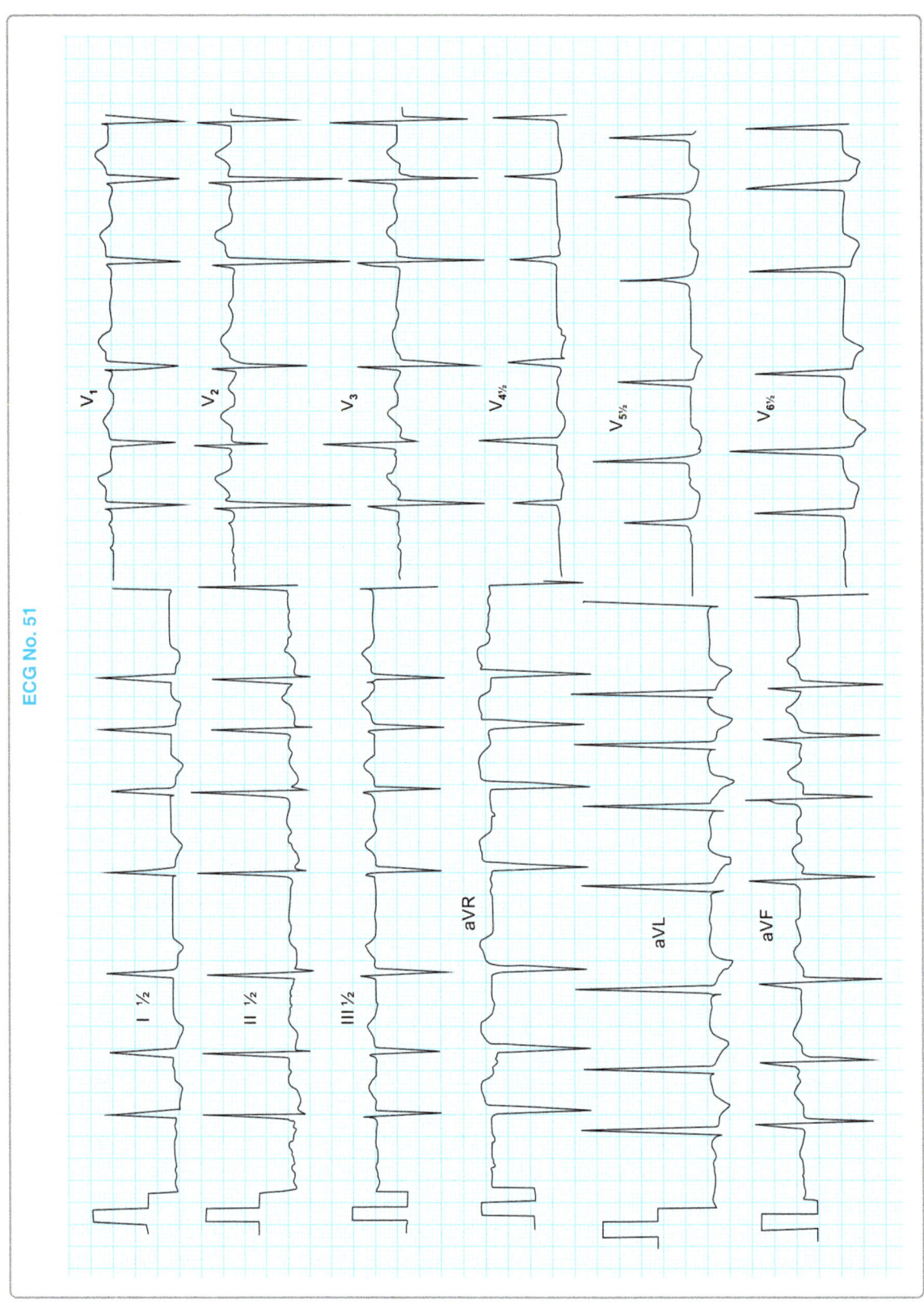

ECG No. 51

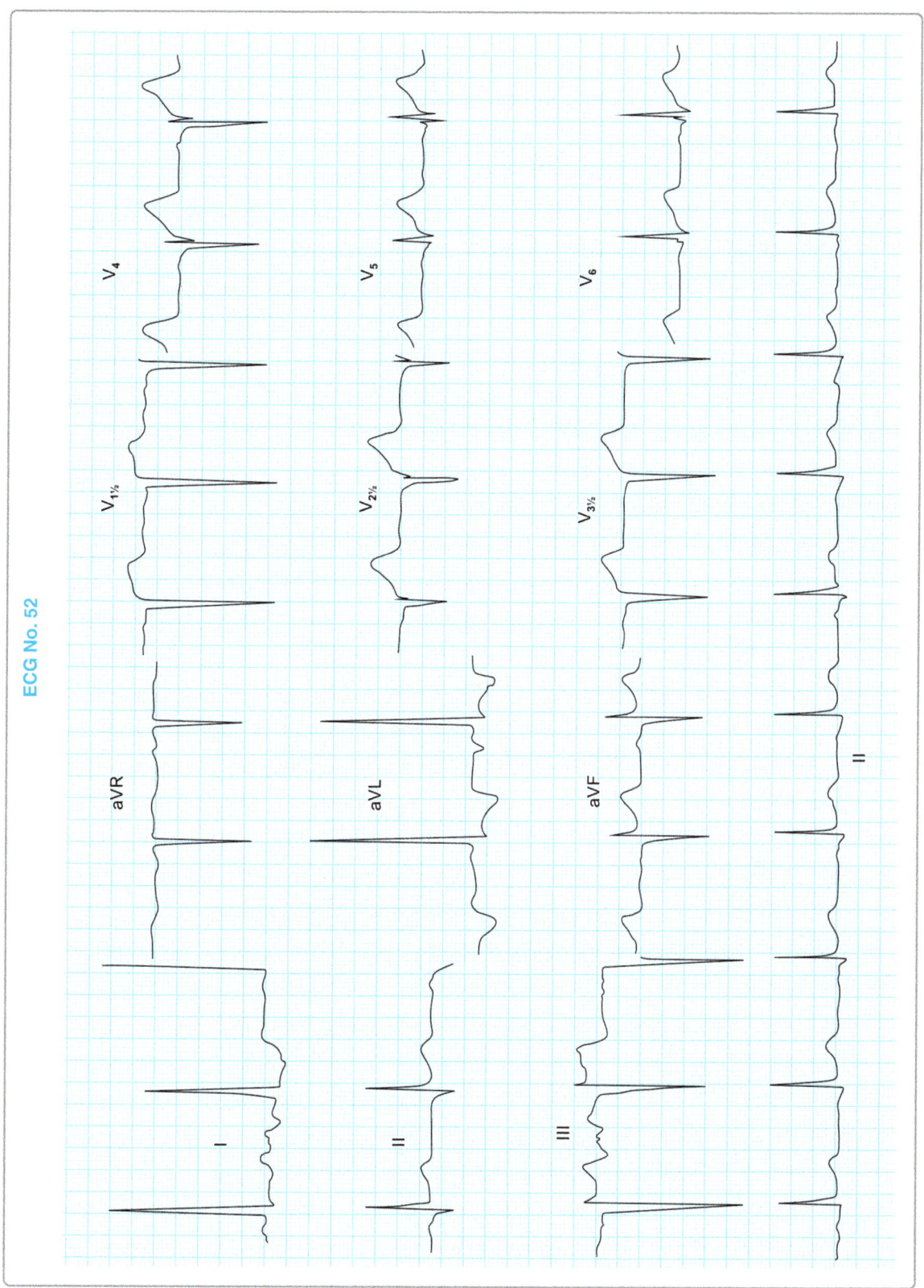

ECG in Medical Practice

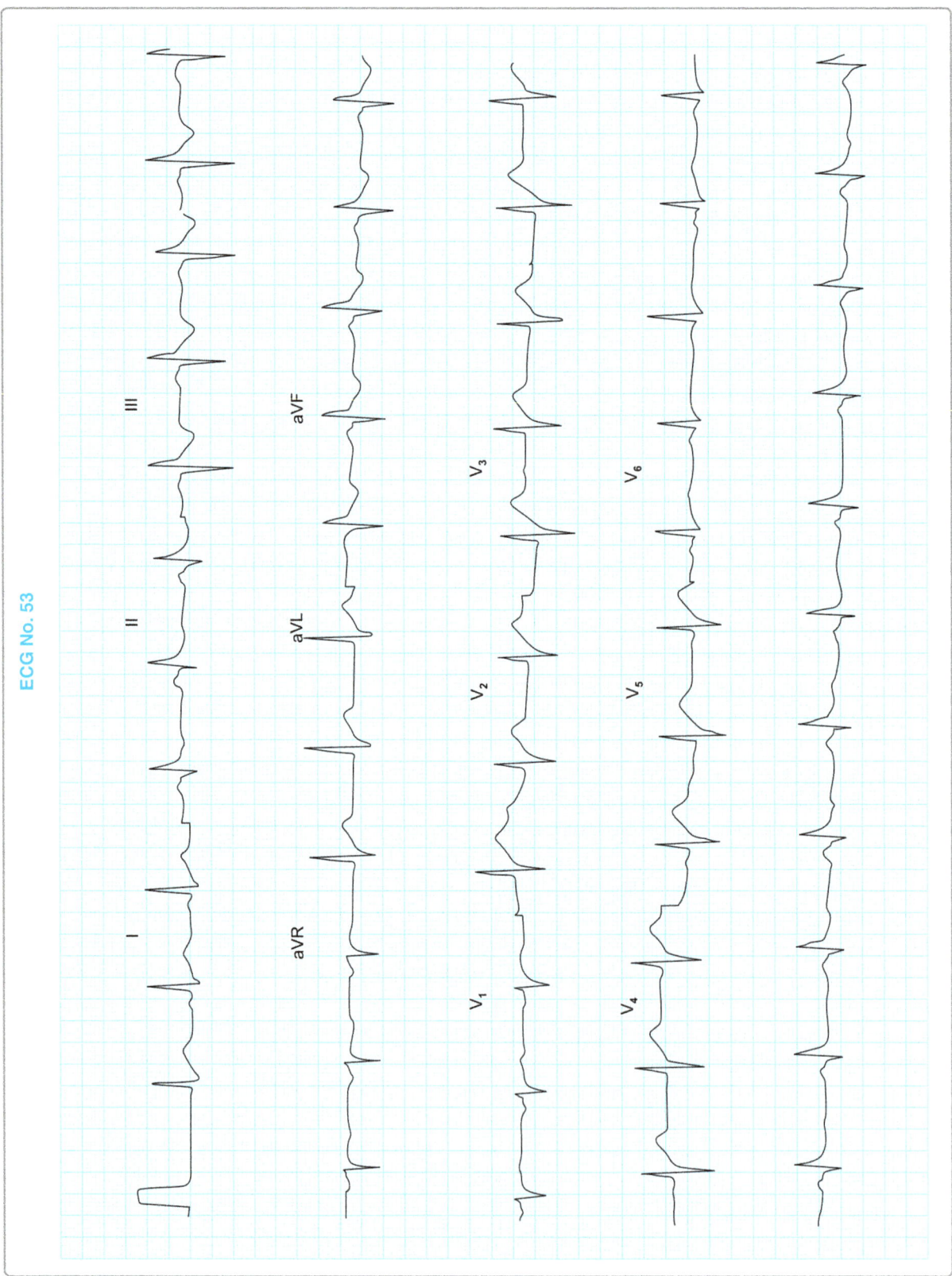

ECG No. 53

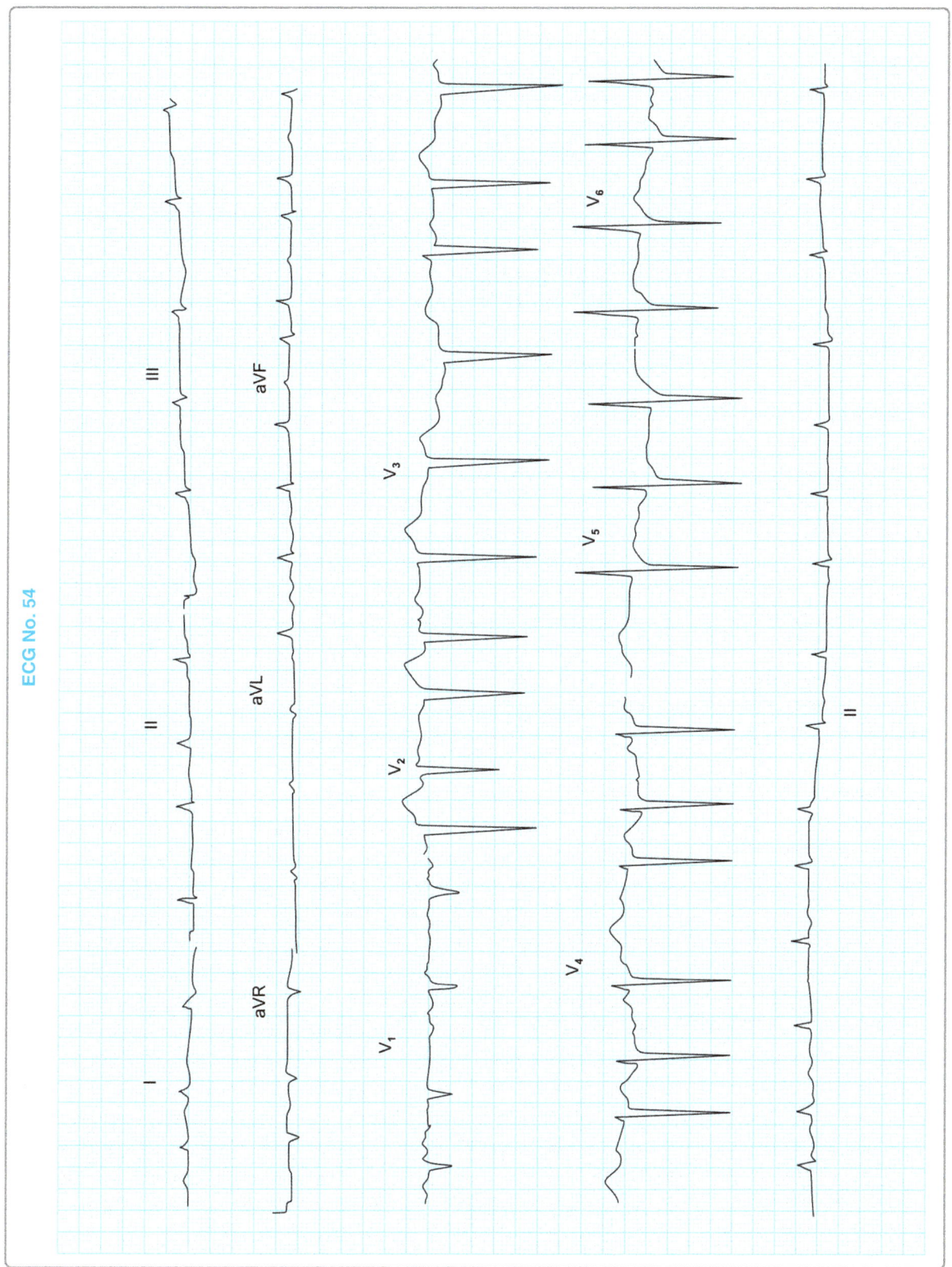

ECG No. 54

ECG in Medical Practice

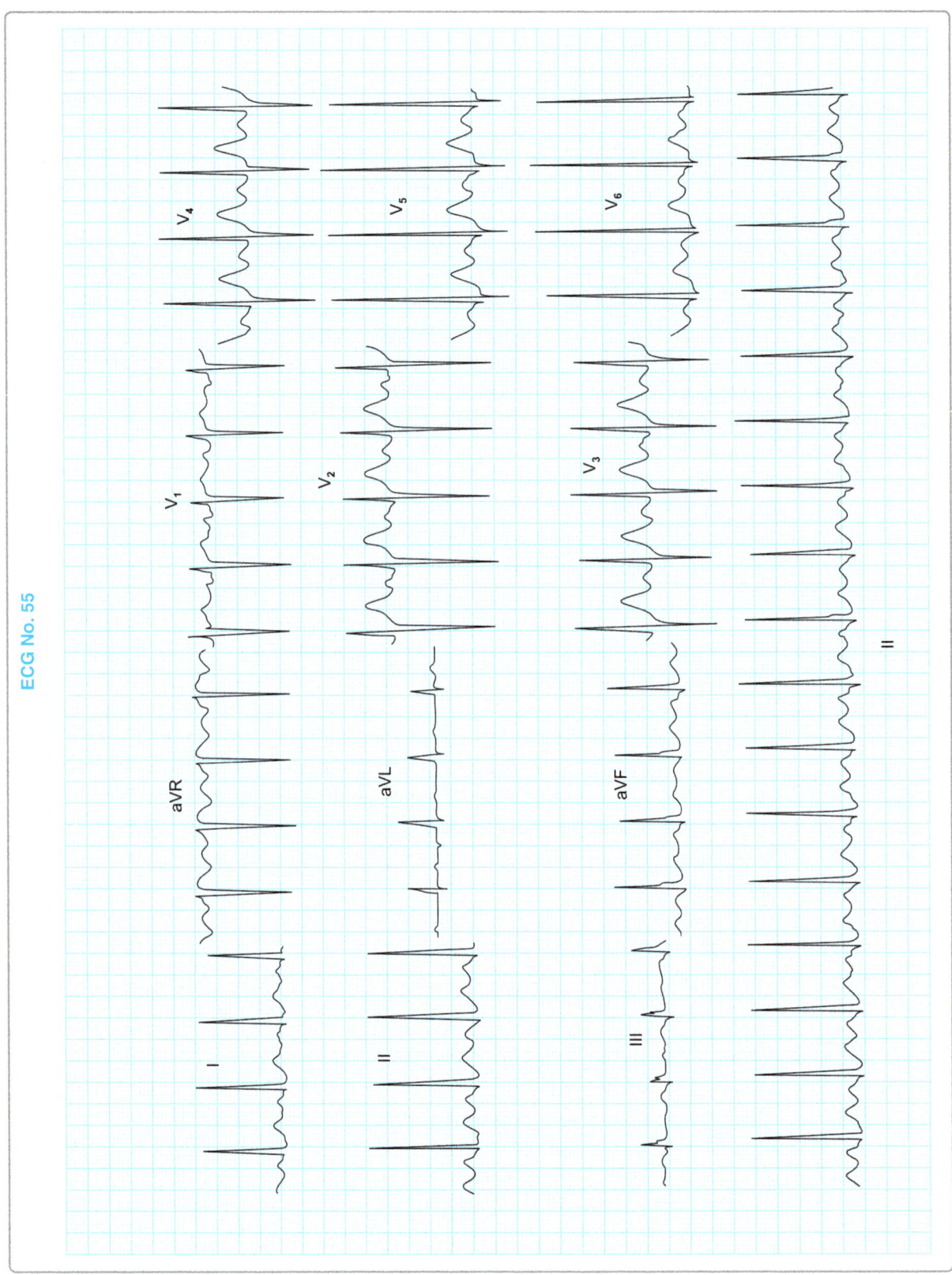

ECG No. 55

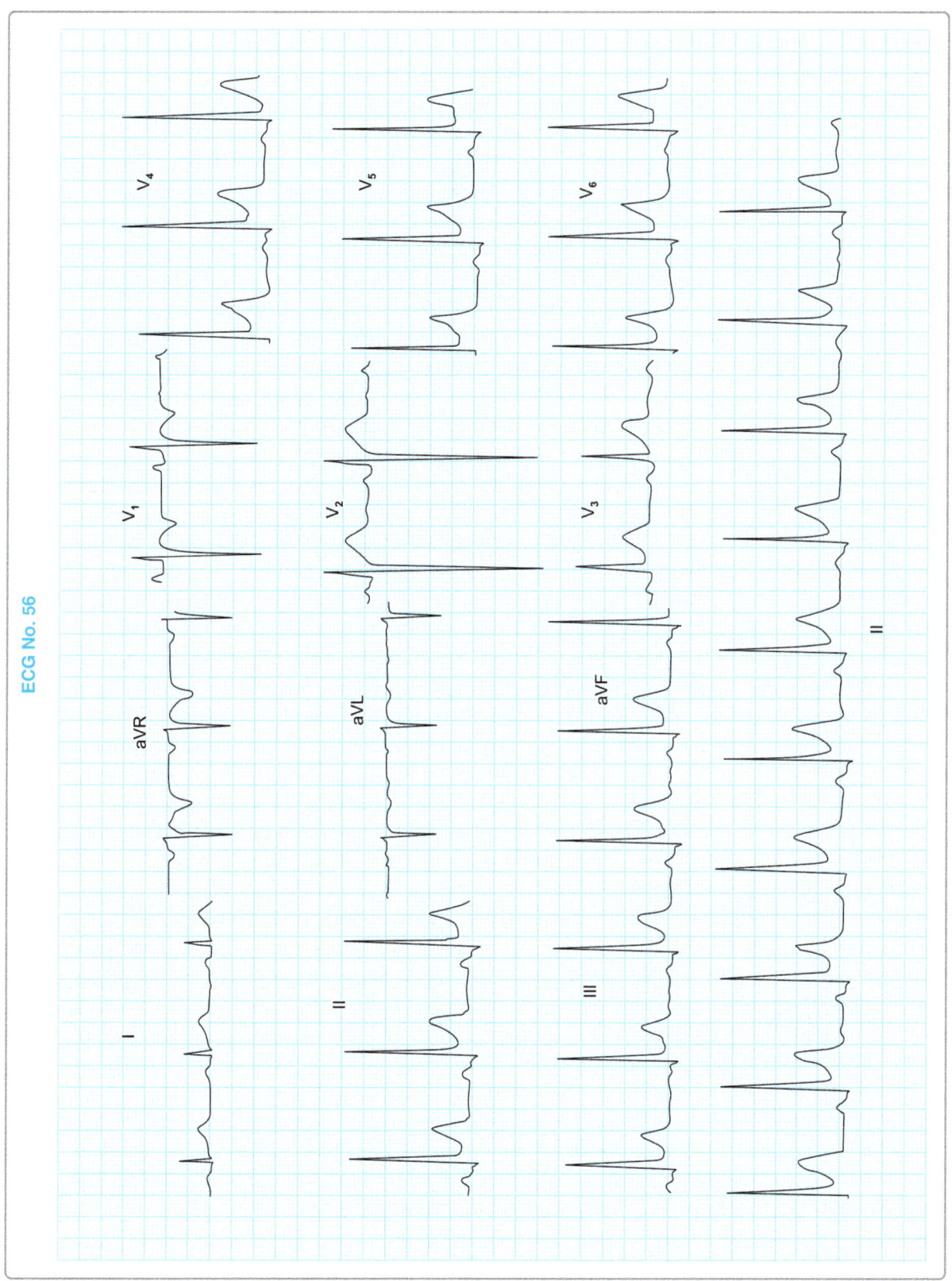

ECG in Medical Practice

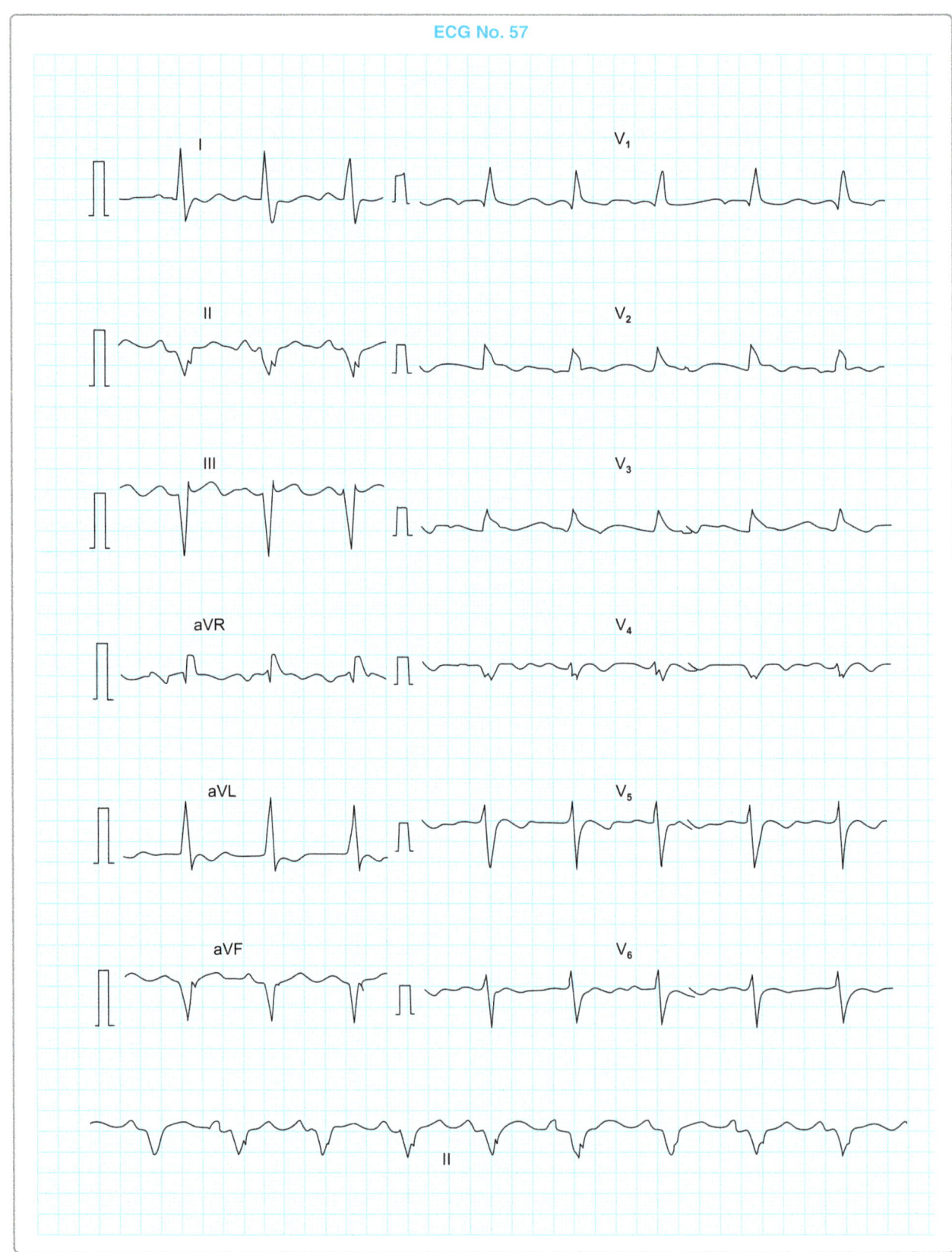

ECG No. 57

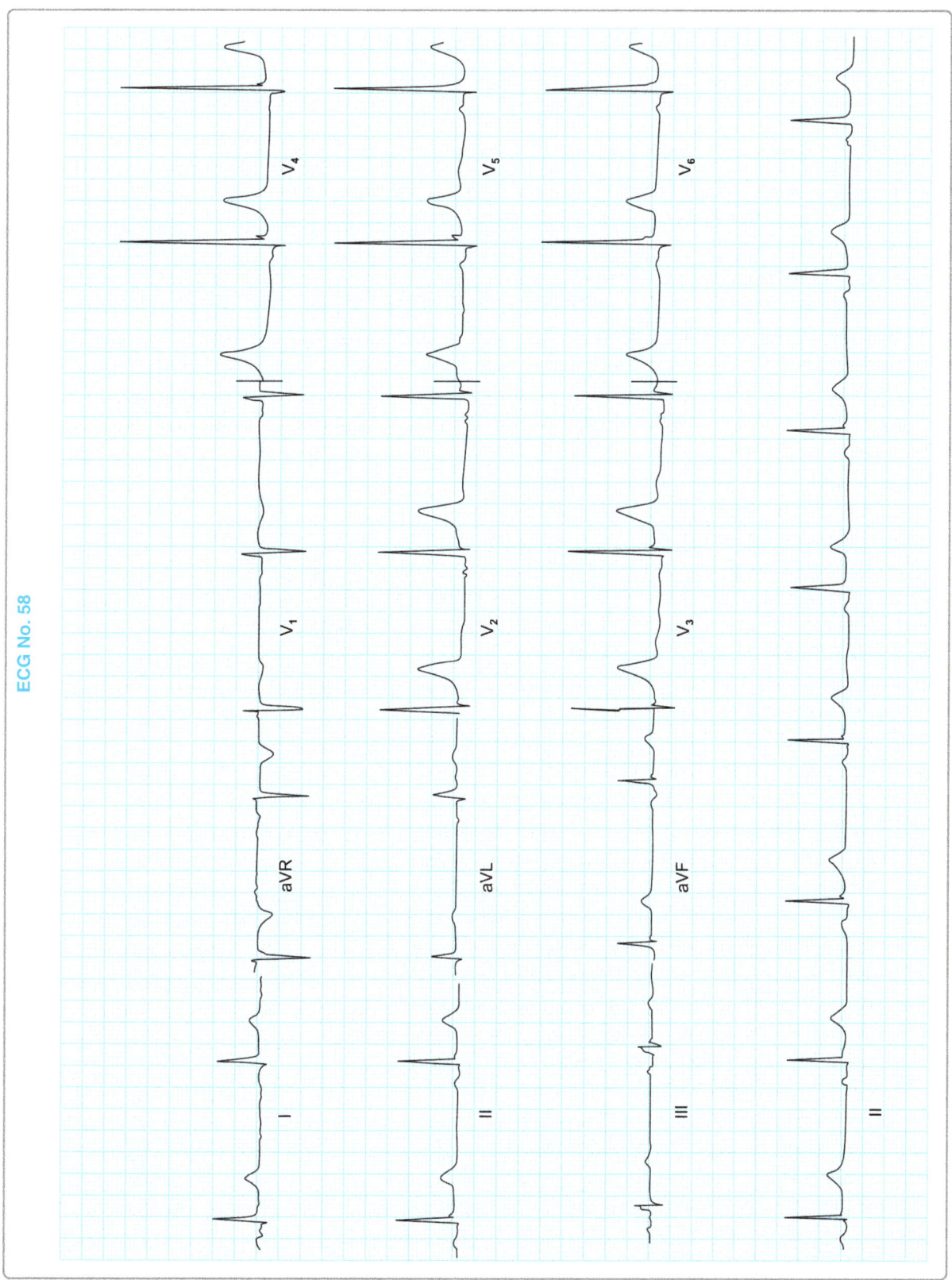

ECG No. 58

ECG in Medical Practice

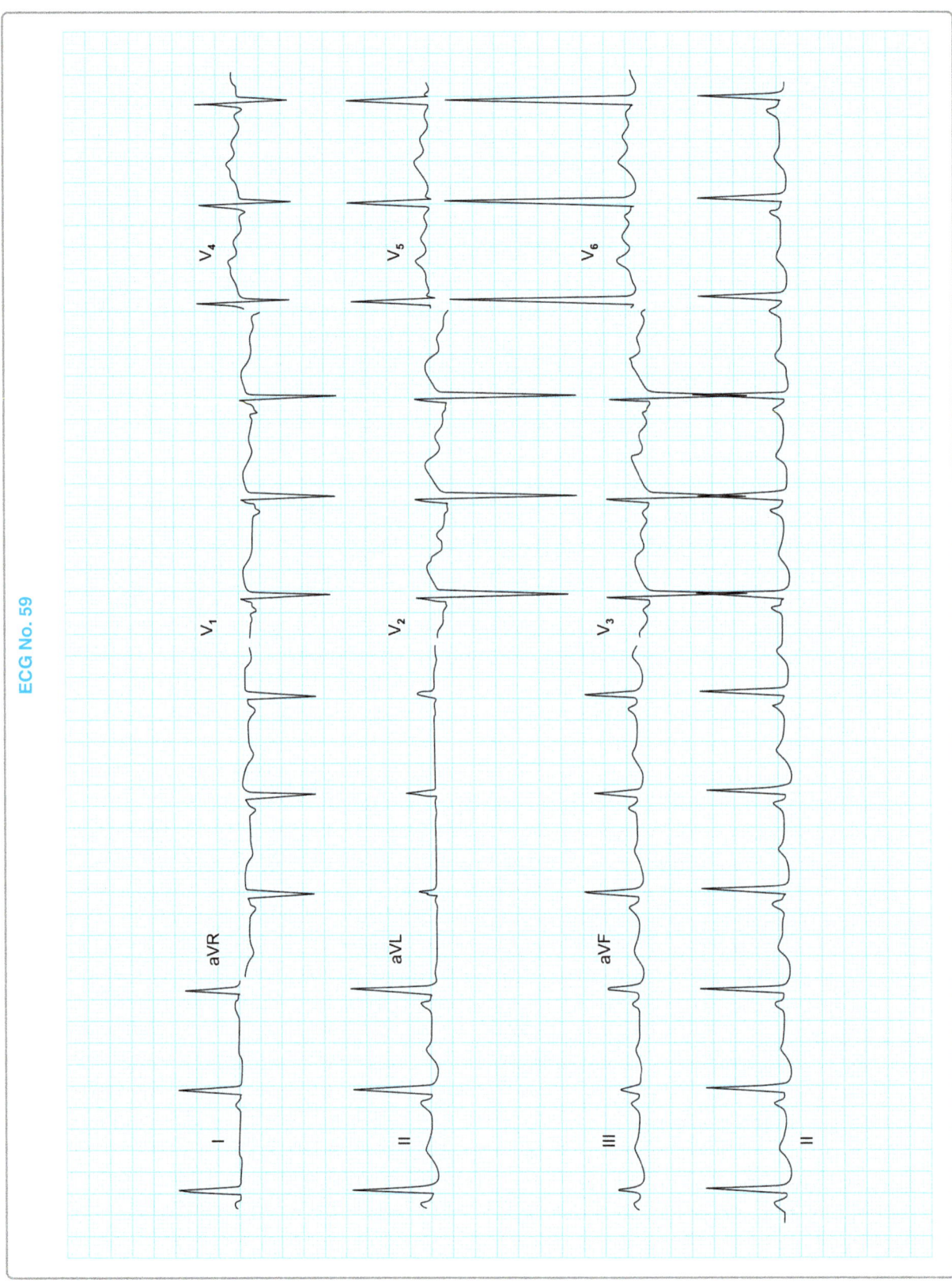

ECG No. 59

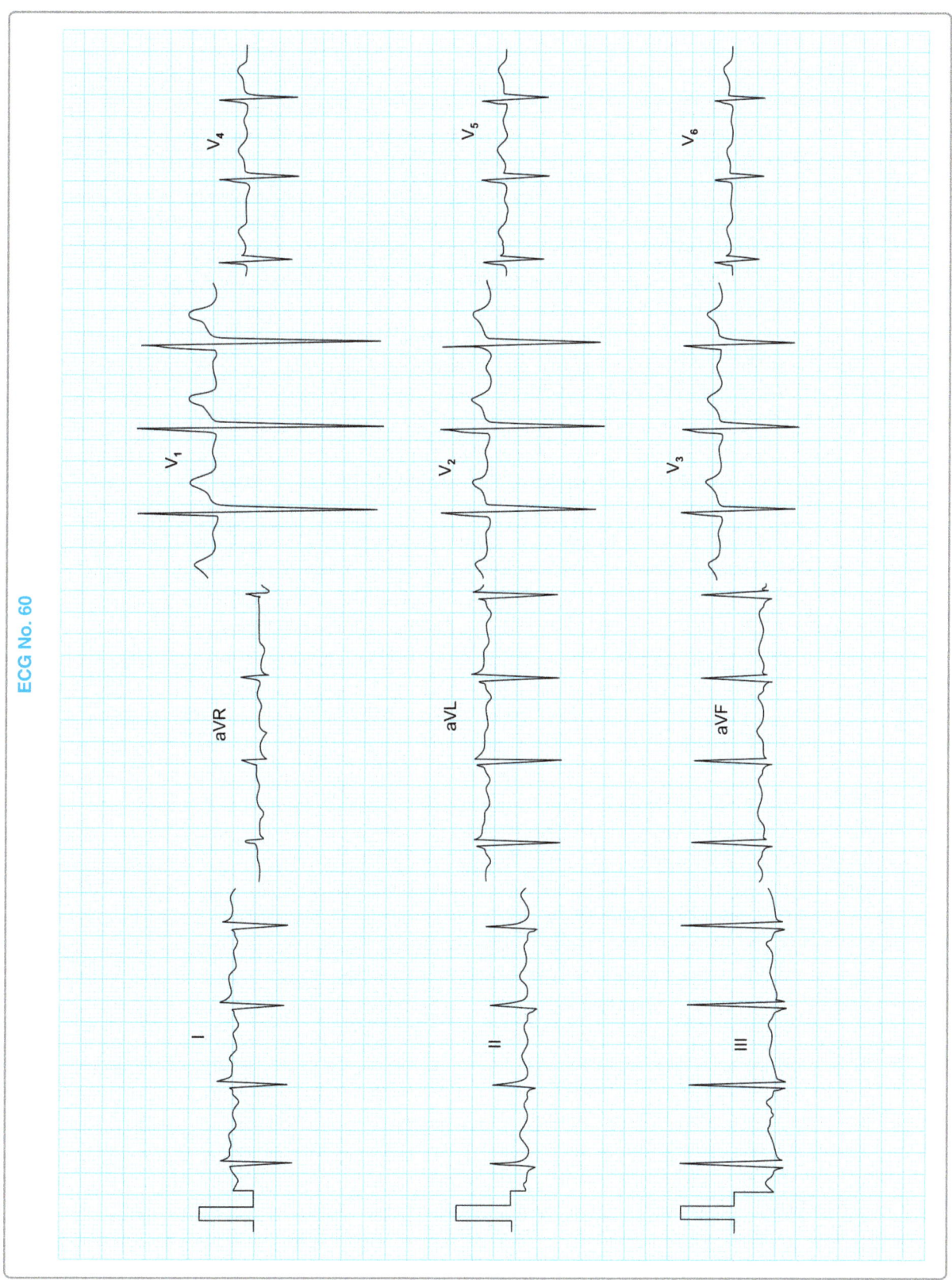

ECG No. 60

ECG in Medical Practice

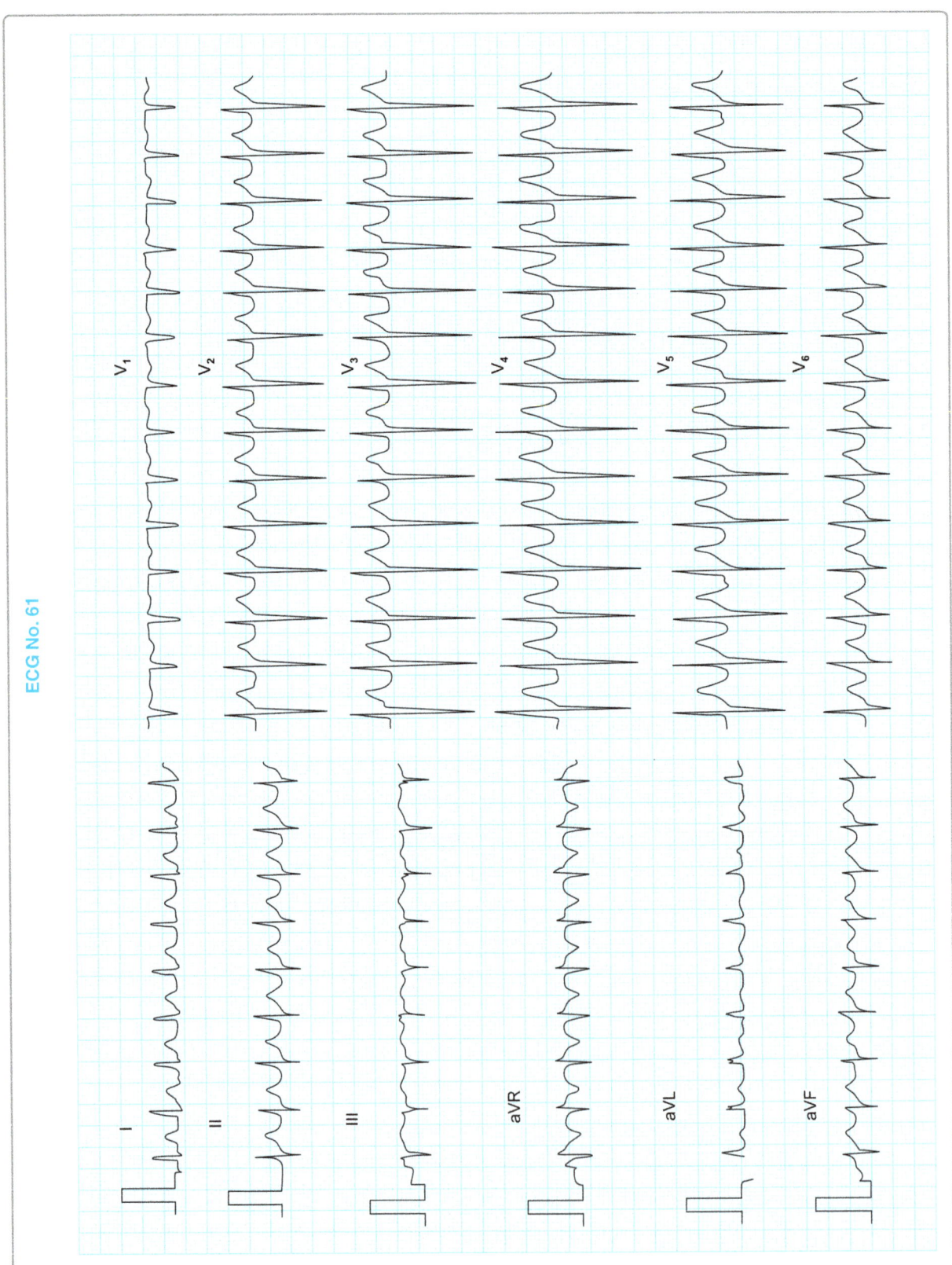

ECG No. 61

ECG No. 62

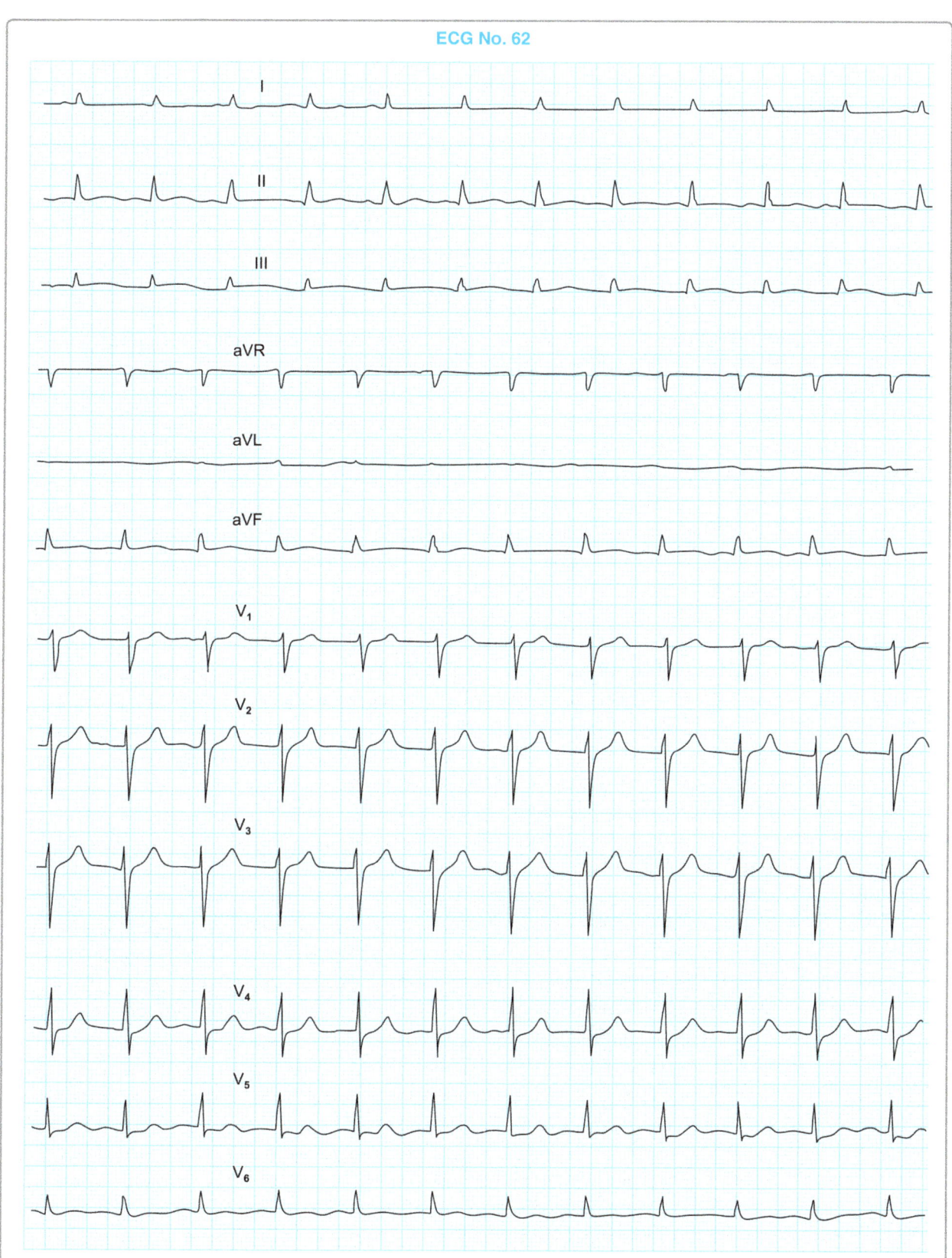

ECG No. 63

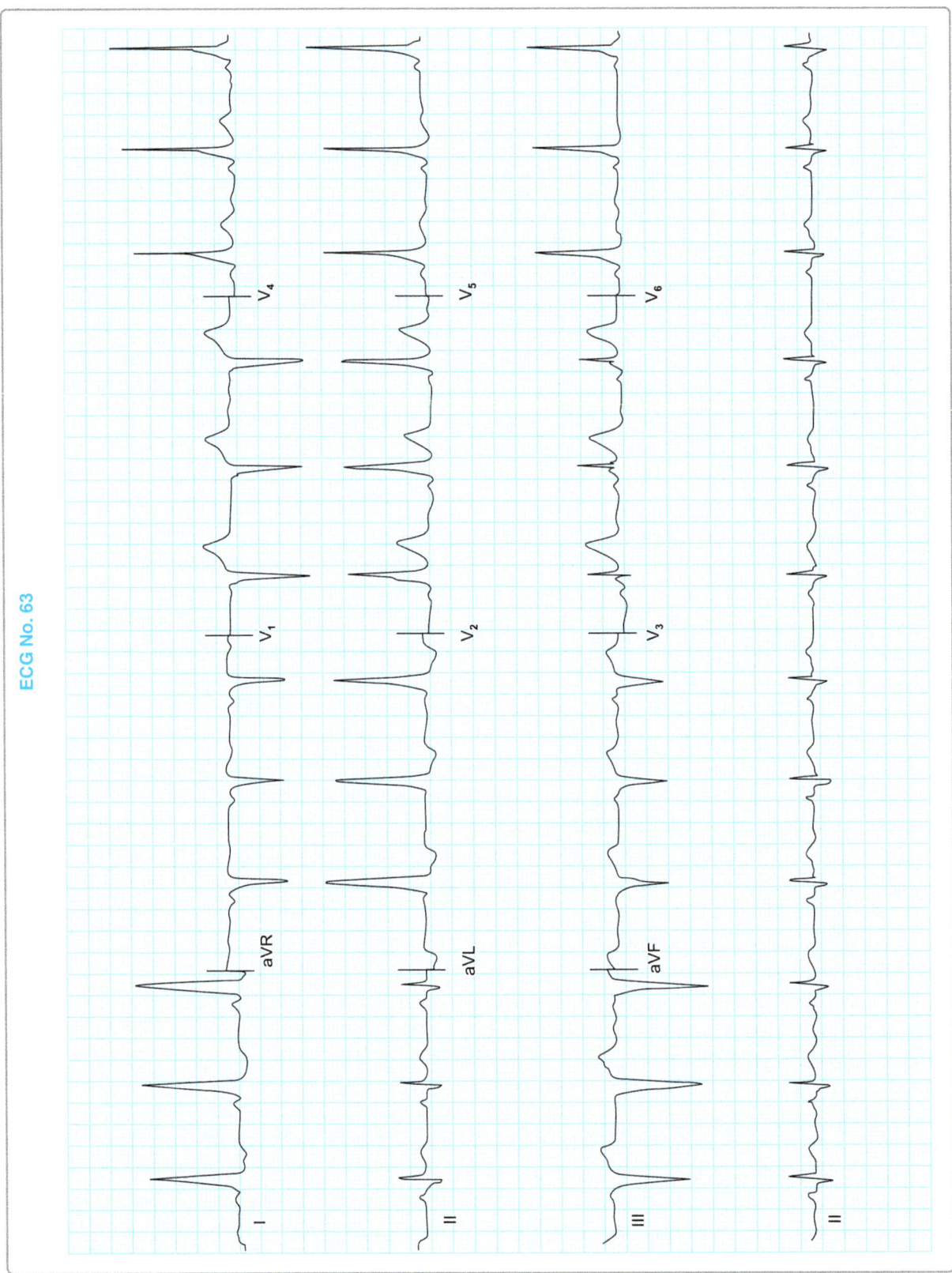

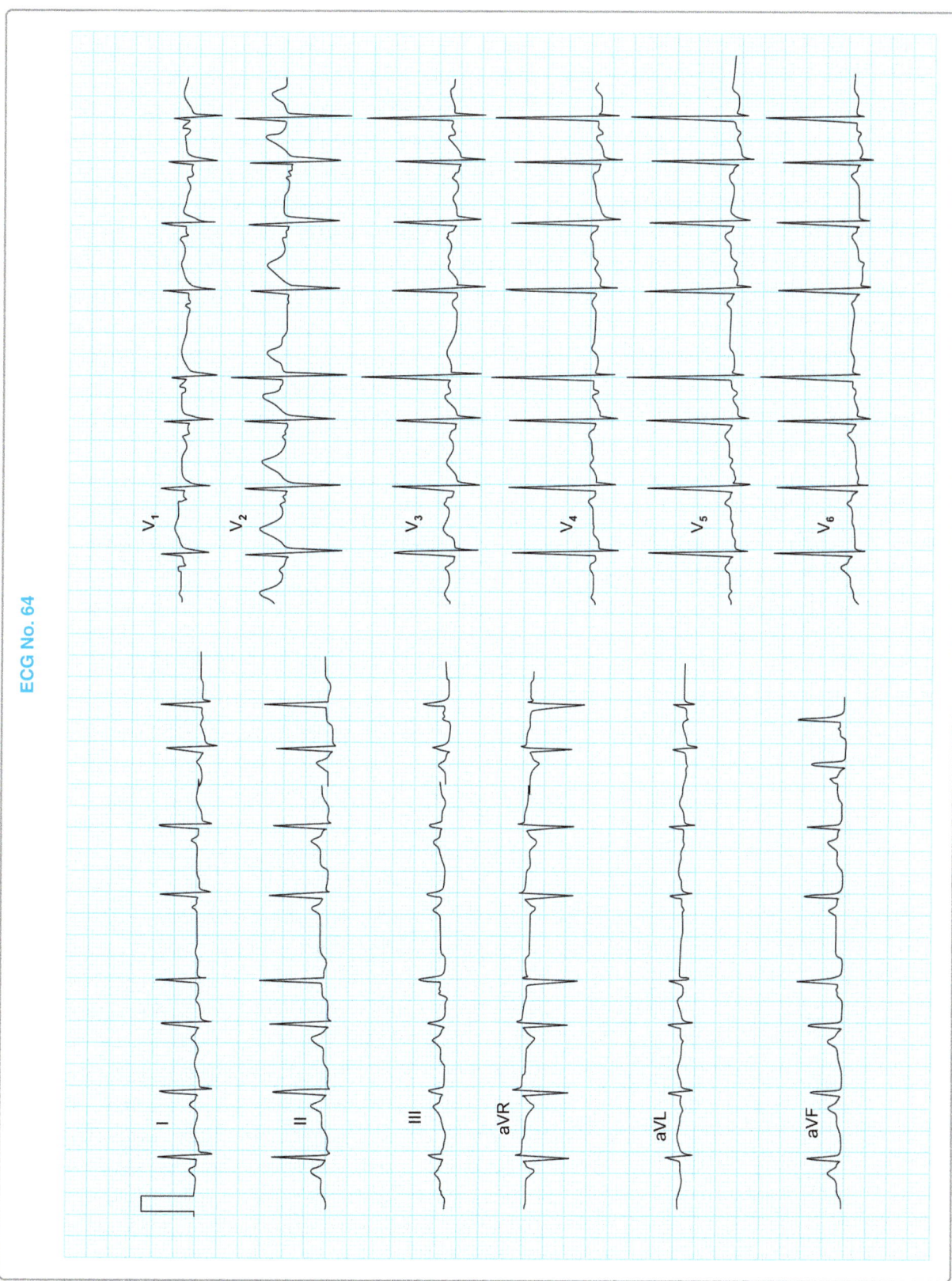

ECG No. 64

ECG No. 65

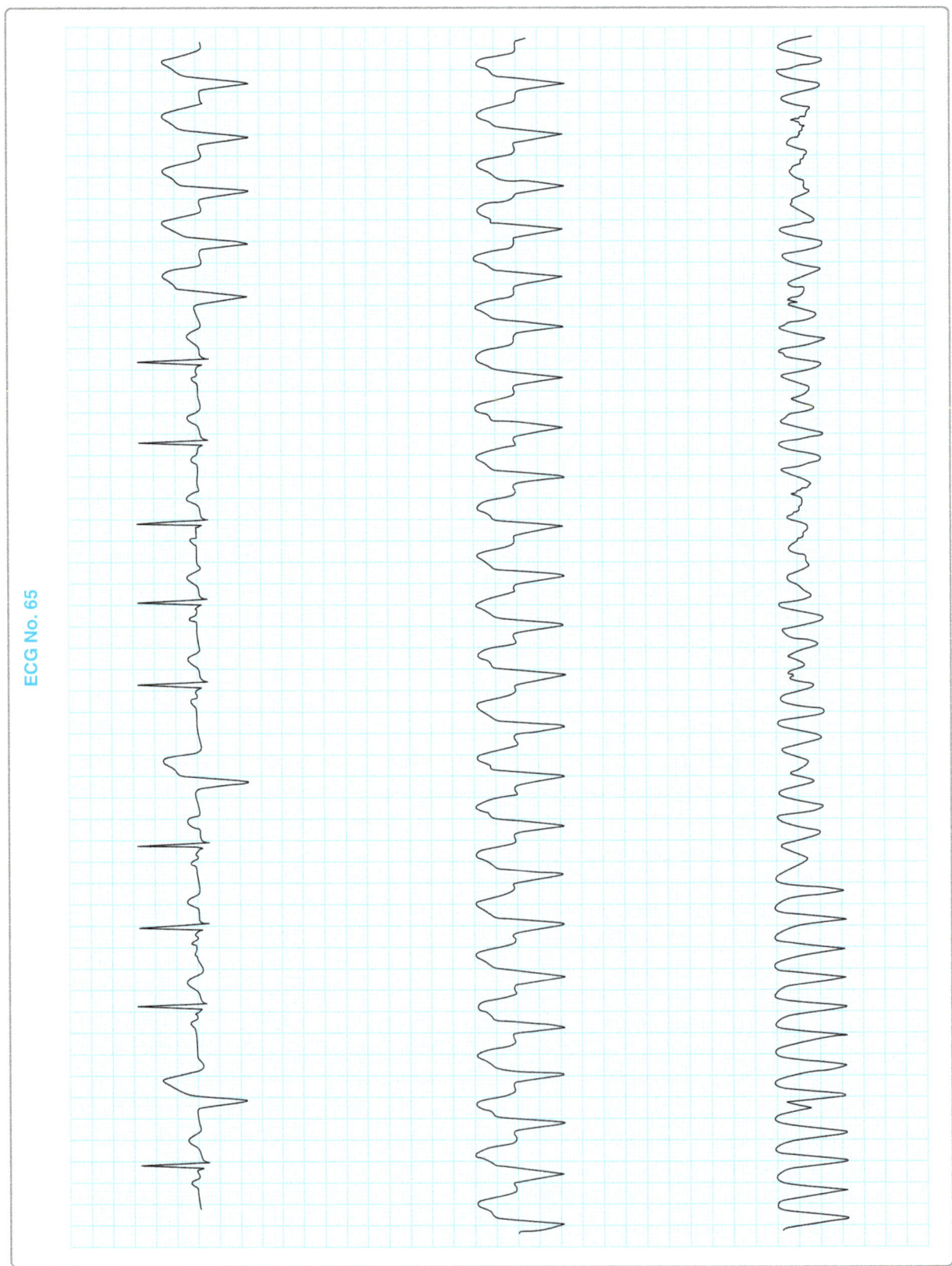

ECG No. 66

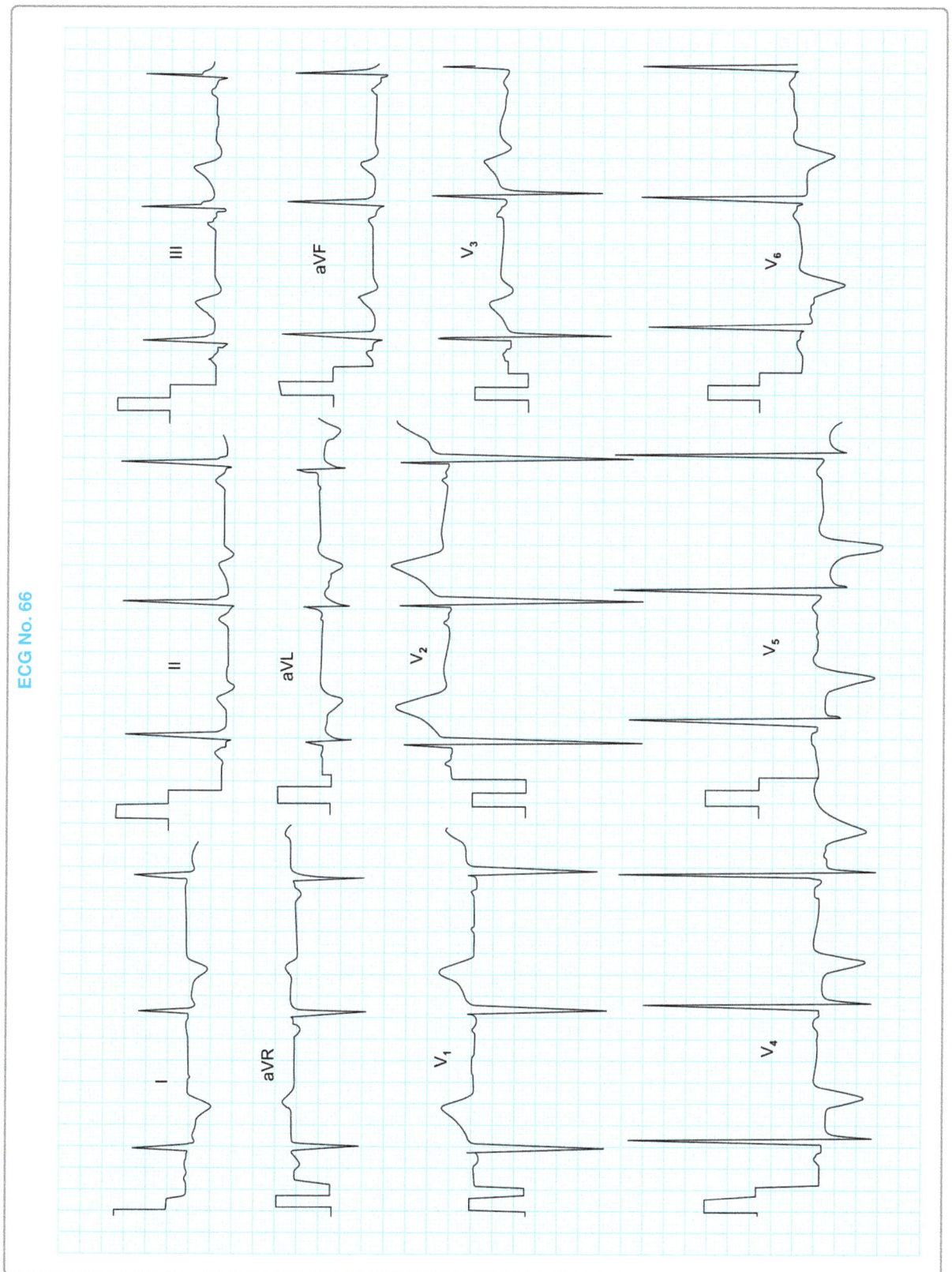

ECG No. 67

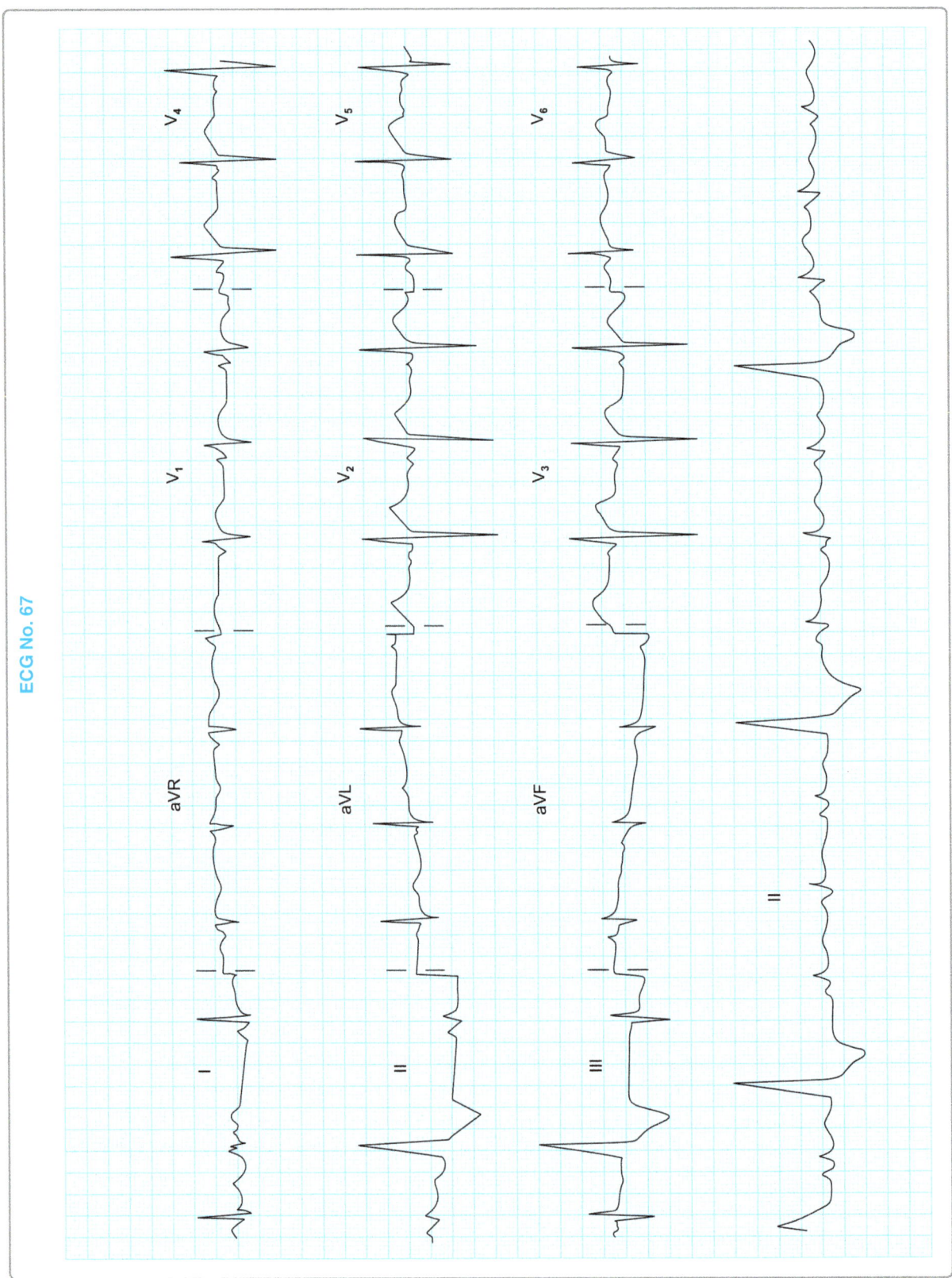

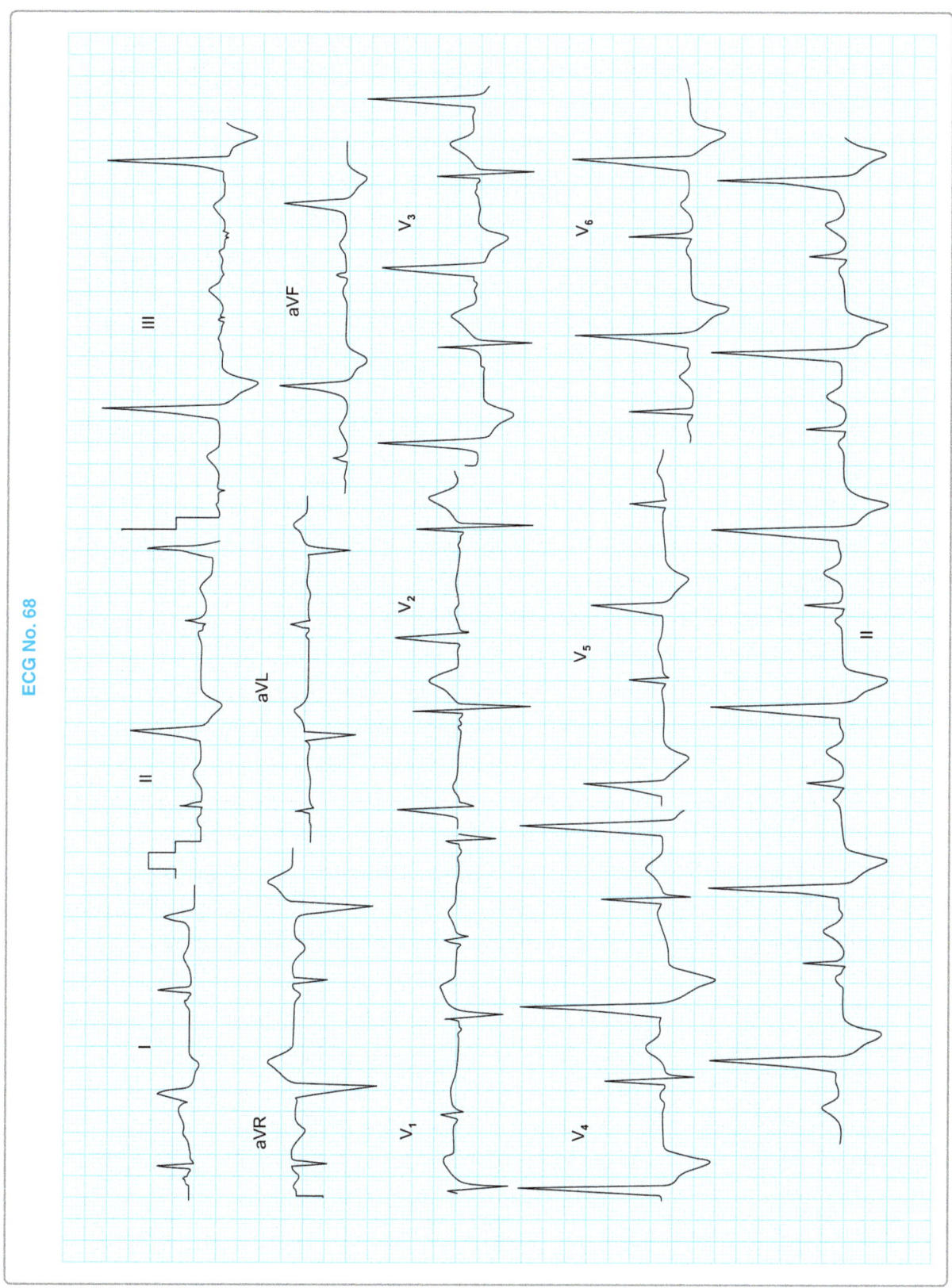

ECG in Medical Practice

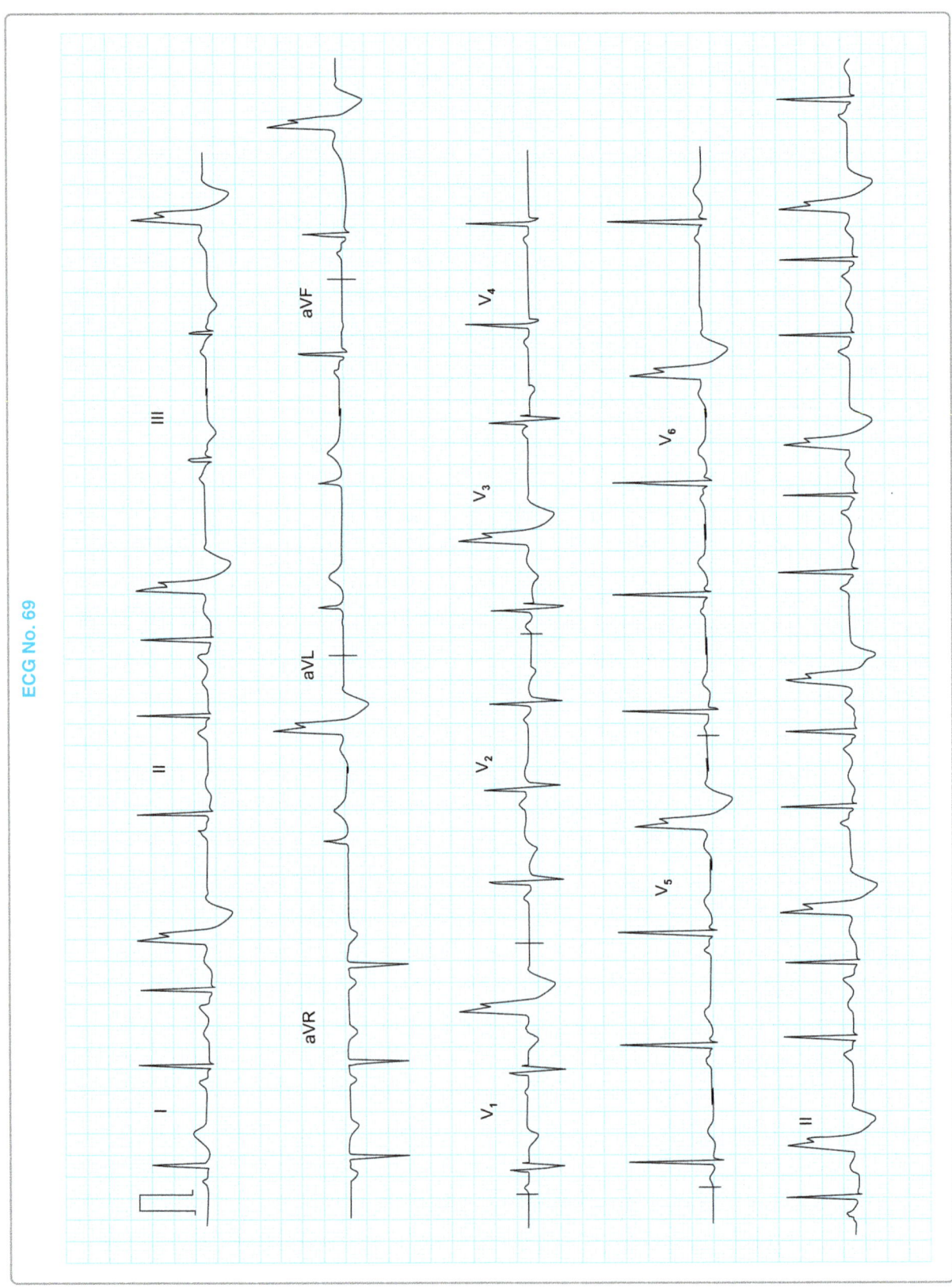

ECG No. 69

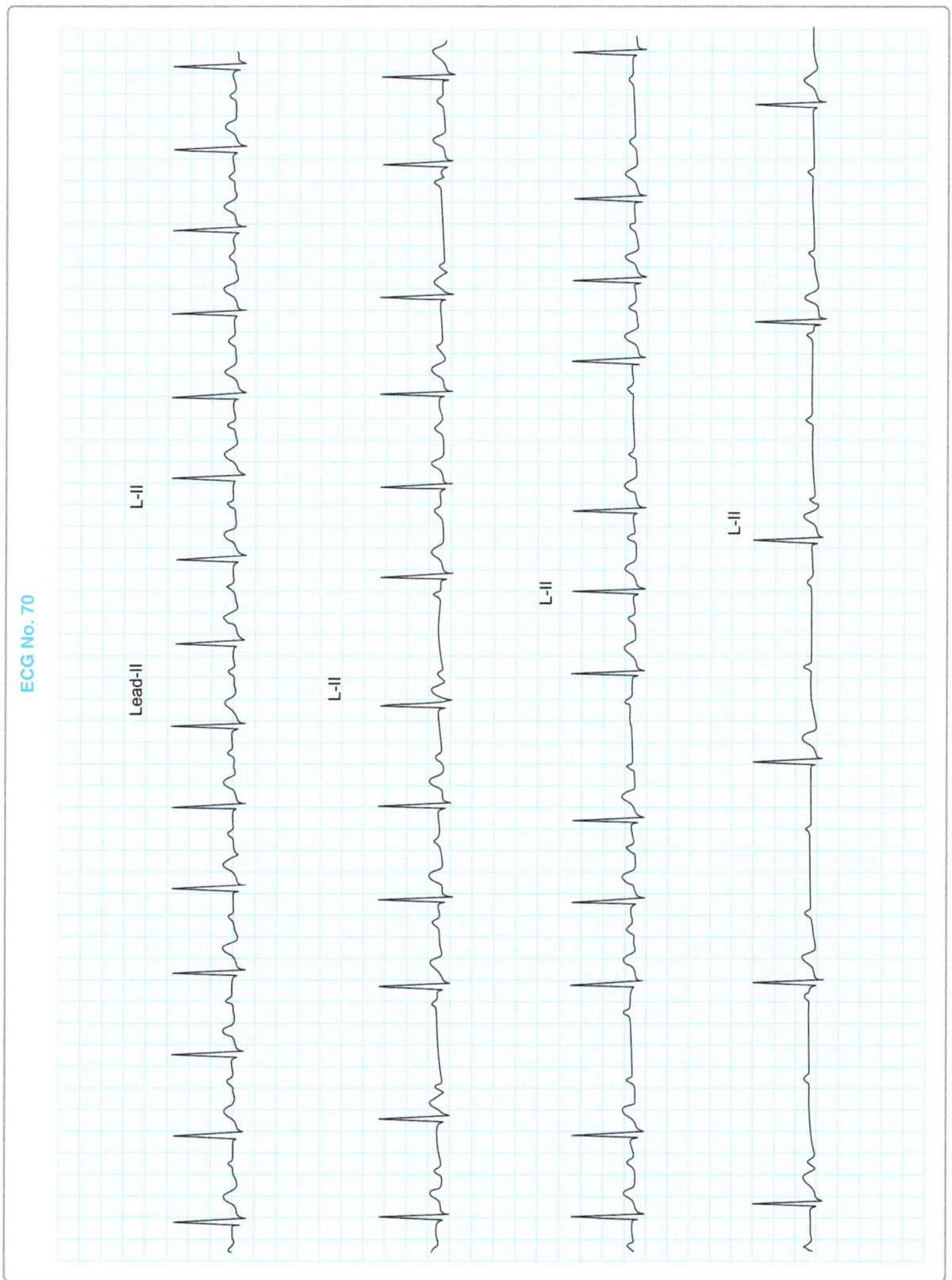

ECG in Medical Practice

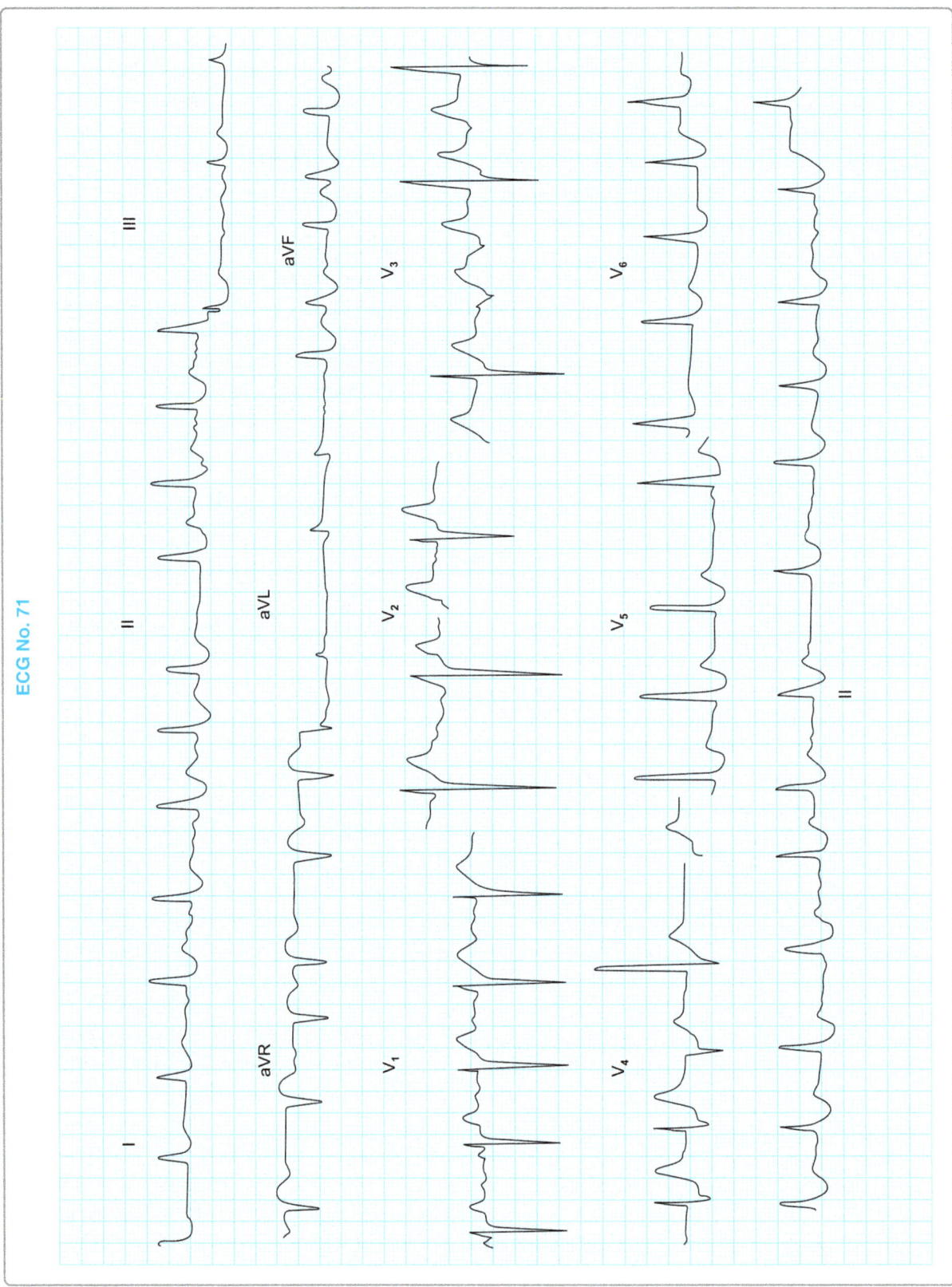

ECG No. 71

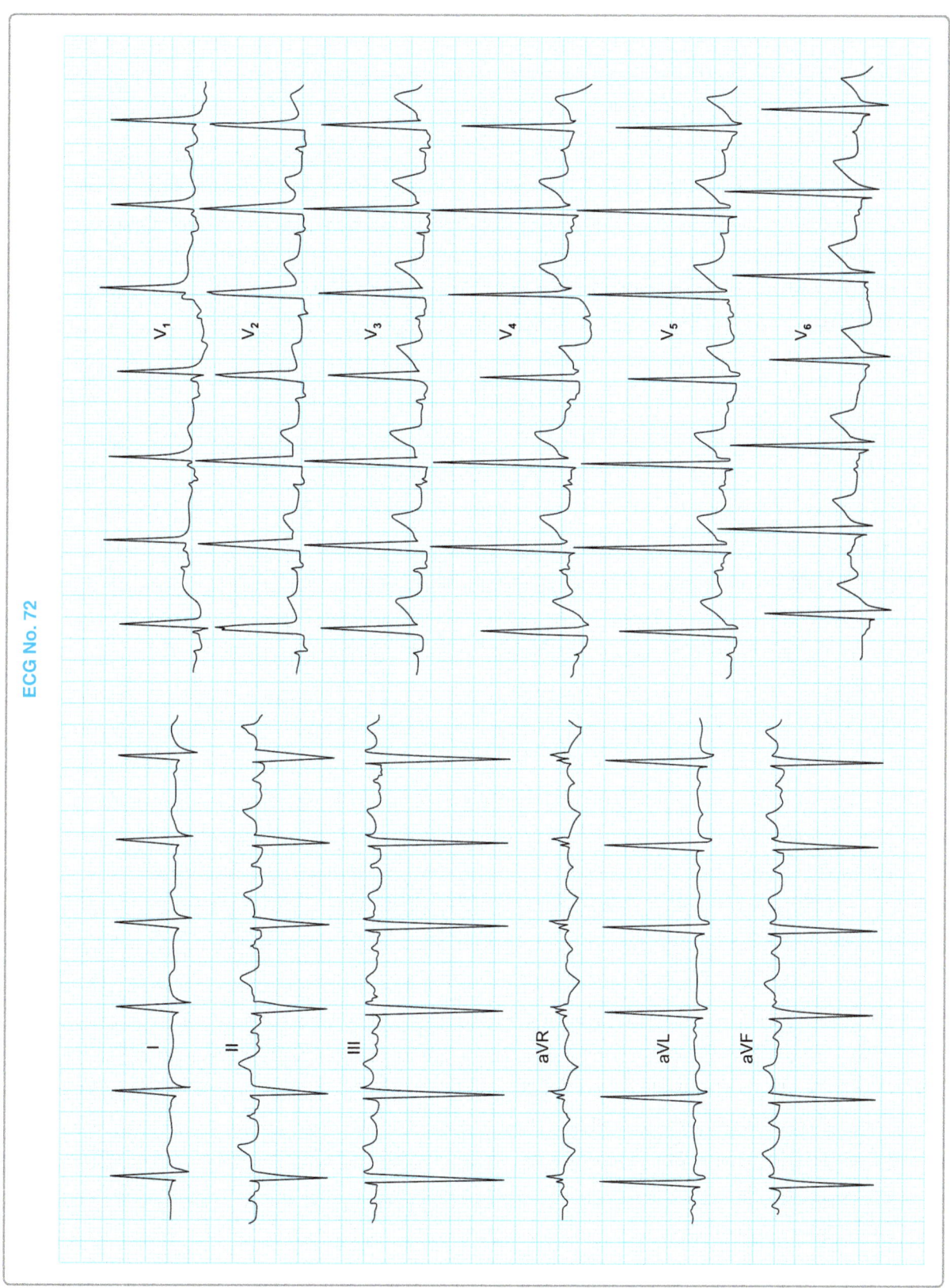

ECG No. 72

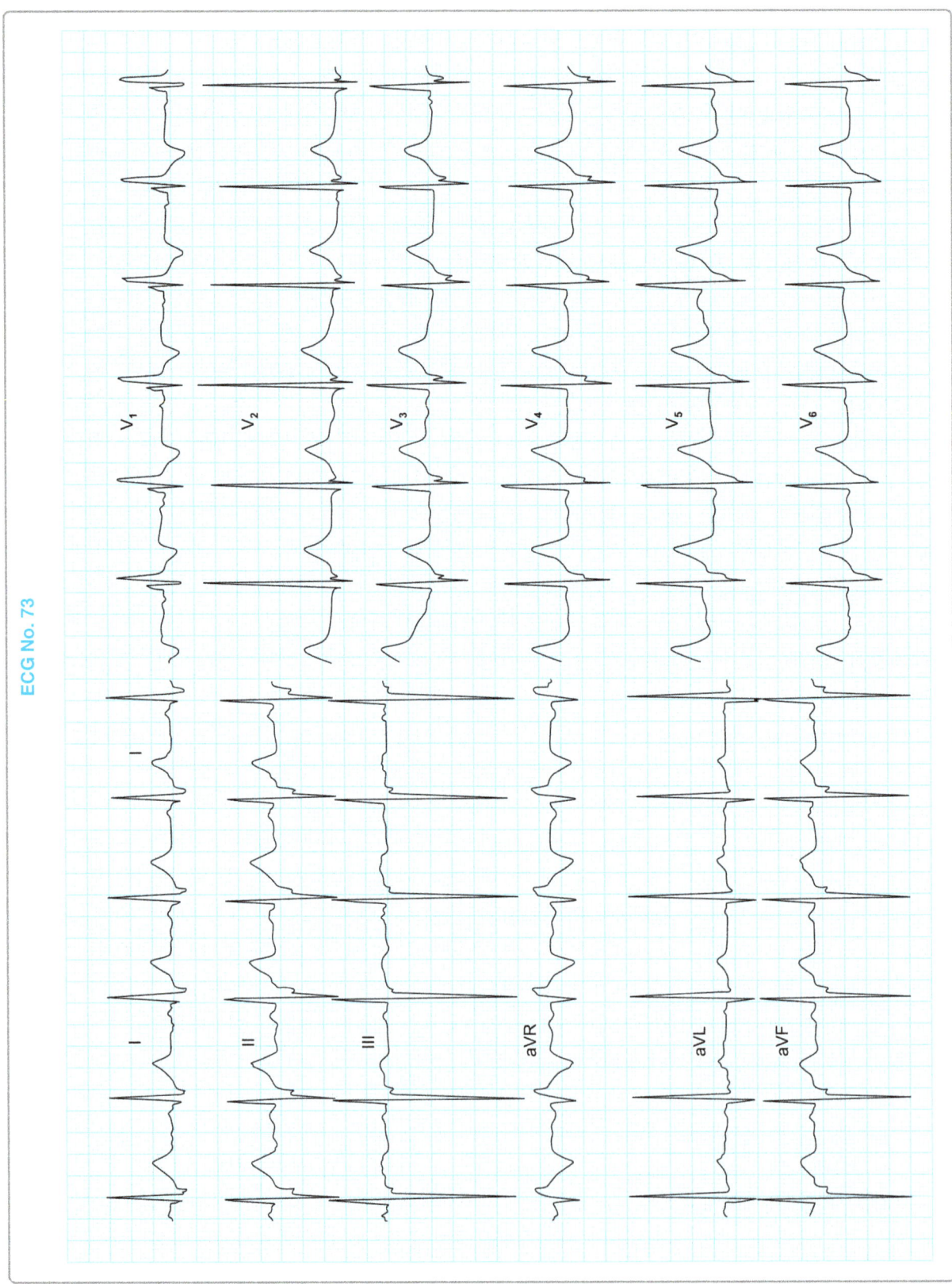

ECG No. 73

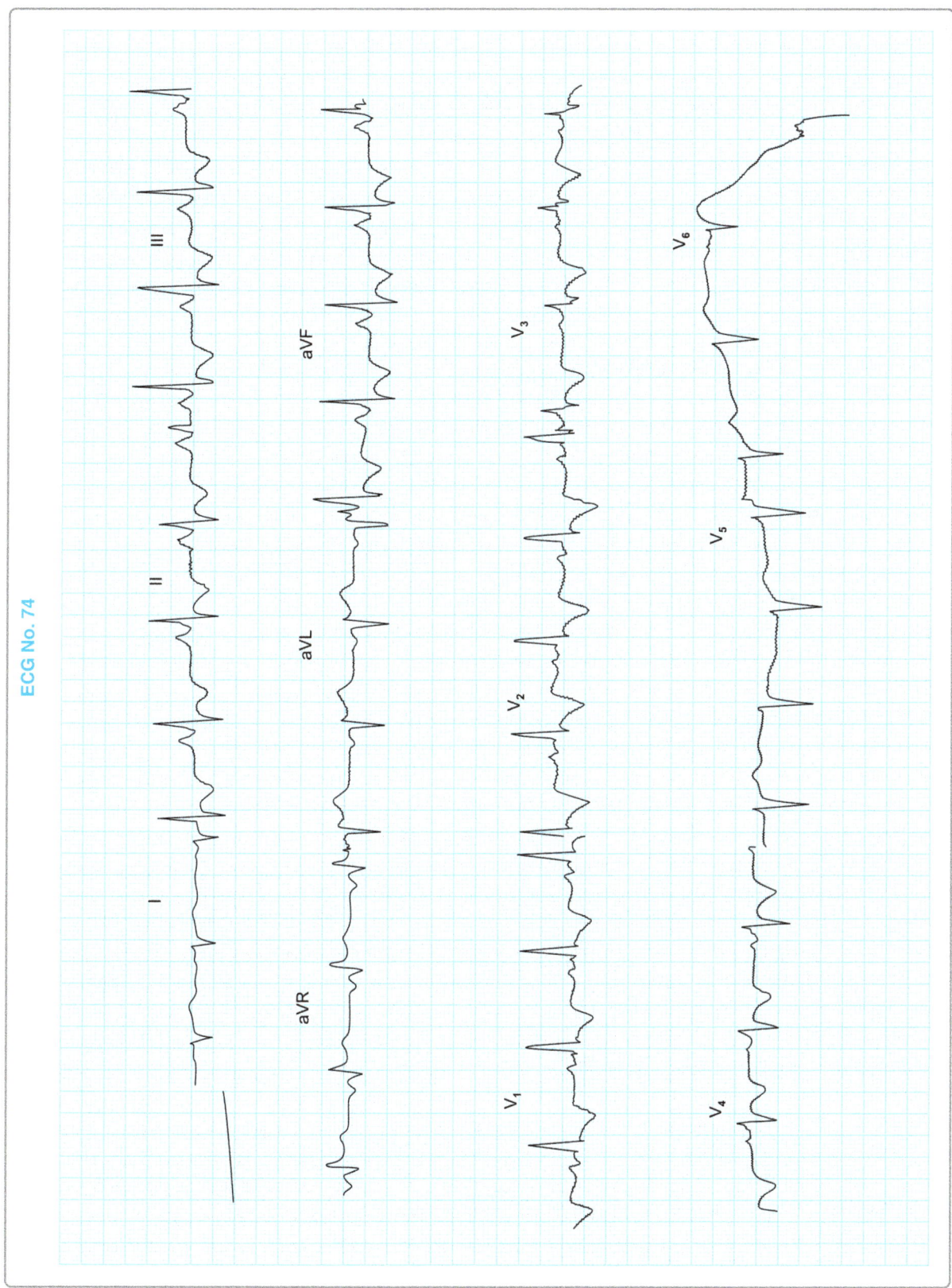

ECG No. 74

ECG in Medical Practice

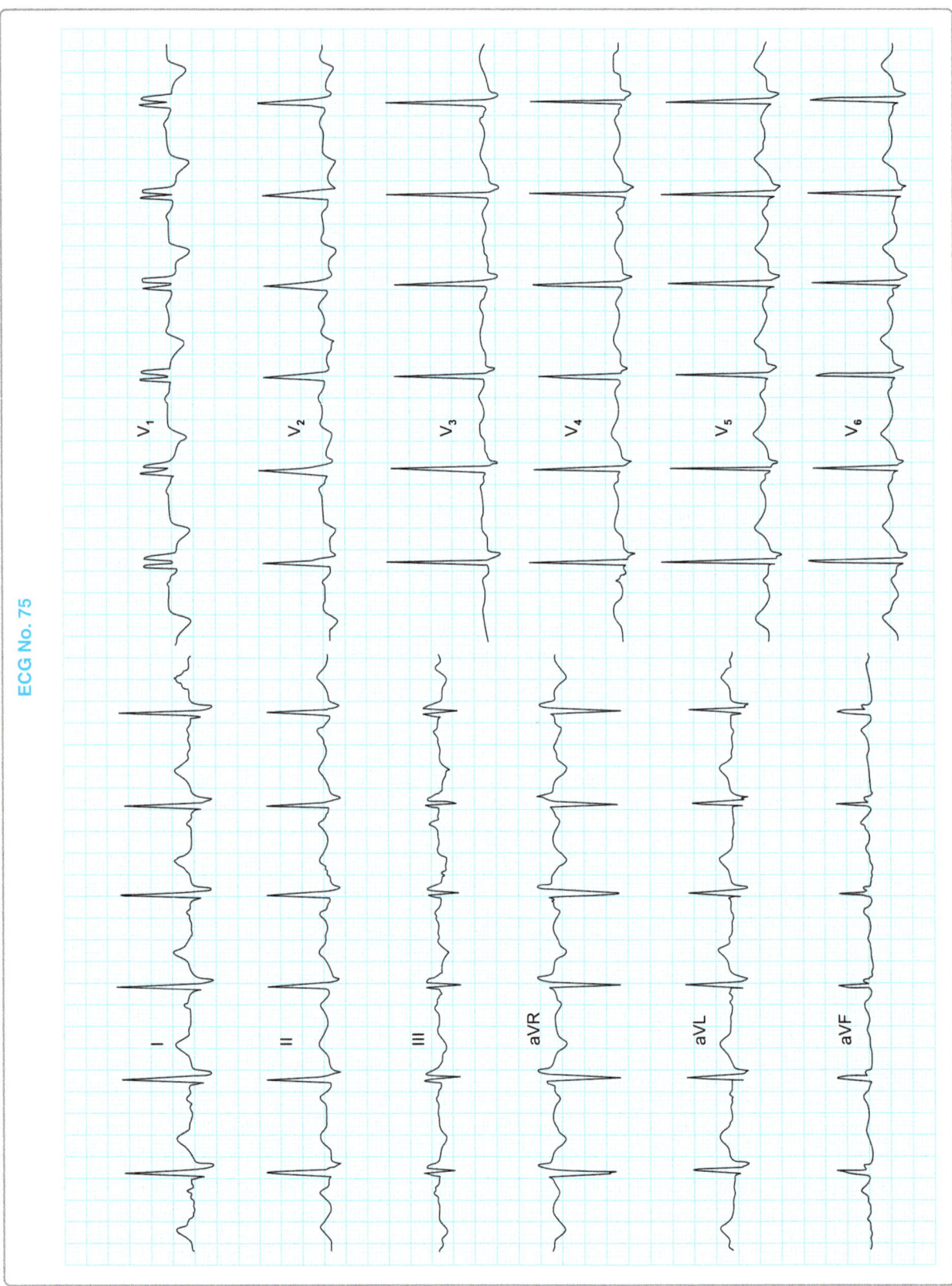

ECG No. 75

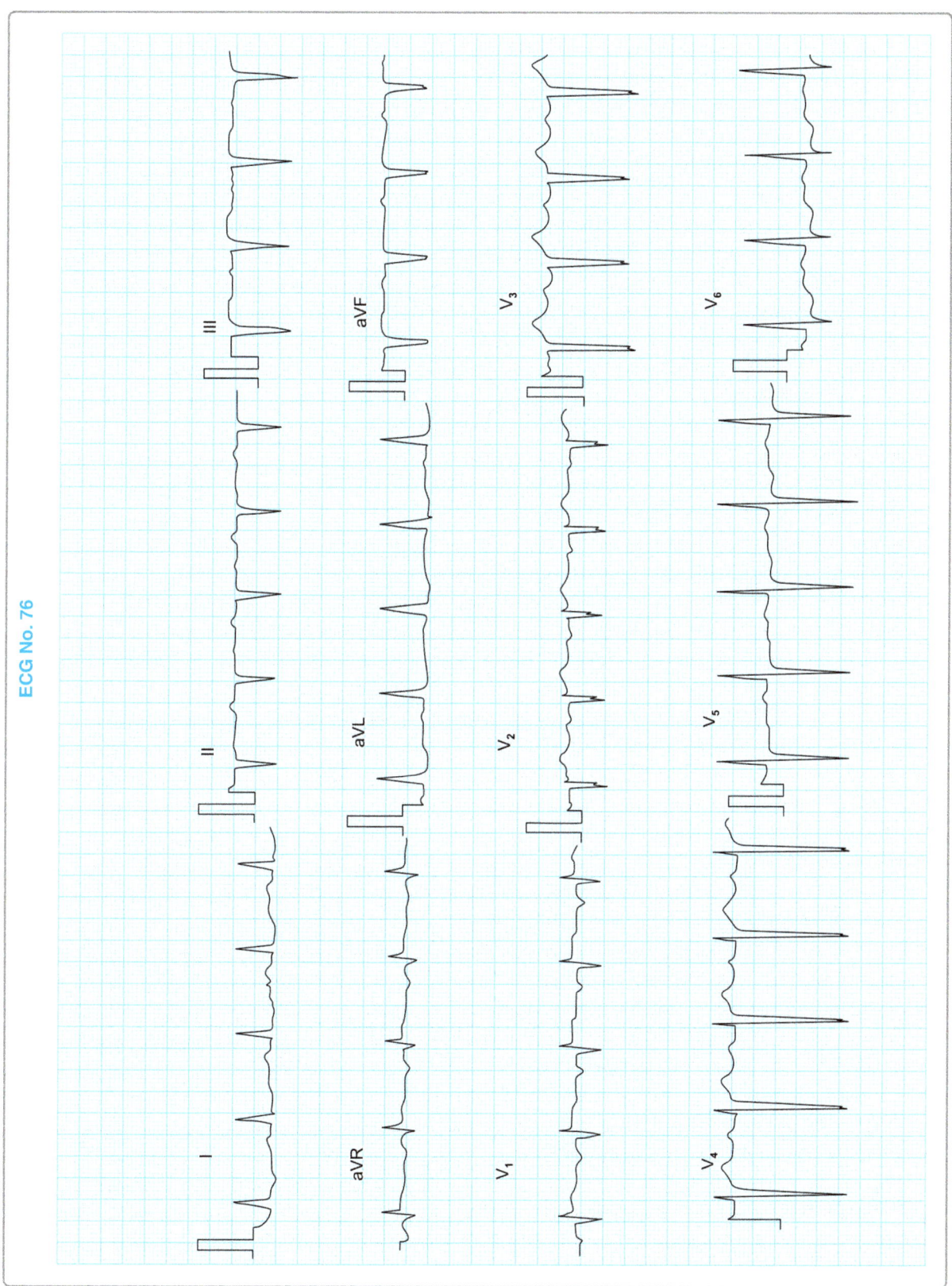

ECG No. 76

ECG in Medical Practice

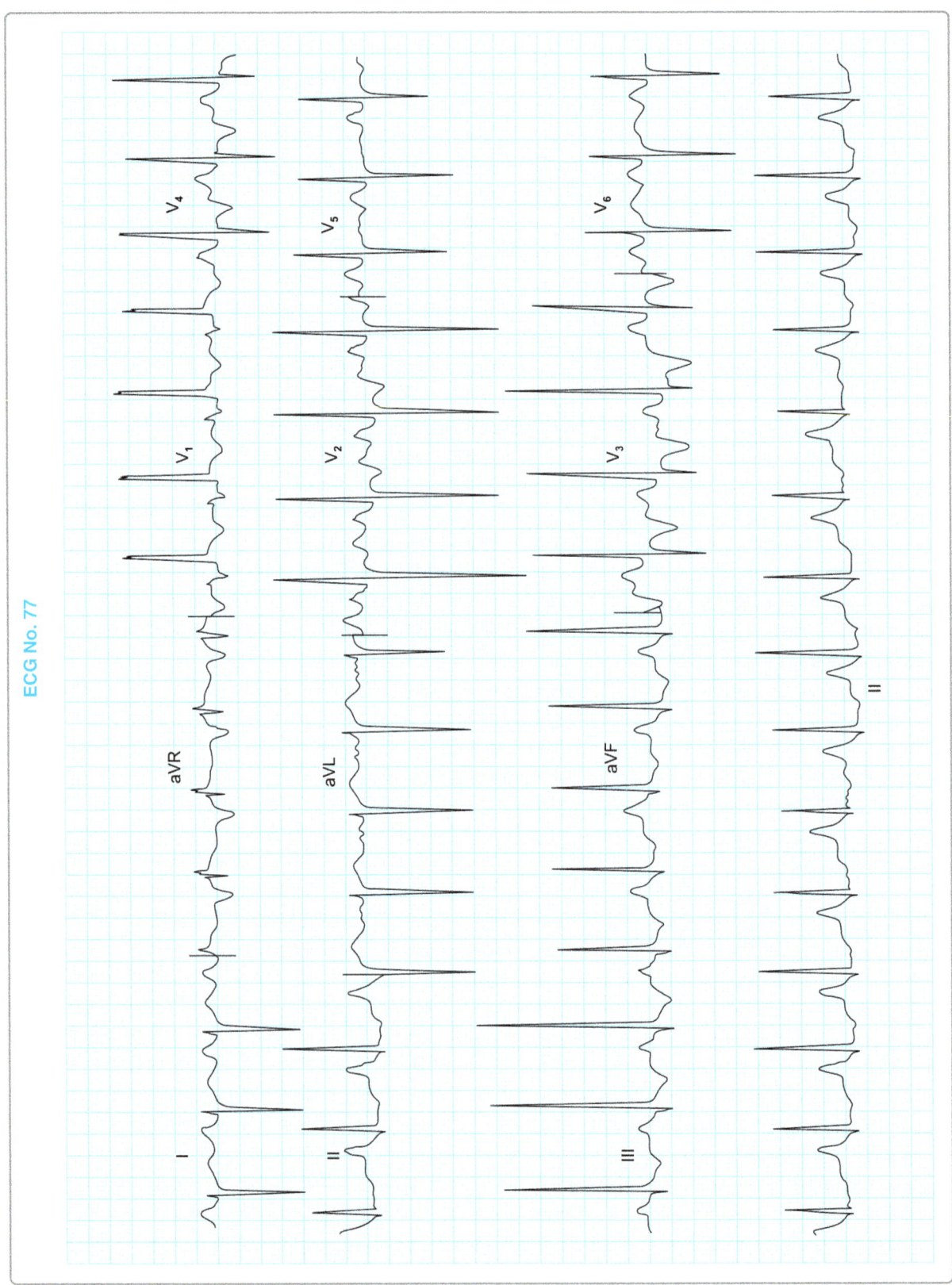

ECG No. 77

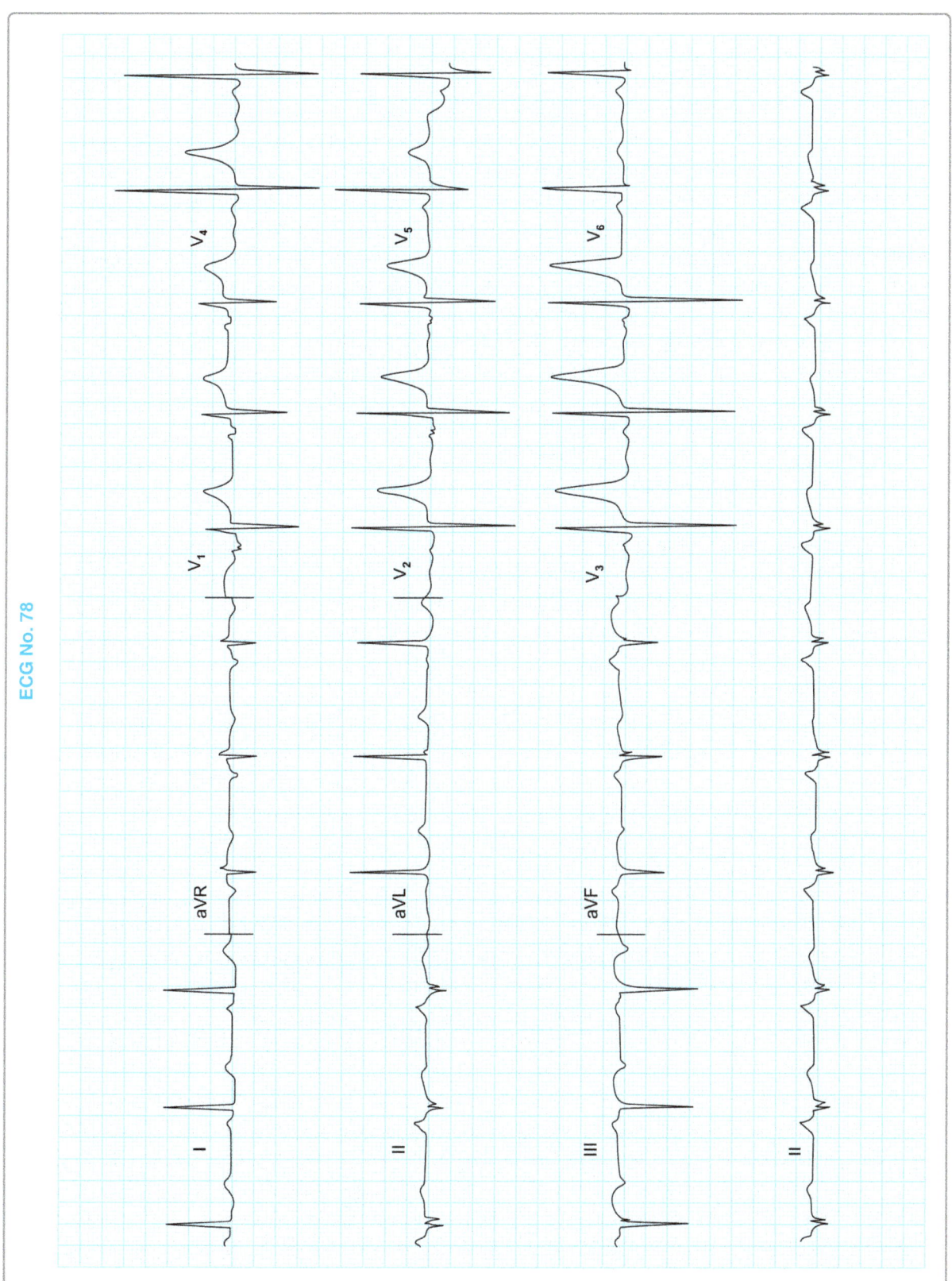

ECG in Medical Practice

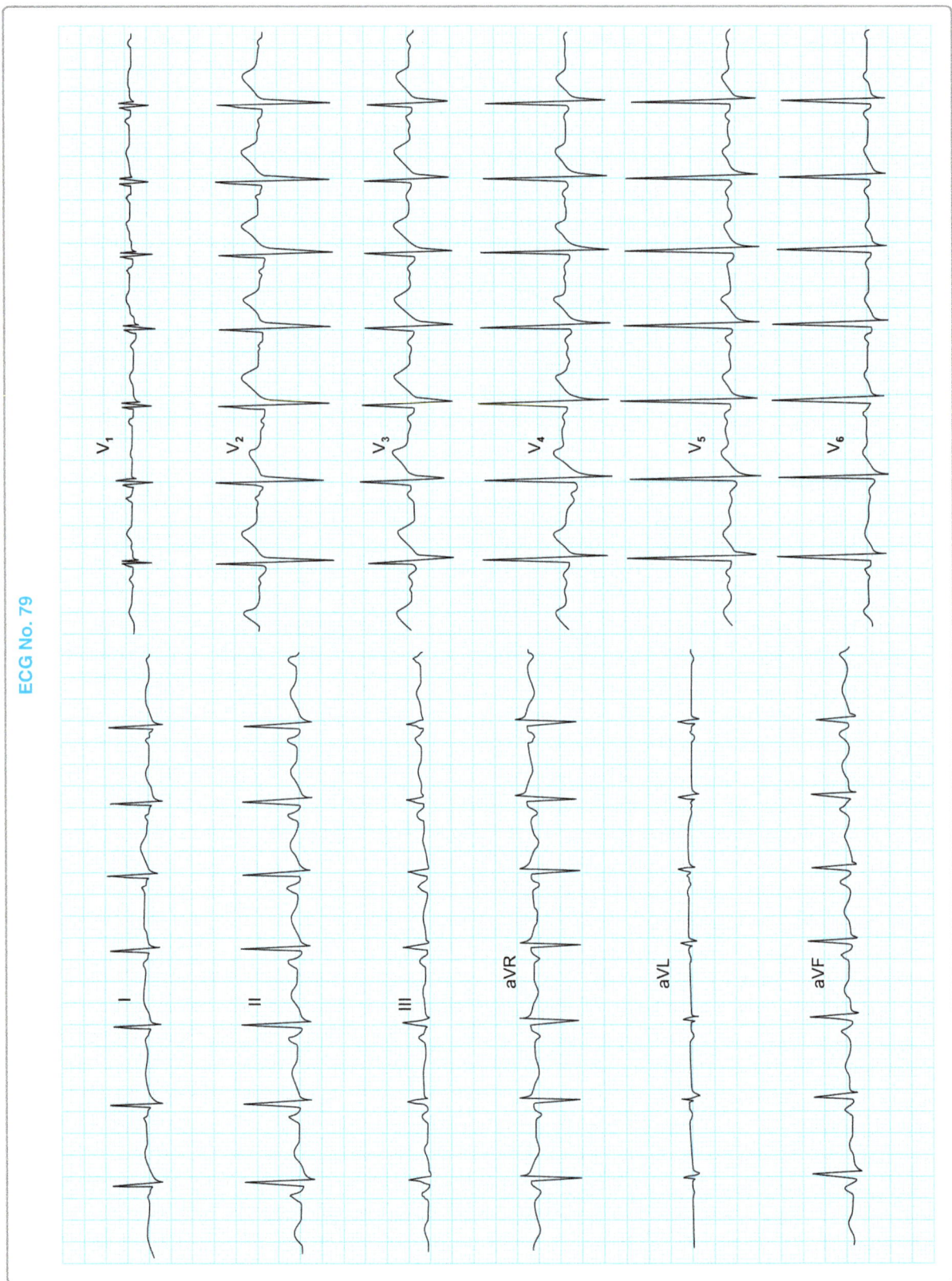

ECG No. 79

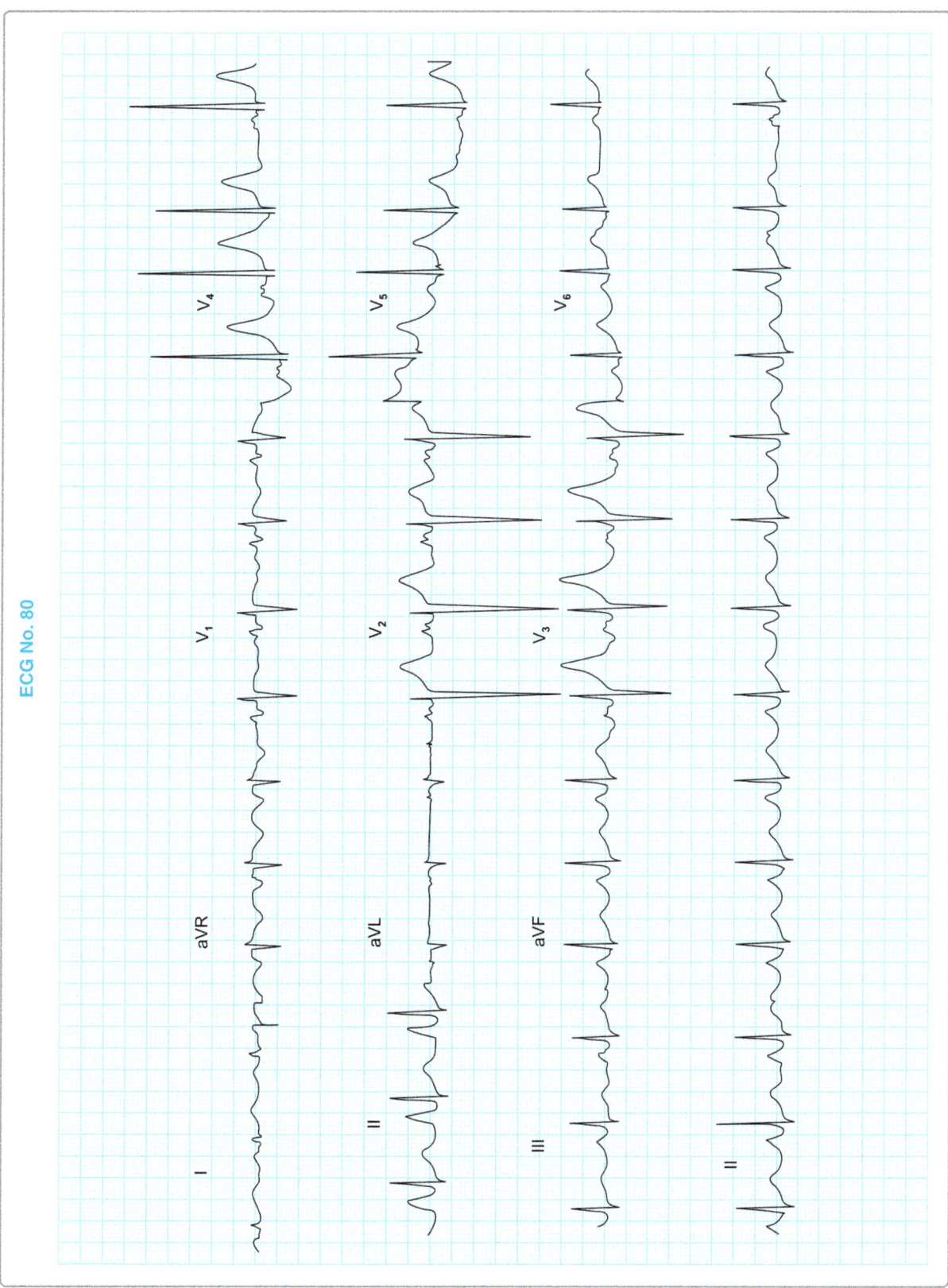

ECG in Medical Practice

ECG No. 81

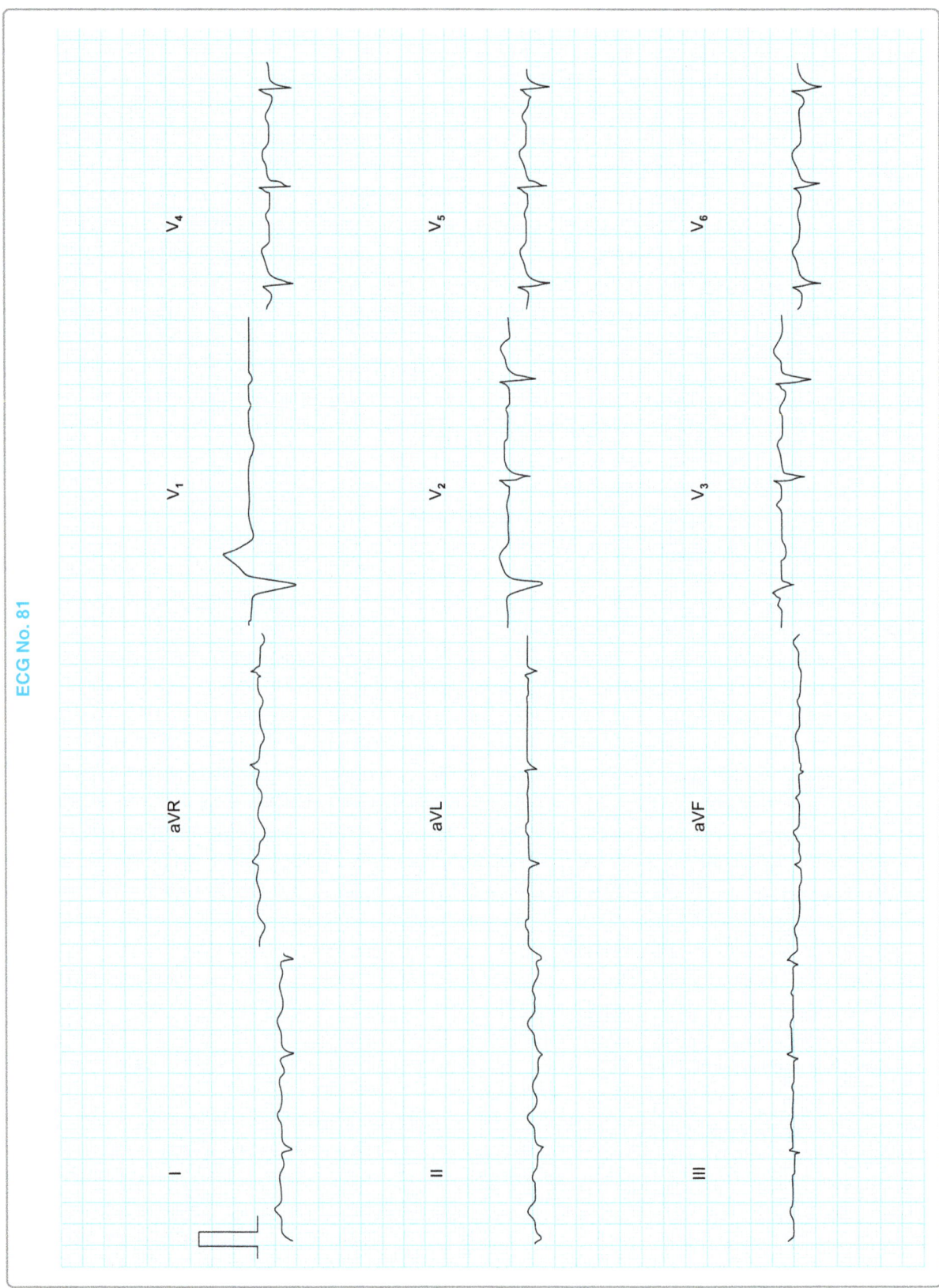

ECG No. 82

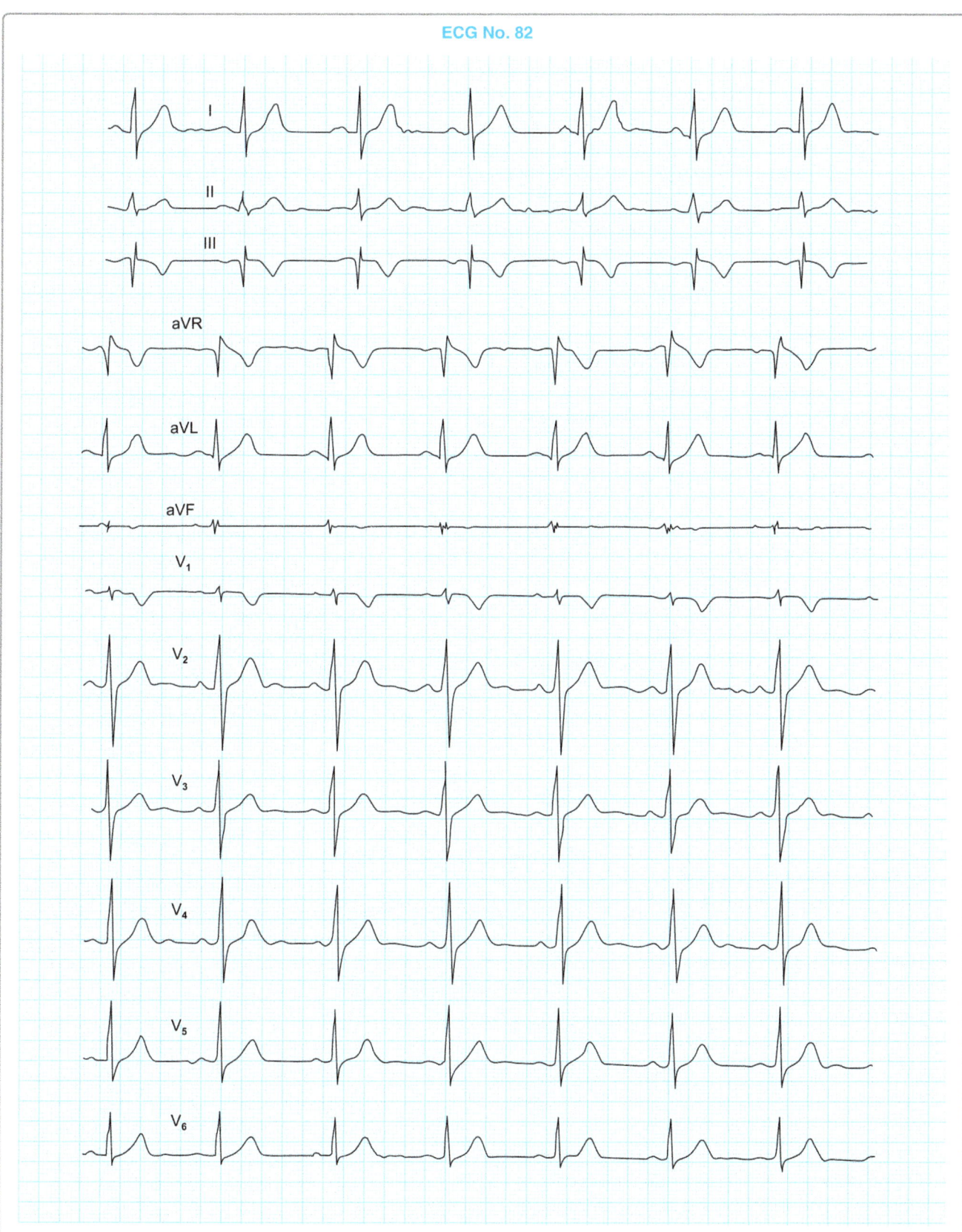

ECG in Medical Practice

ECG No. 83

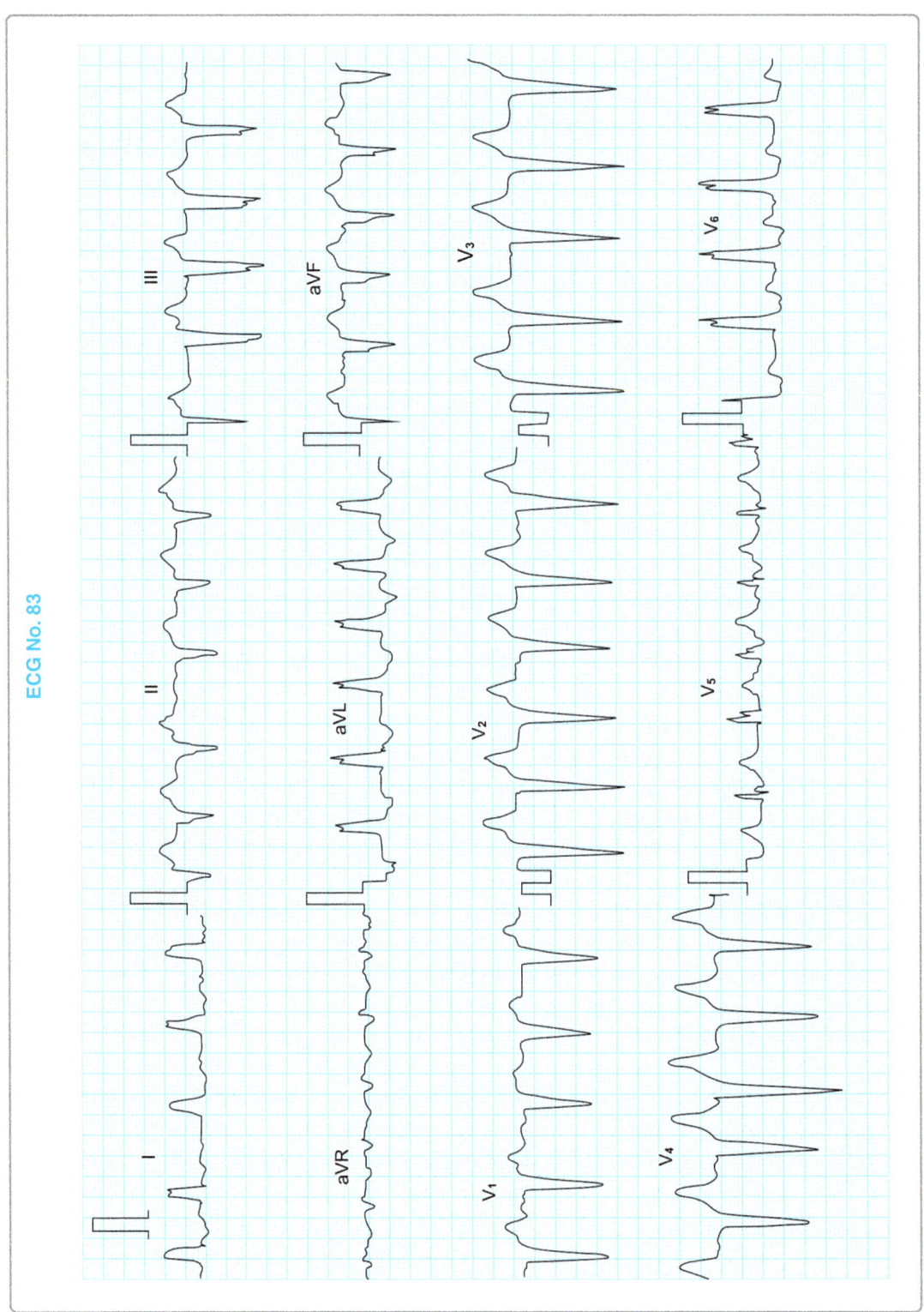

ECG No. 84

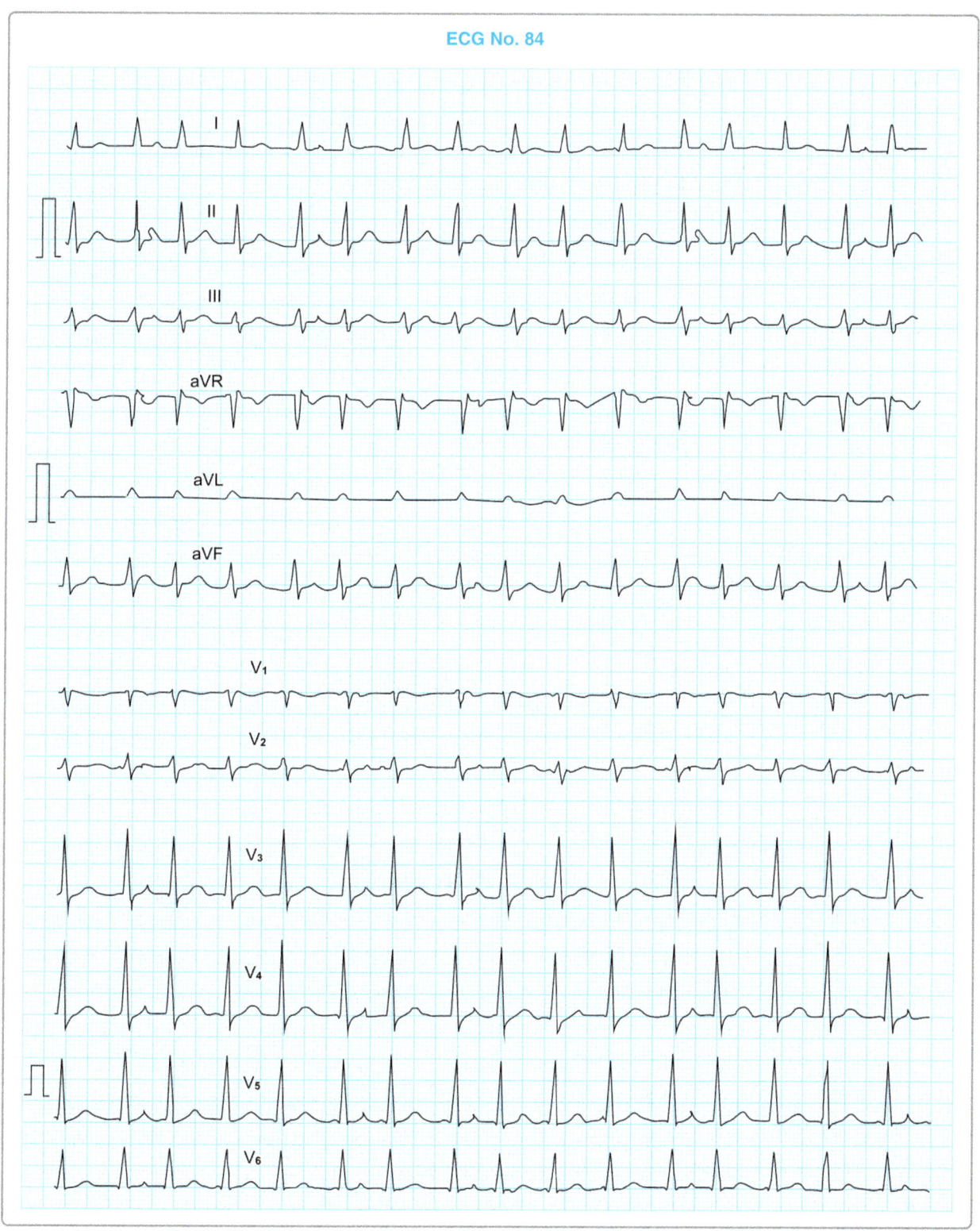

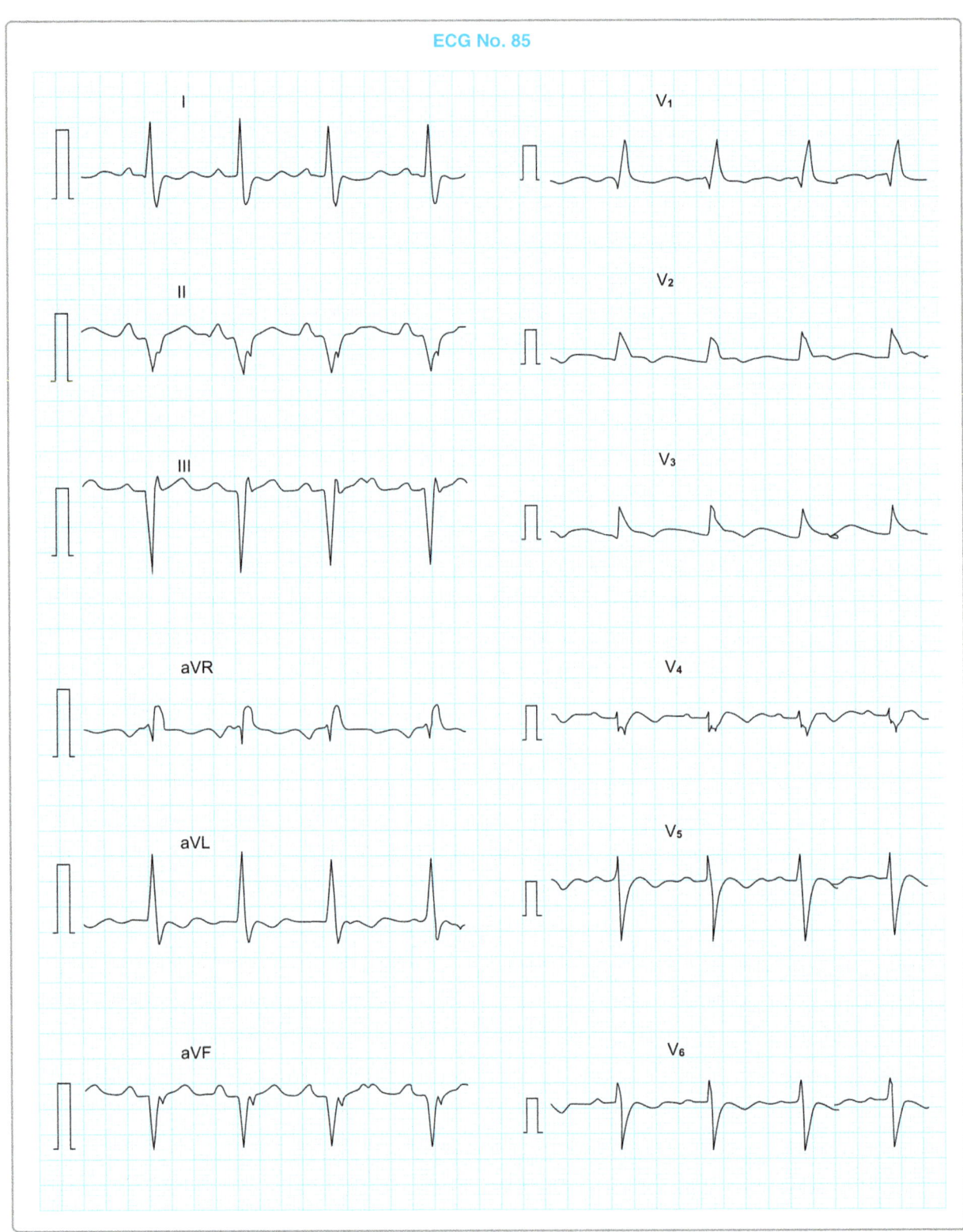

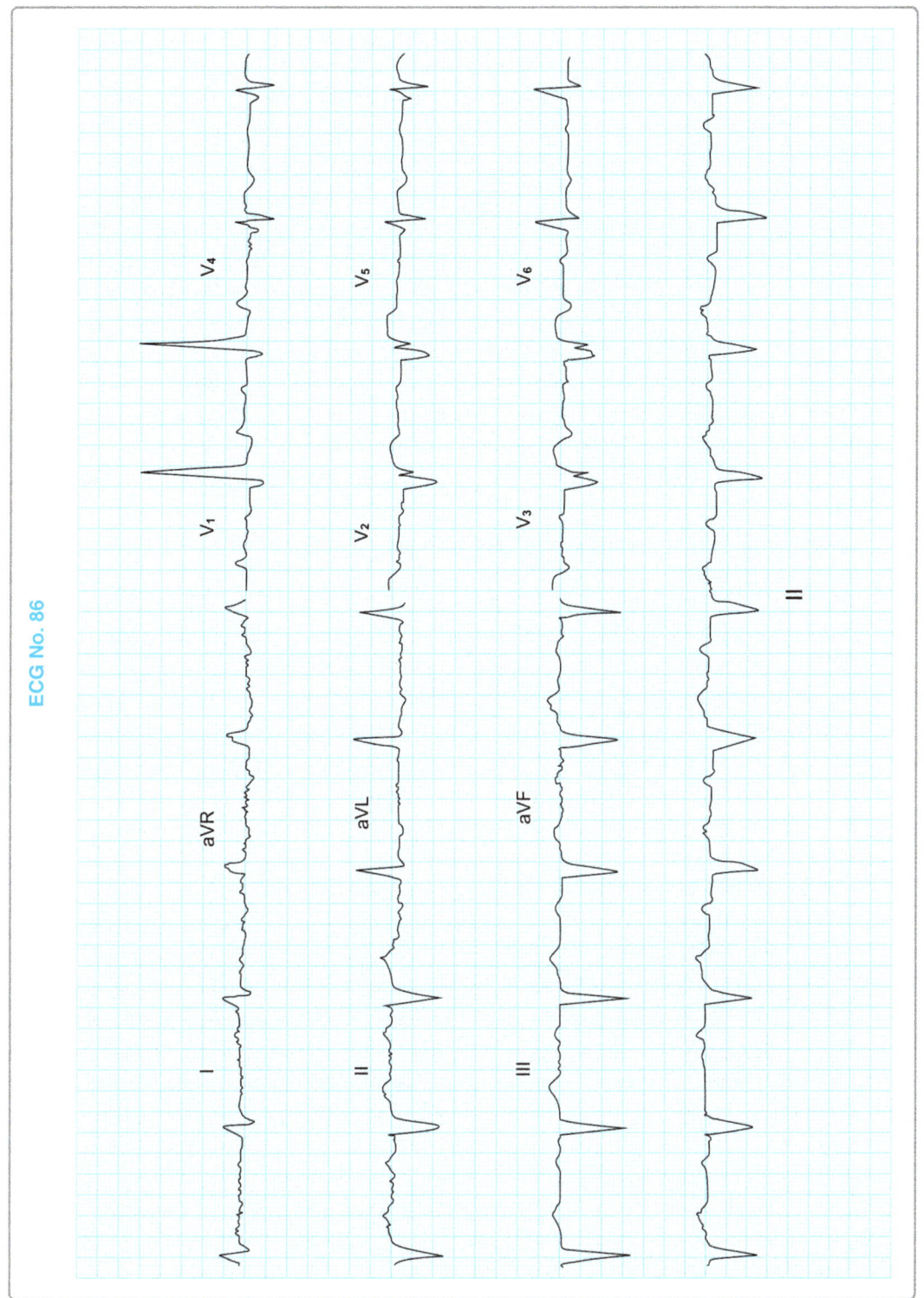

ECG No. 86

ECG in Medical Practice

ECG No. 87

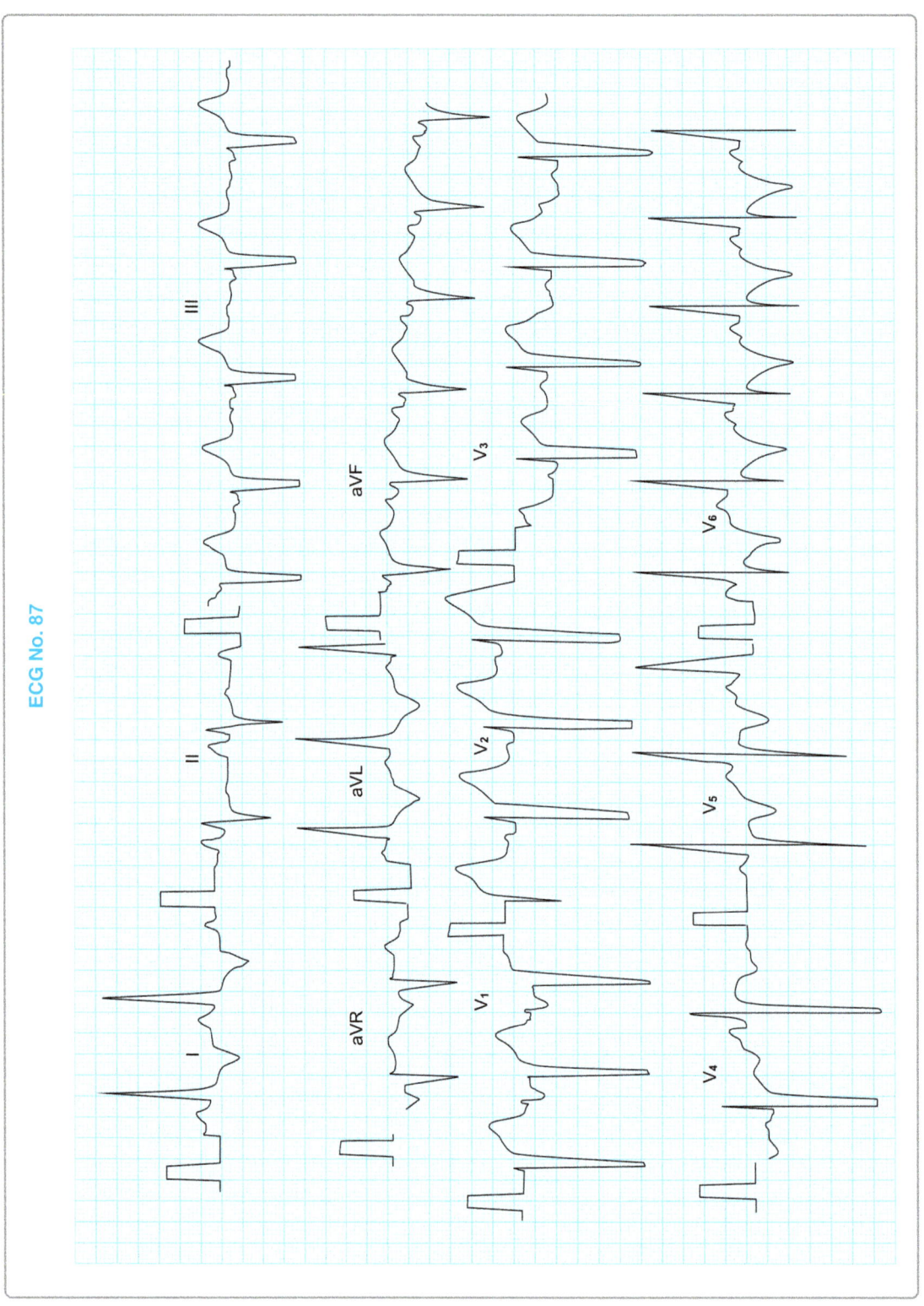

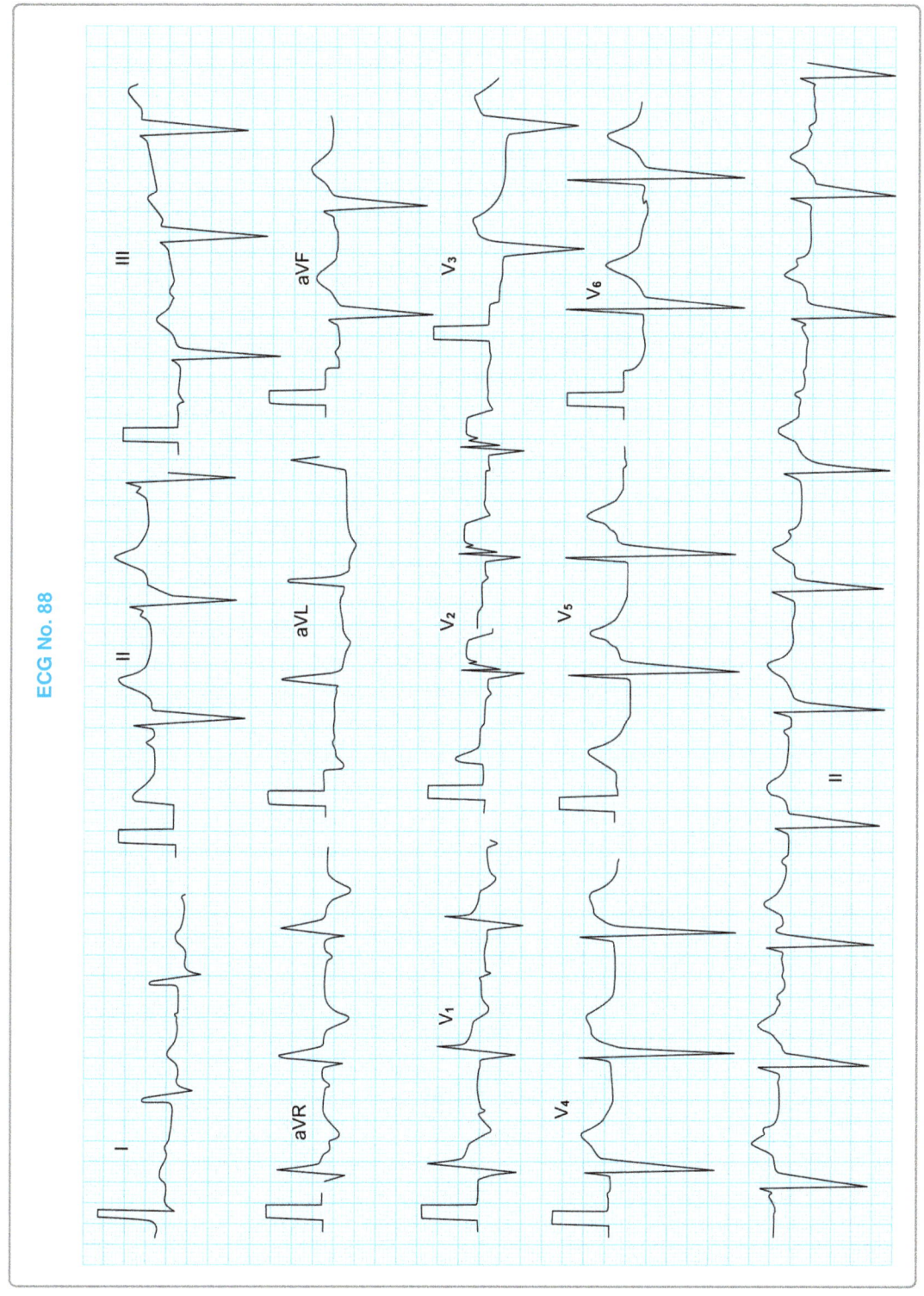

ECG in Medical Practice

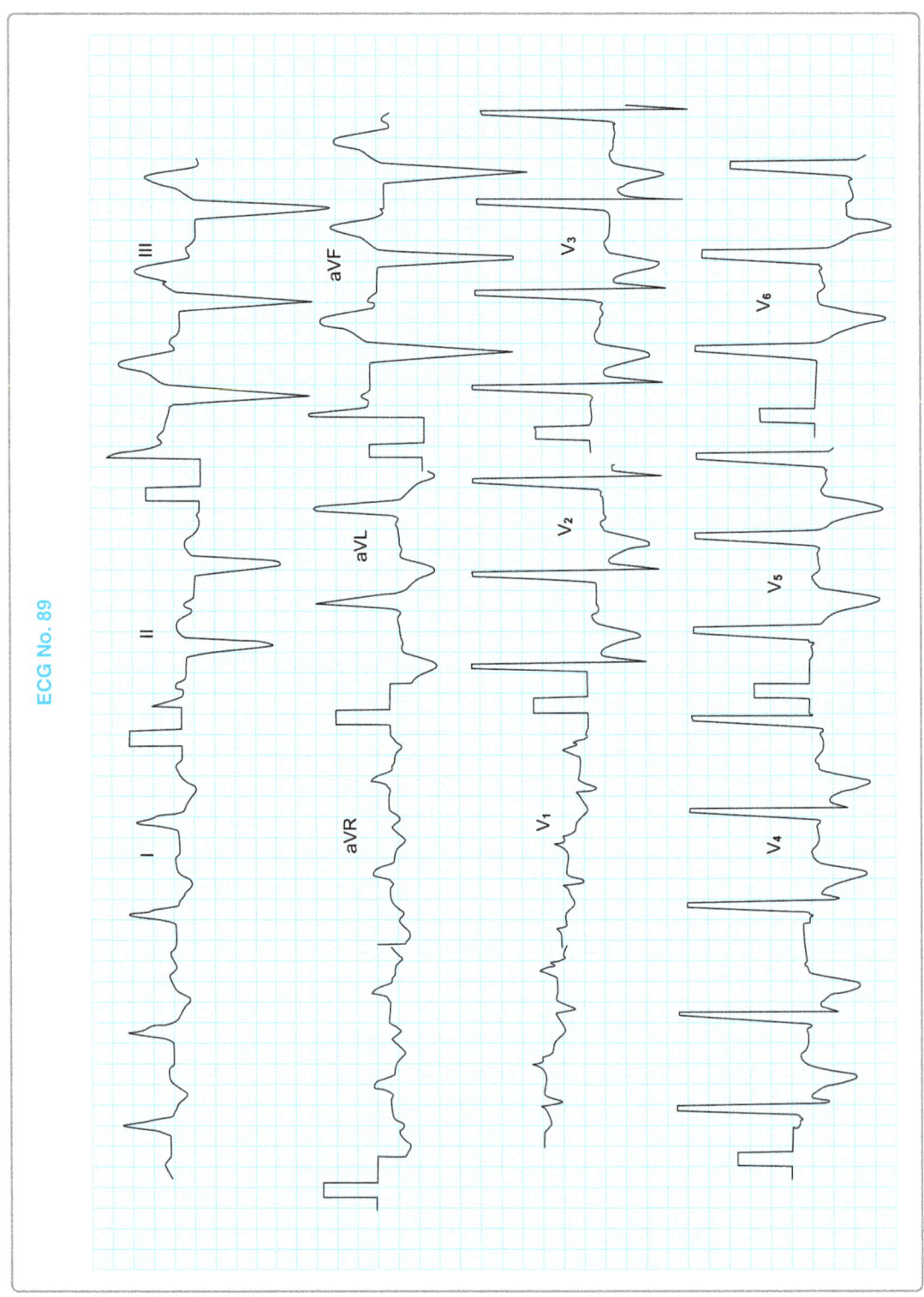

ECG No. 89

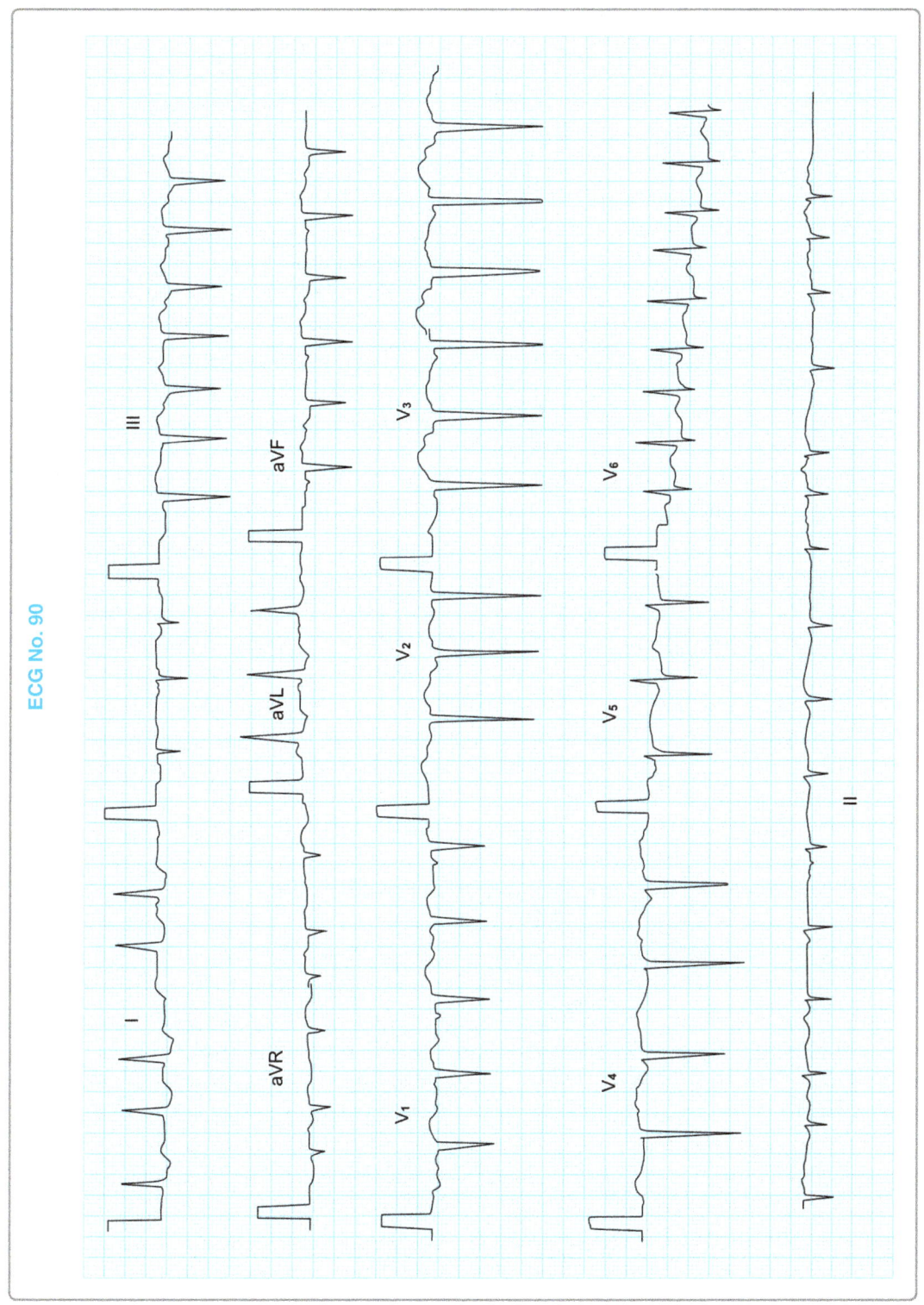

ECG in Medical Practice

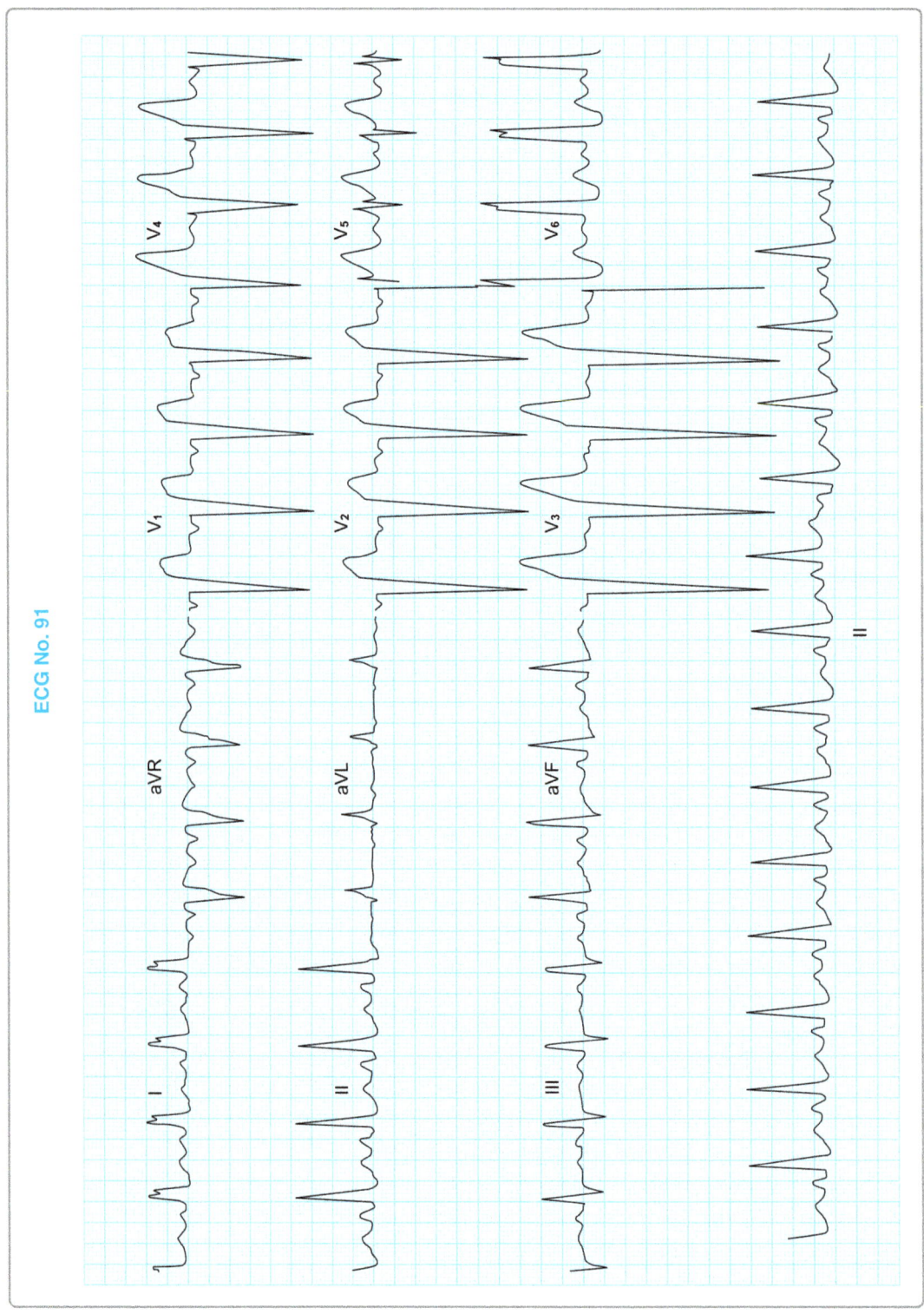

ECG No. 91

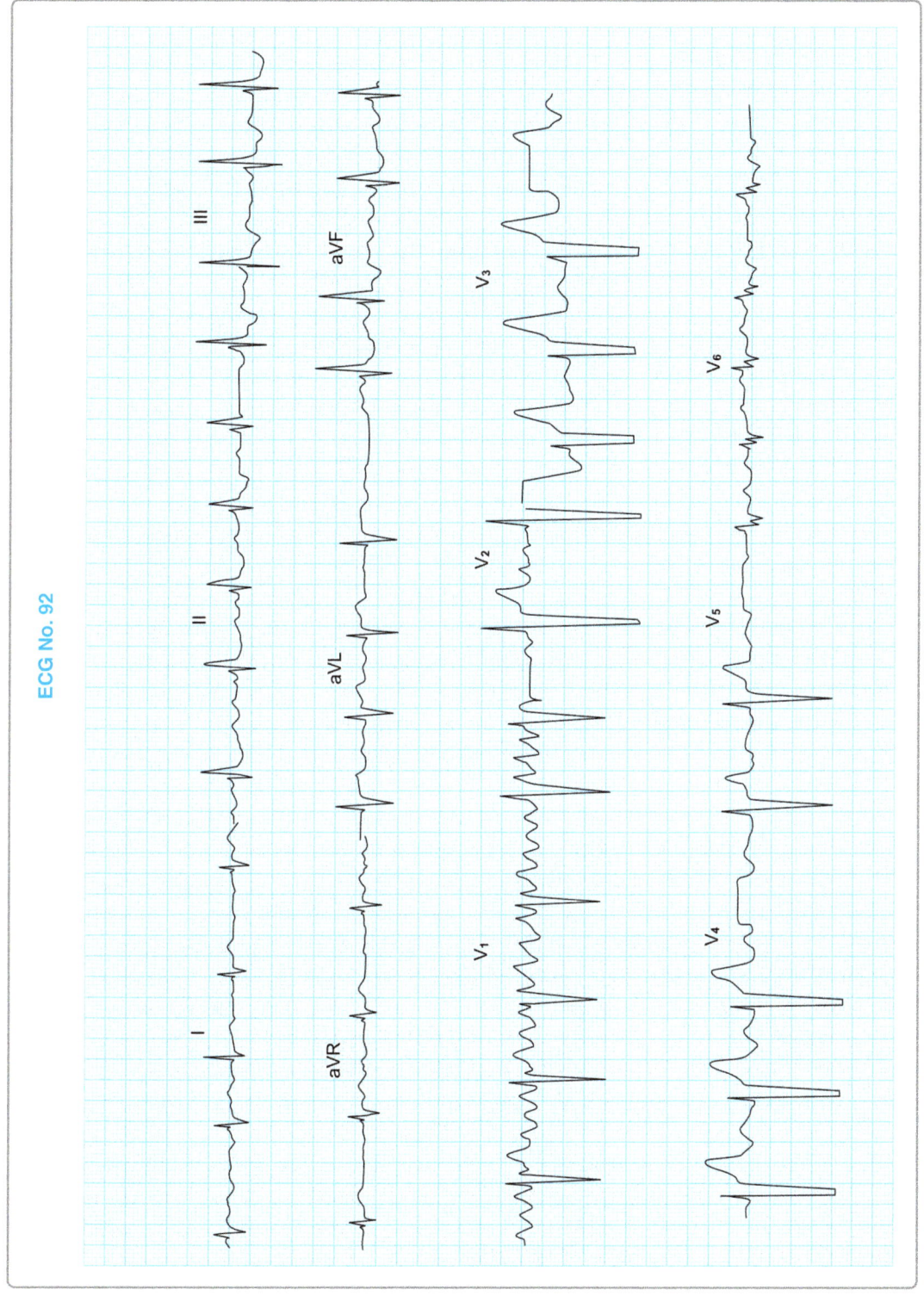

ECG No. 92

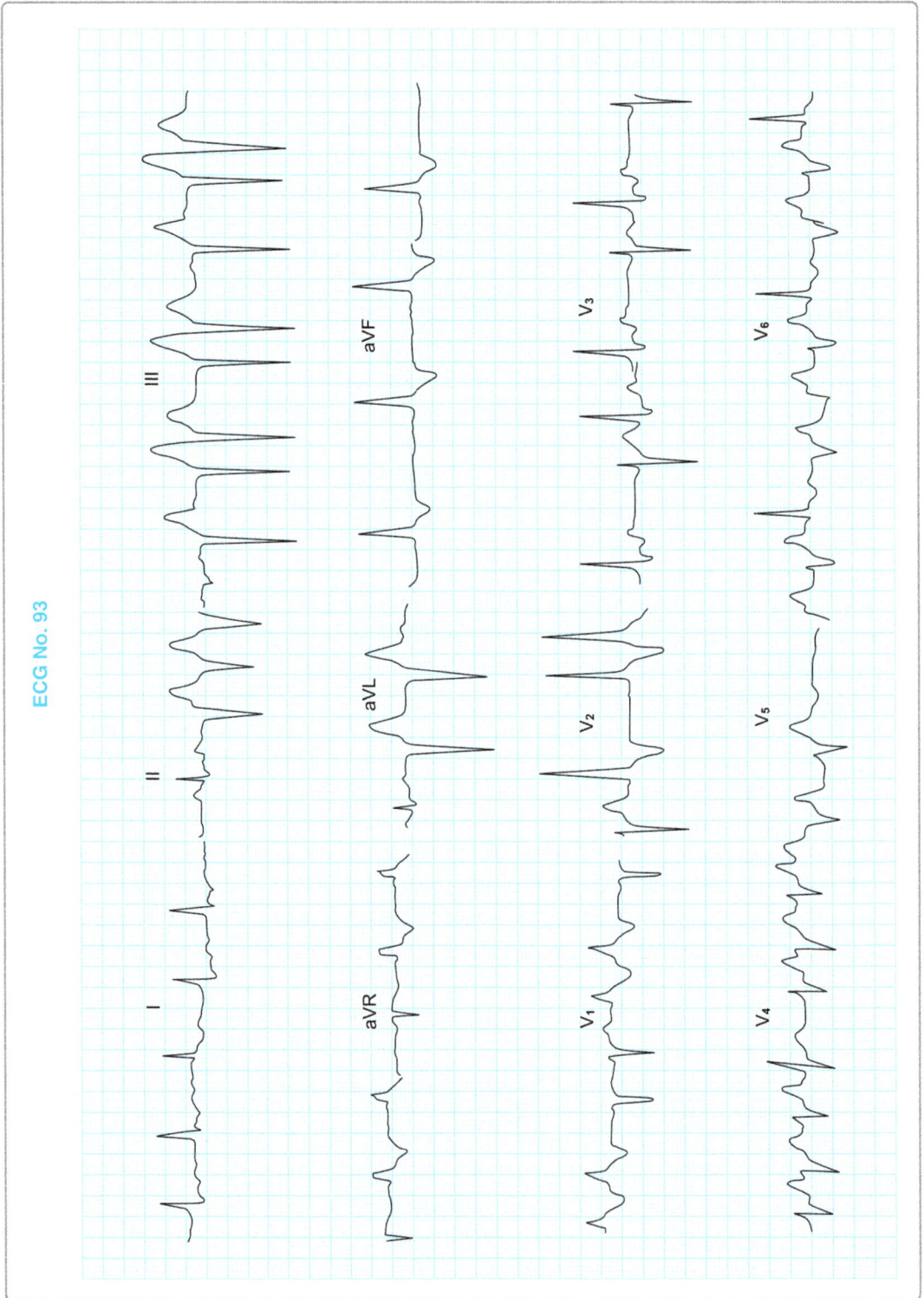

ECG No. 93

ECG No. 94

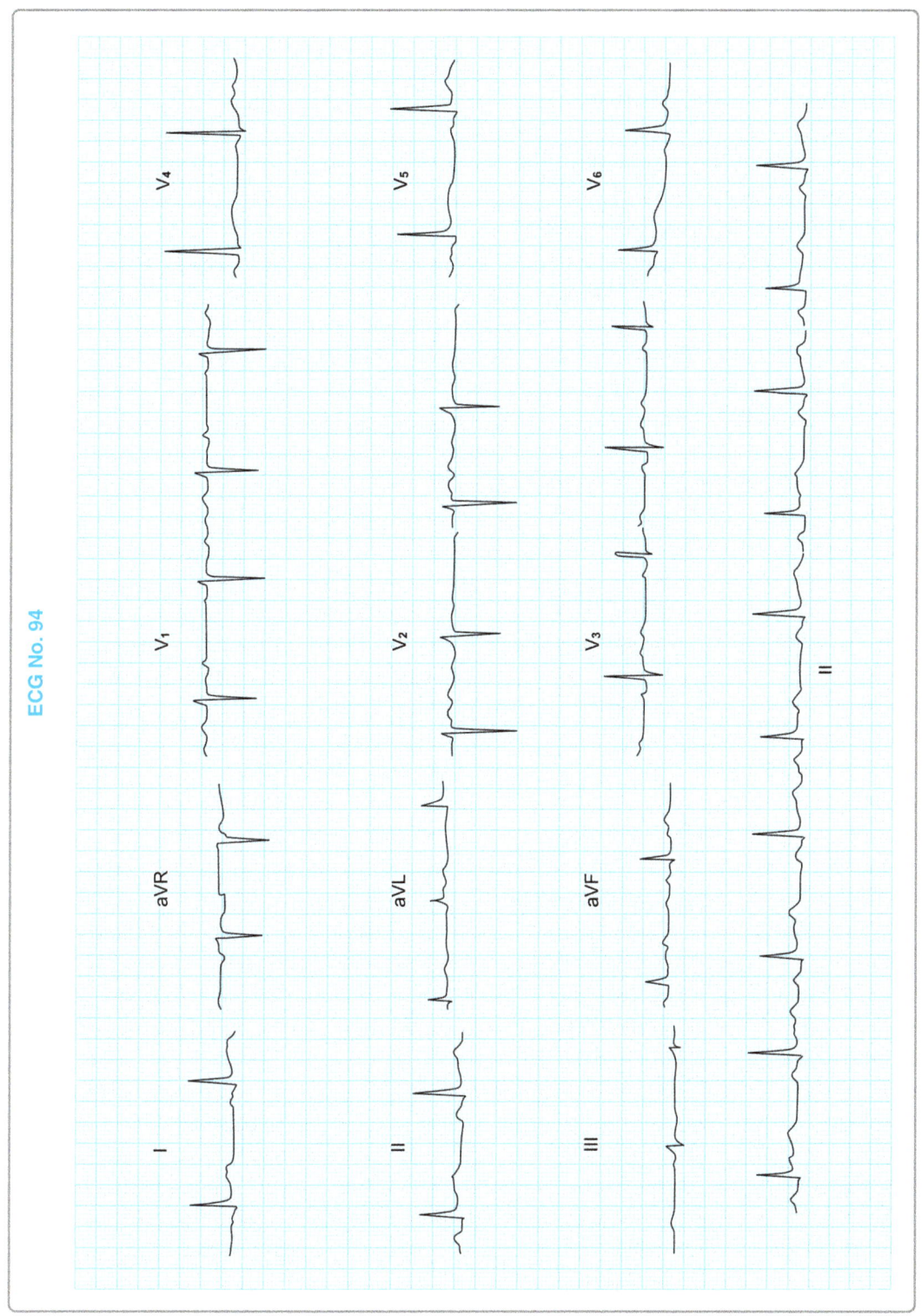

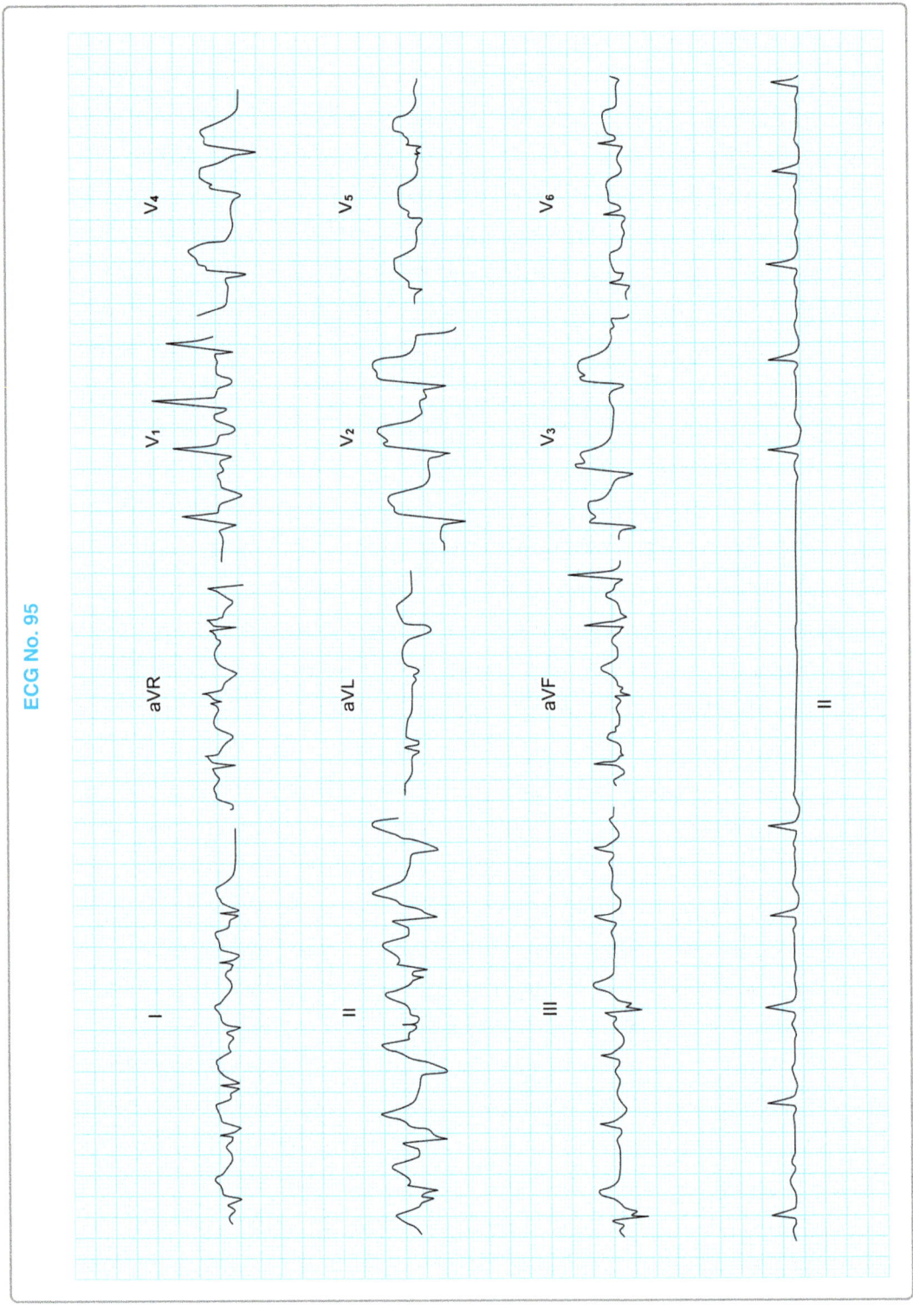

ECG No. 95

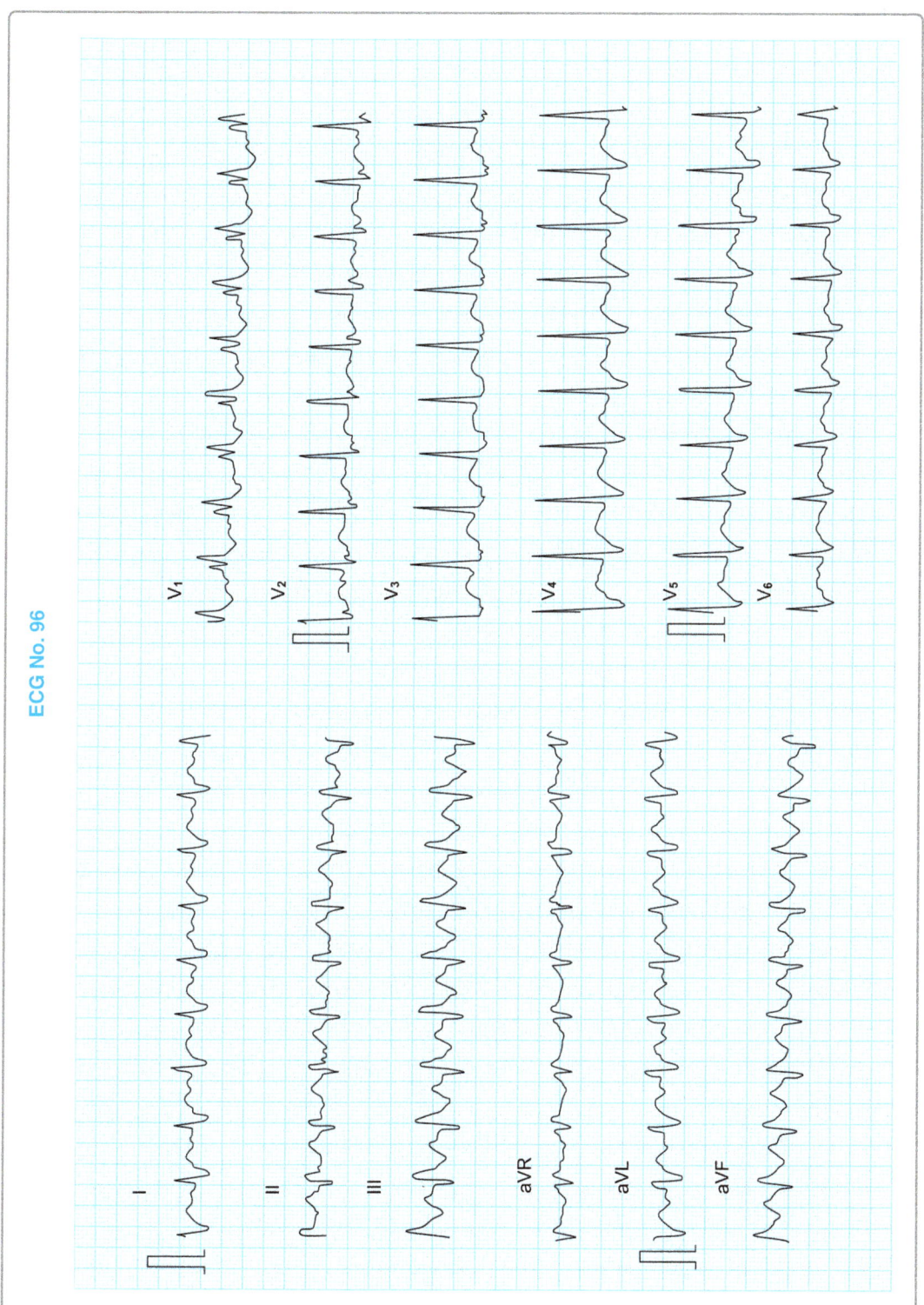

ECG in Medical Practice

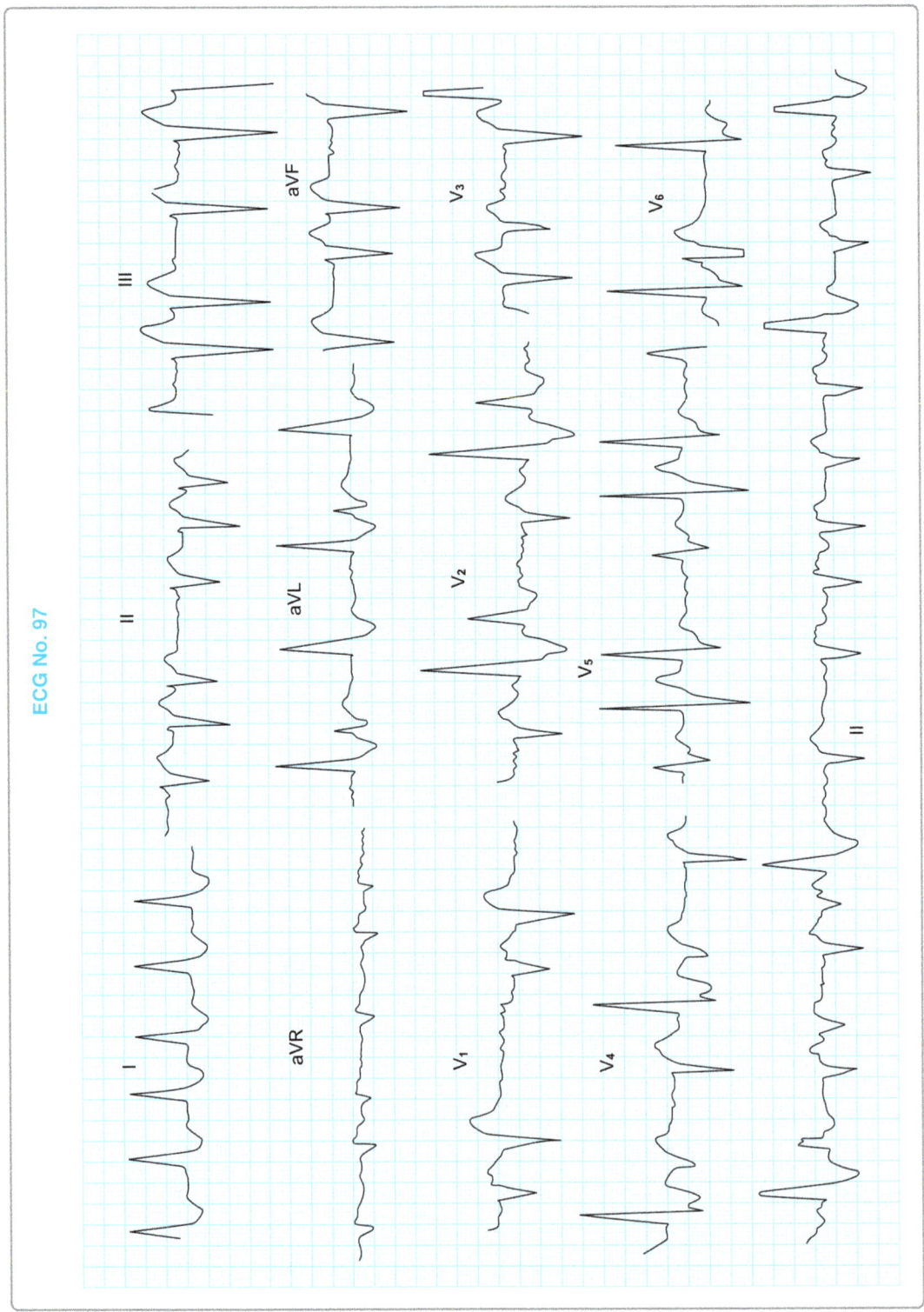

ECG No. 97

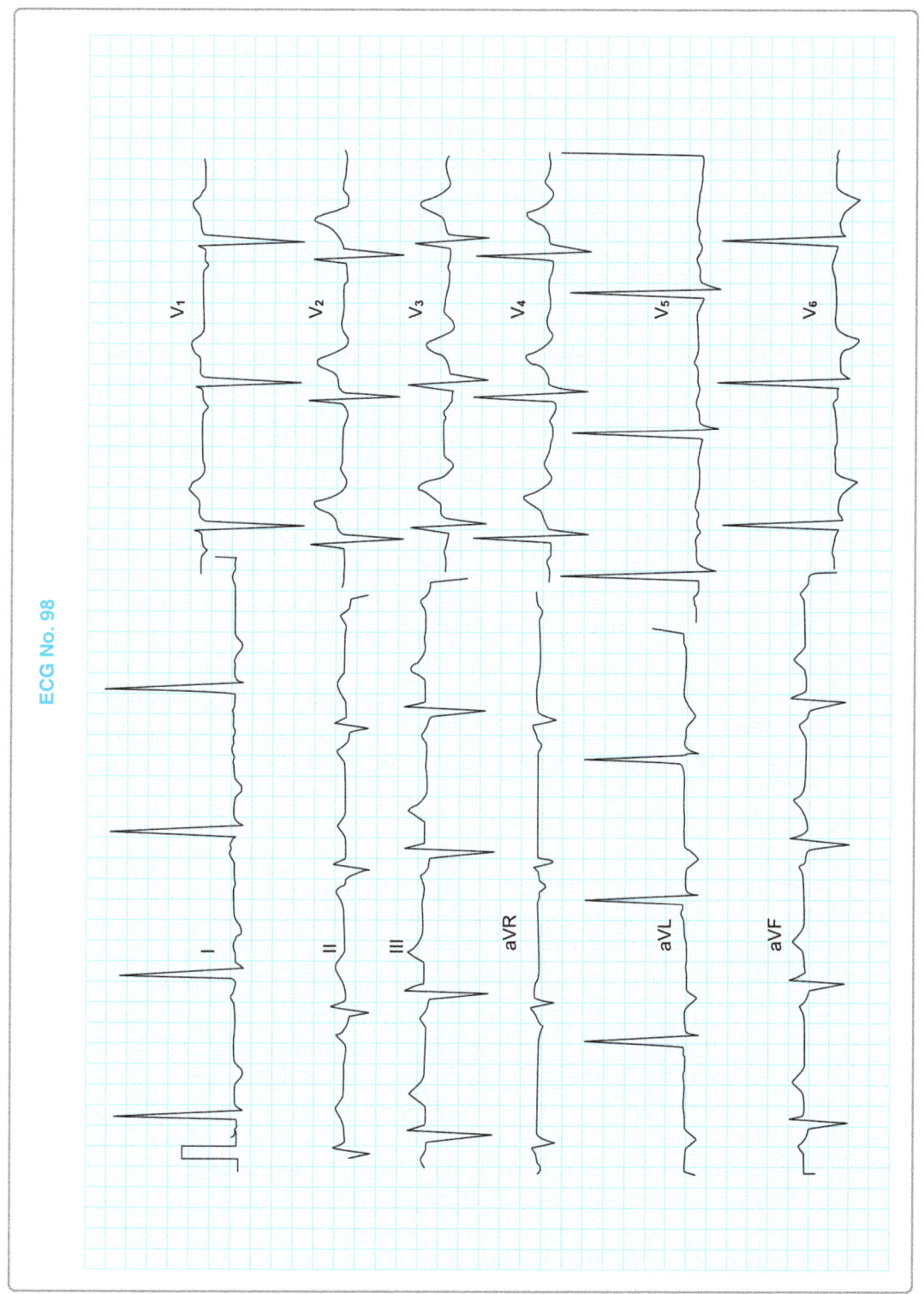

ECG in Medical Practice

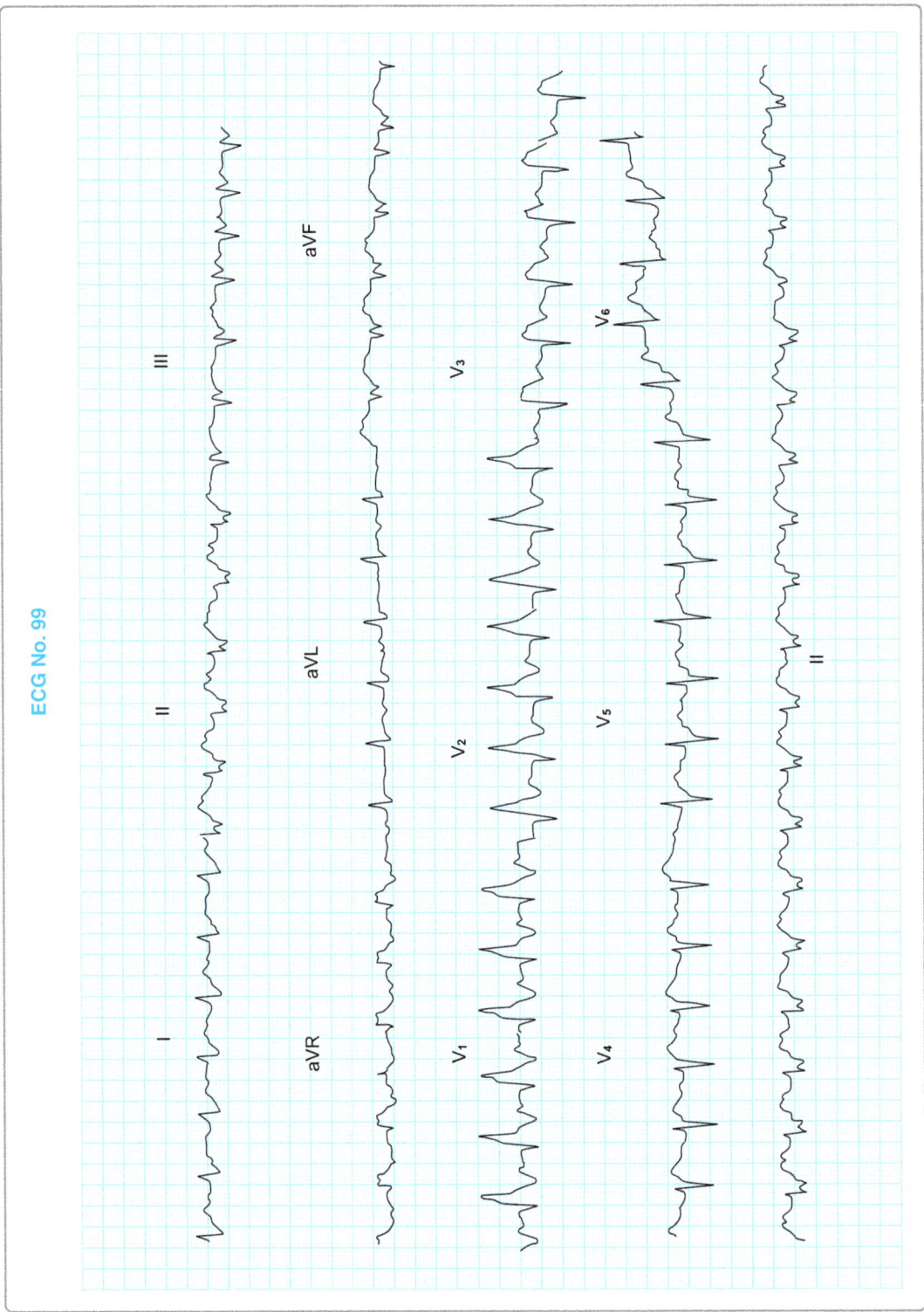

ECG No. 99

ECG No. 100

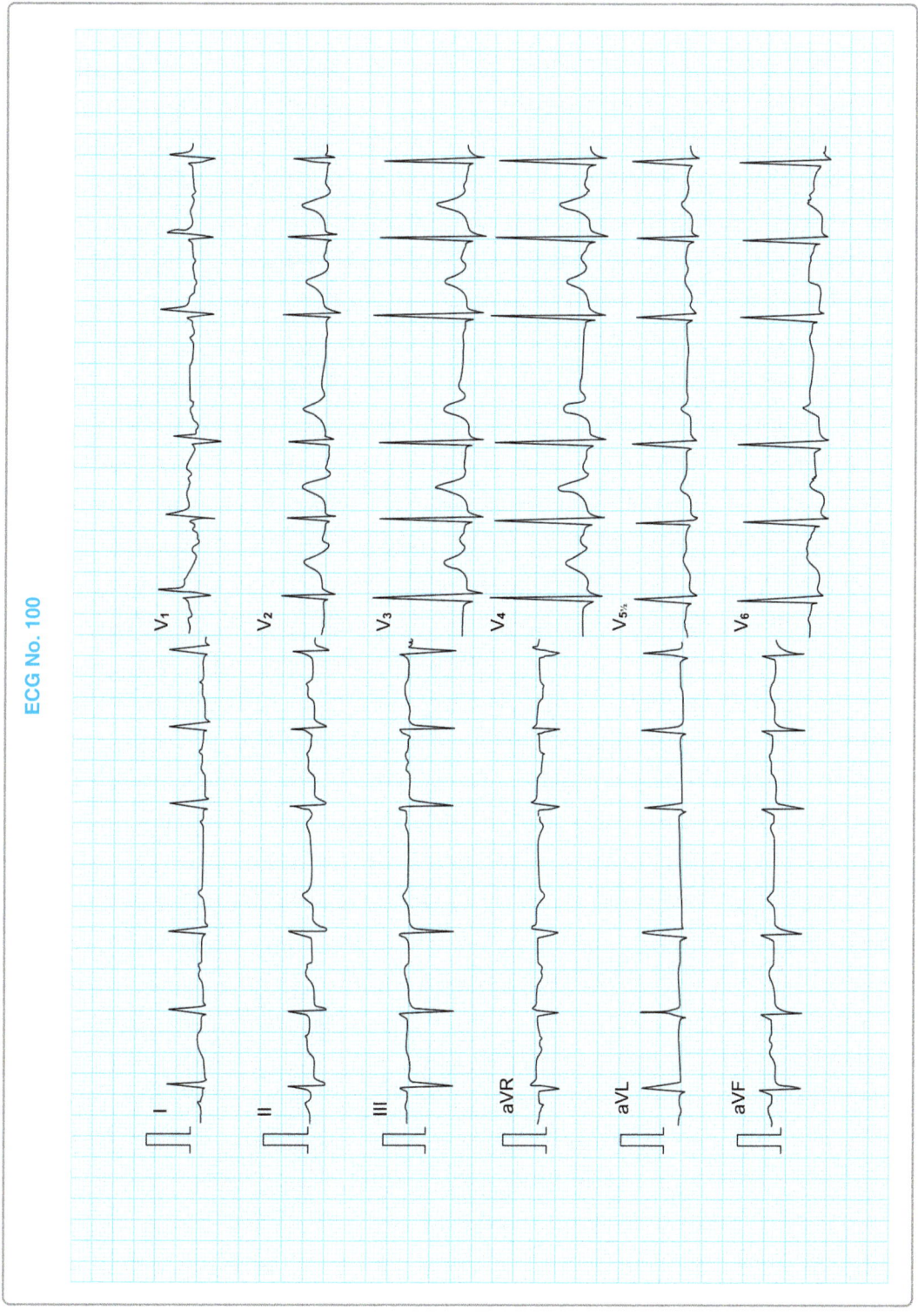

ECG in Medical Practice

ECG No. 101

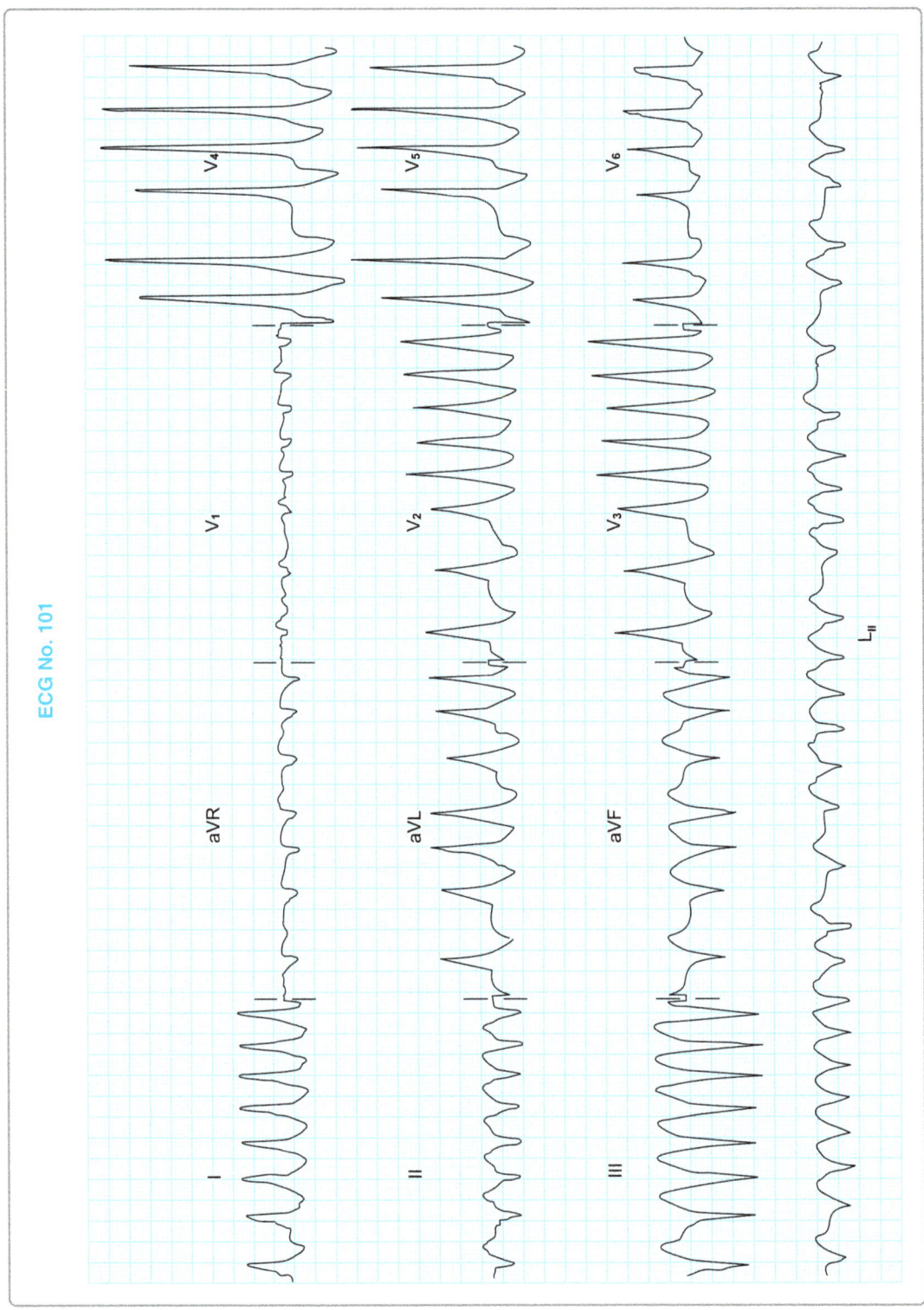

ECG No. 102

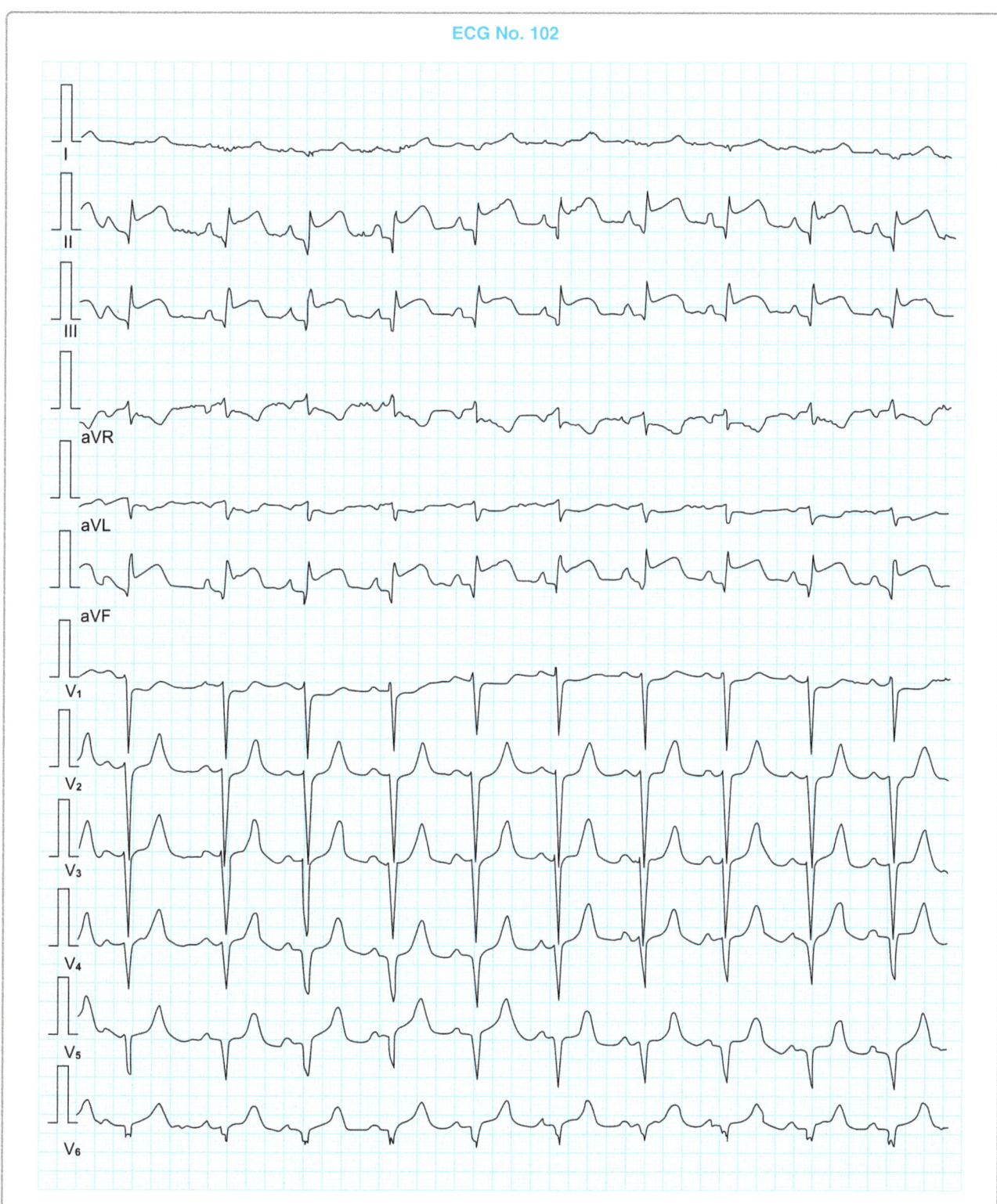

ECG in Medical Practice

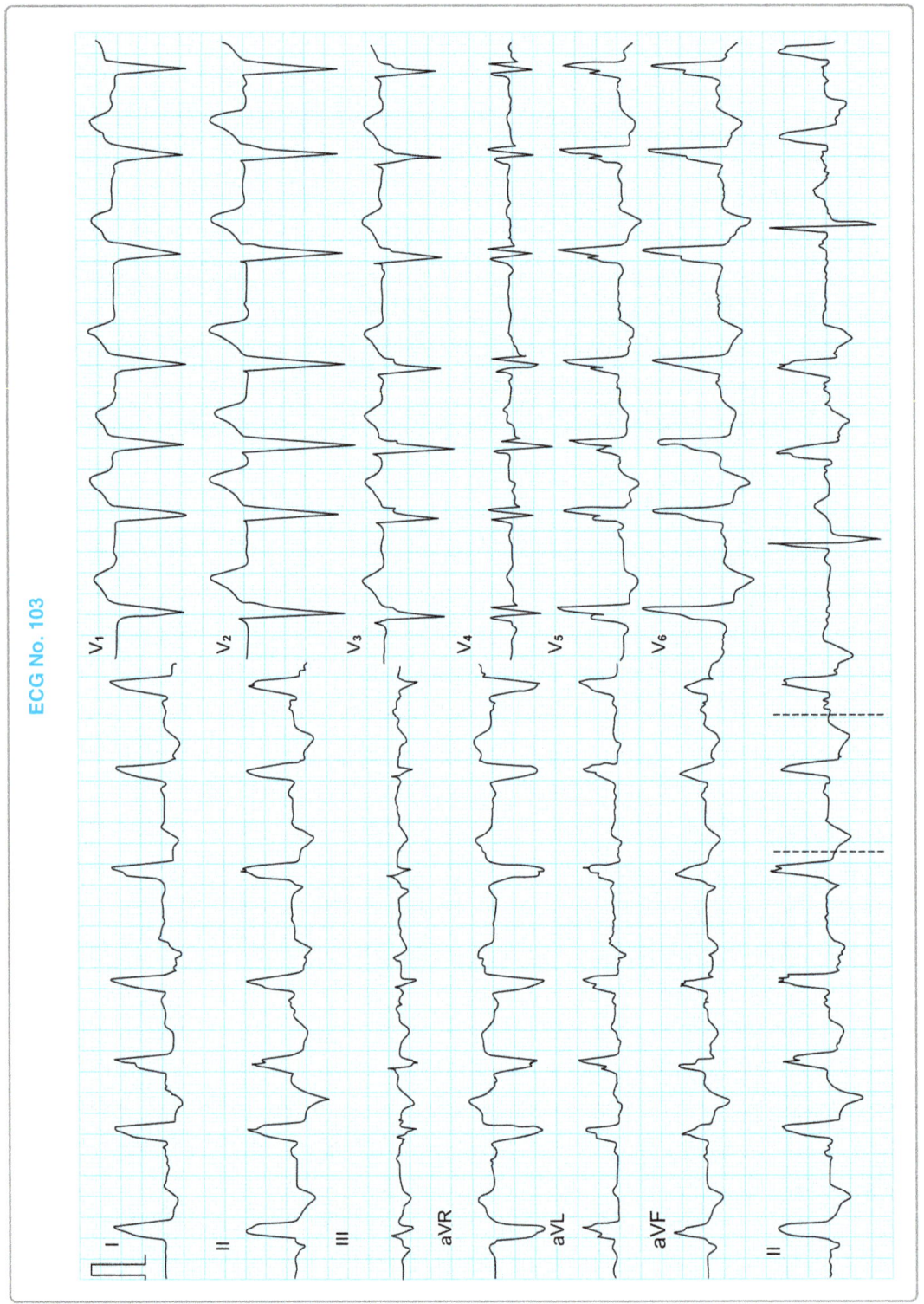

ECG No. 103

Chapter 3: 151 Tracings of ECG

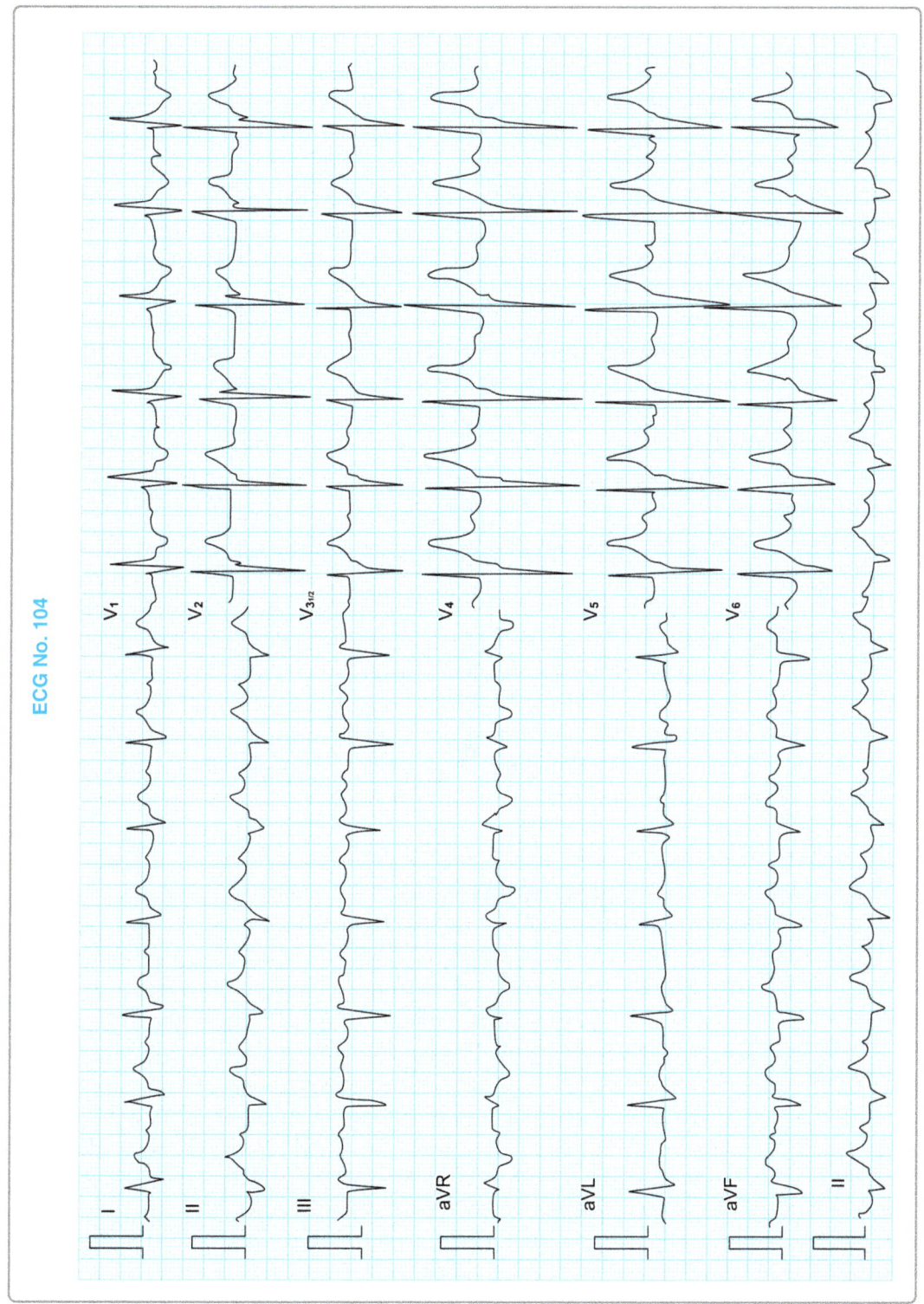

ECG No. 104

ECG in Medical Practice

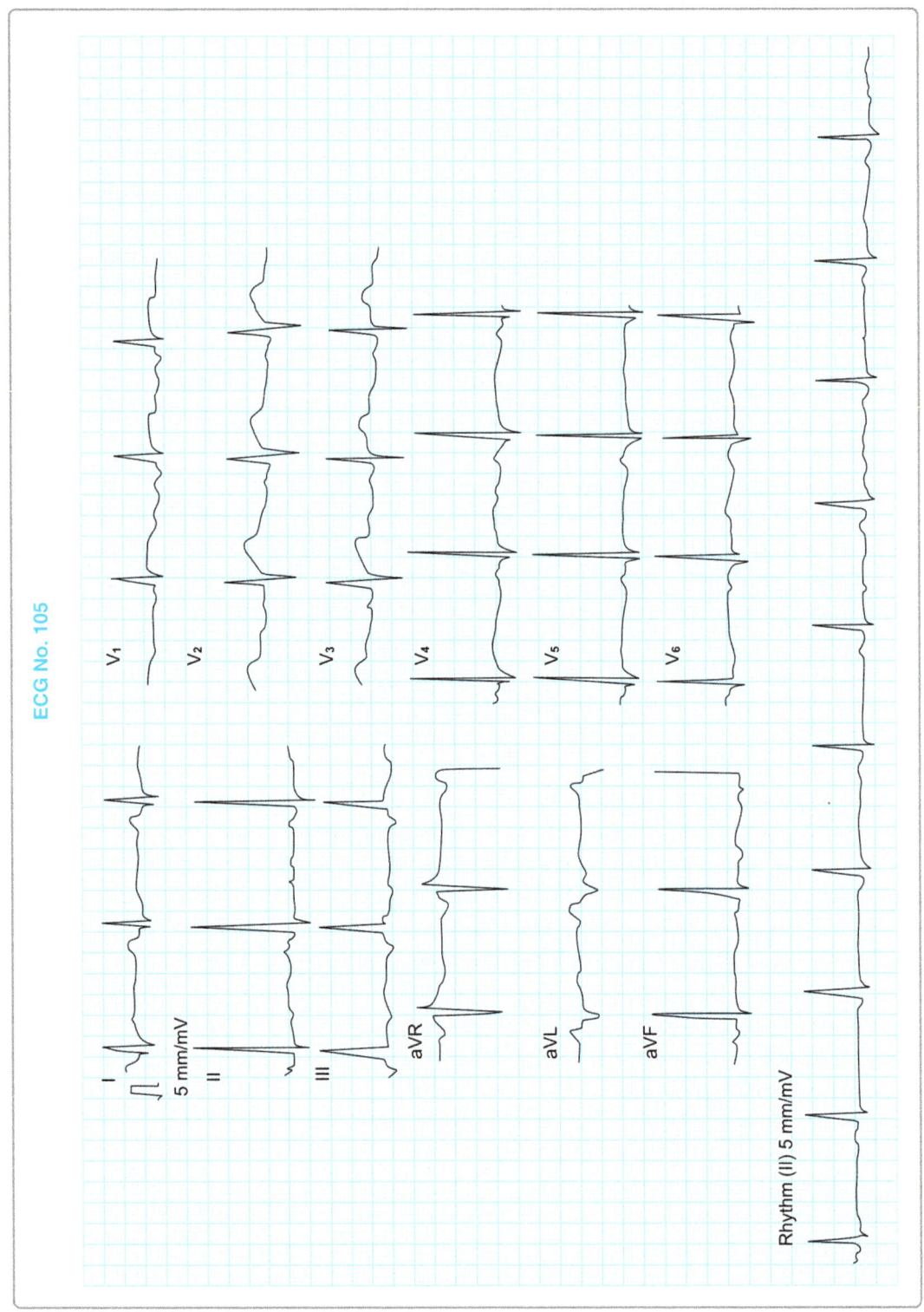

ECG No. 105

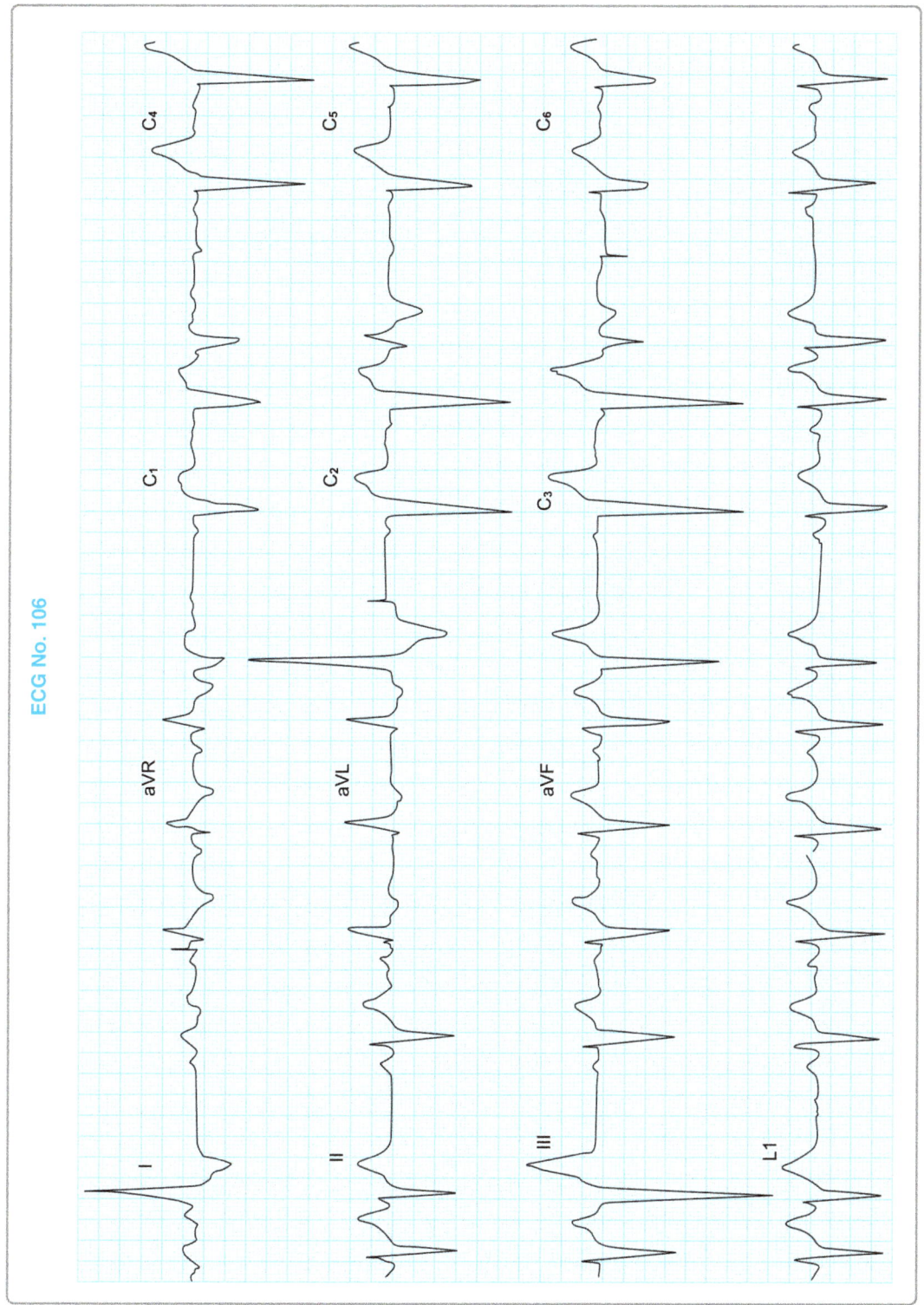

ECG in Medical Practice

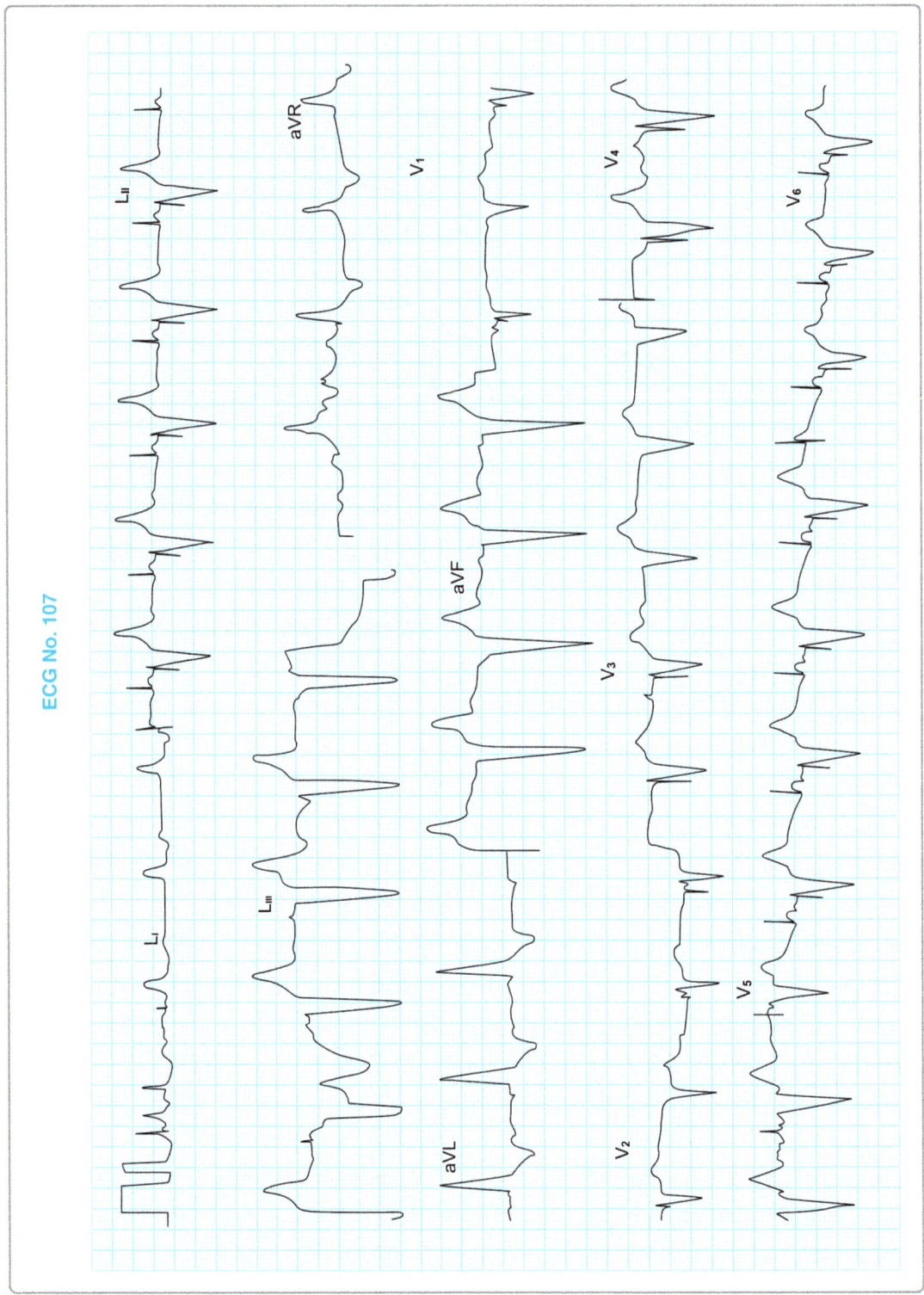

ECG No. 107

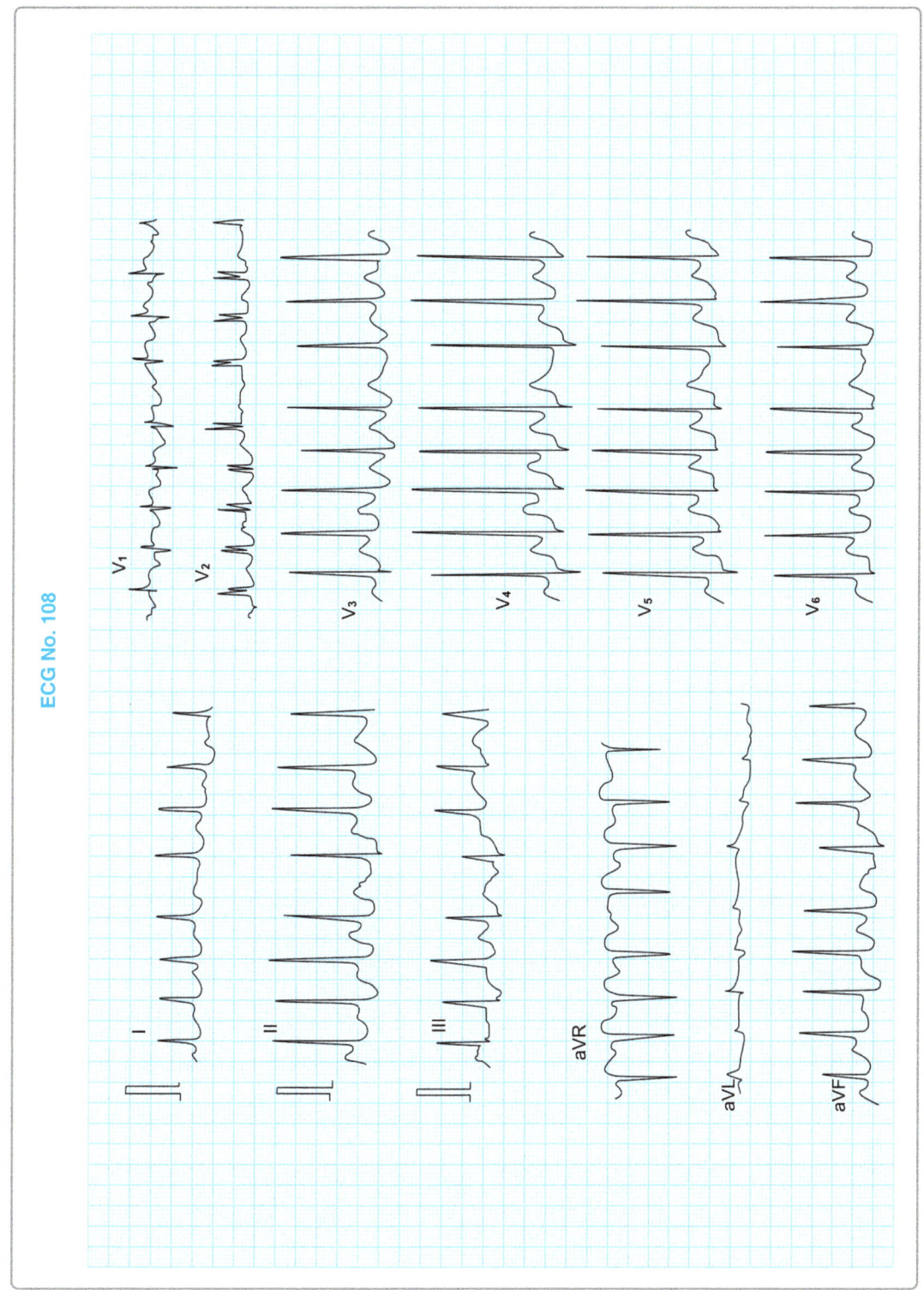

ECG No. 108

ECG in Medical Practice

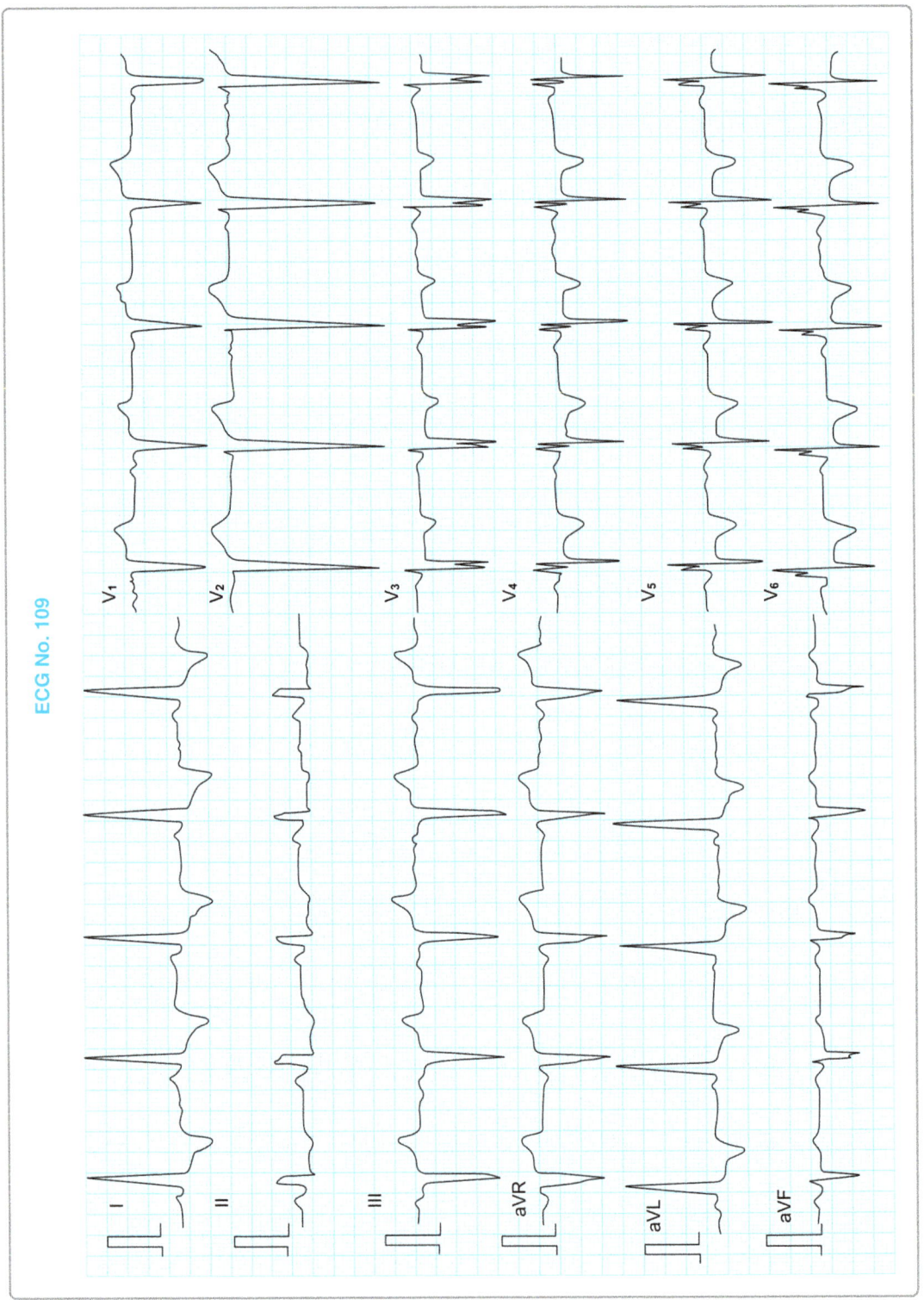

ECG No. 109

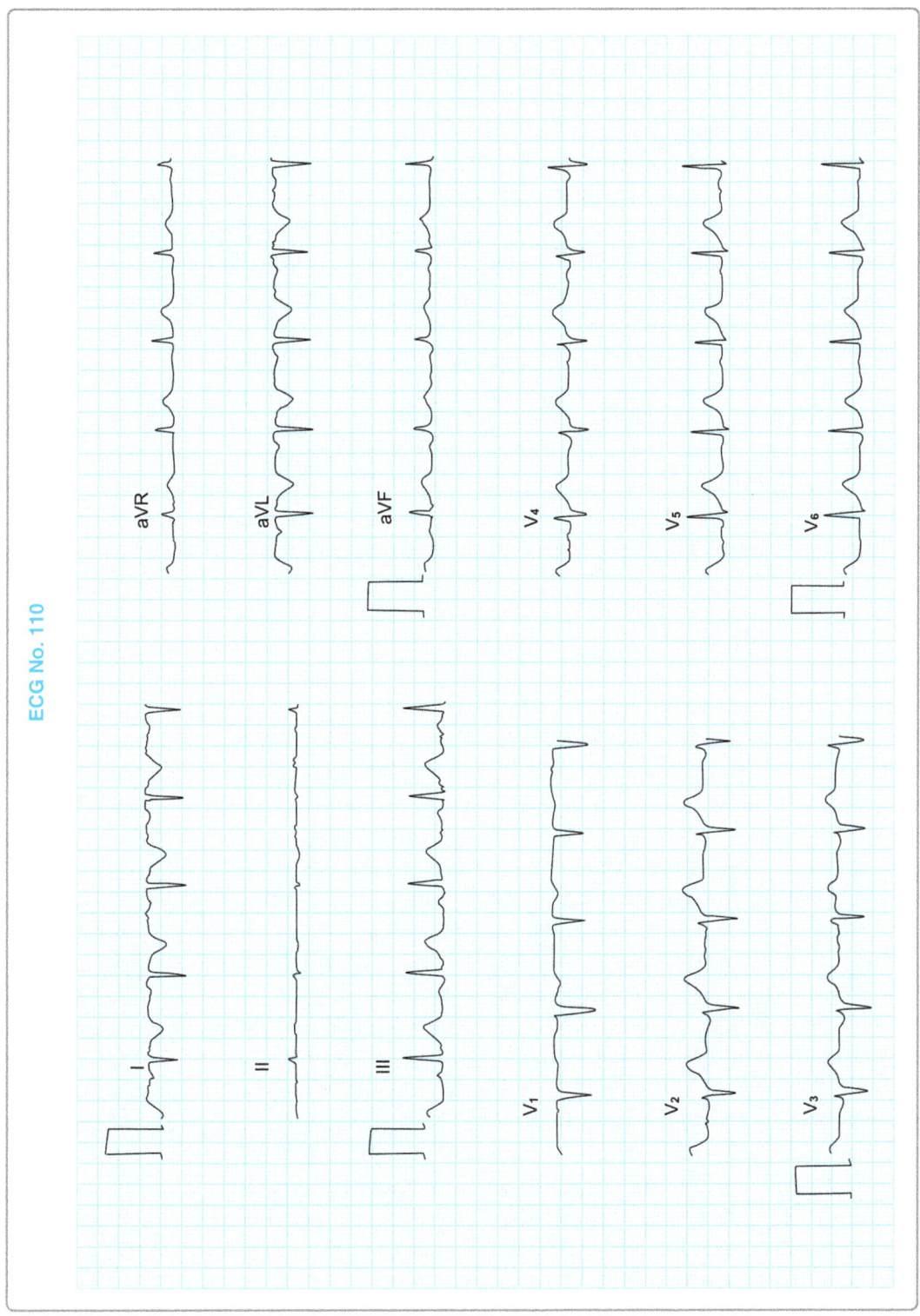

ECG No. 111

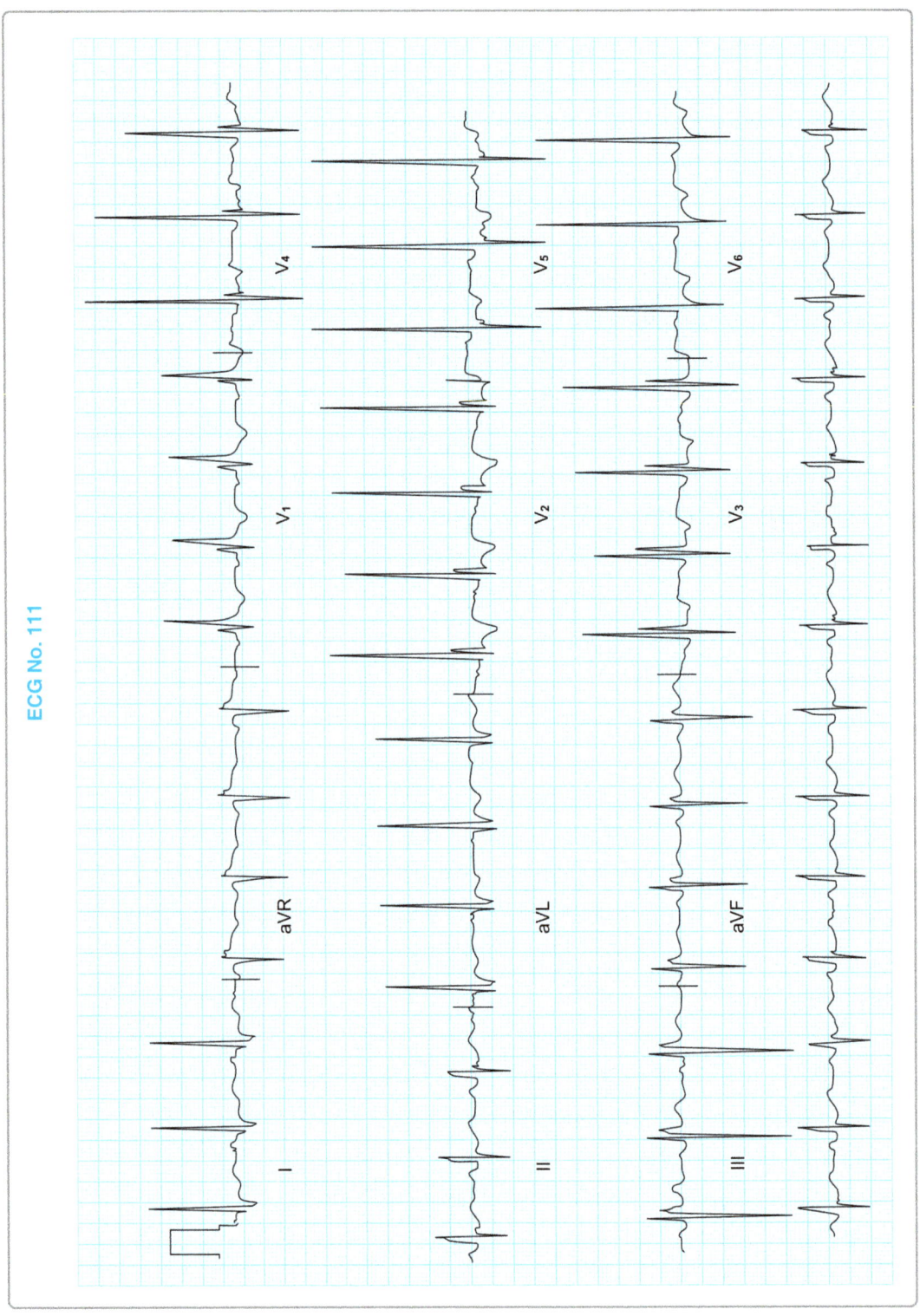

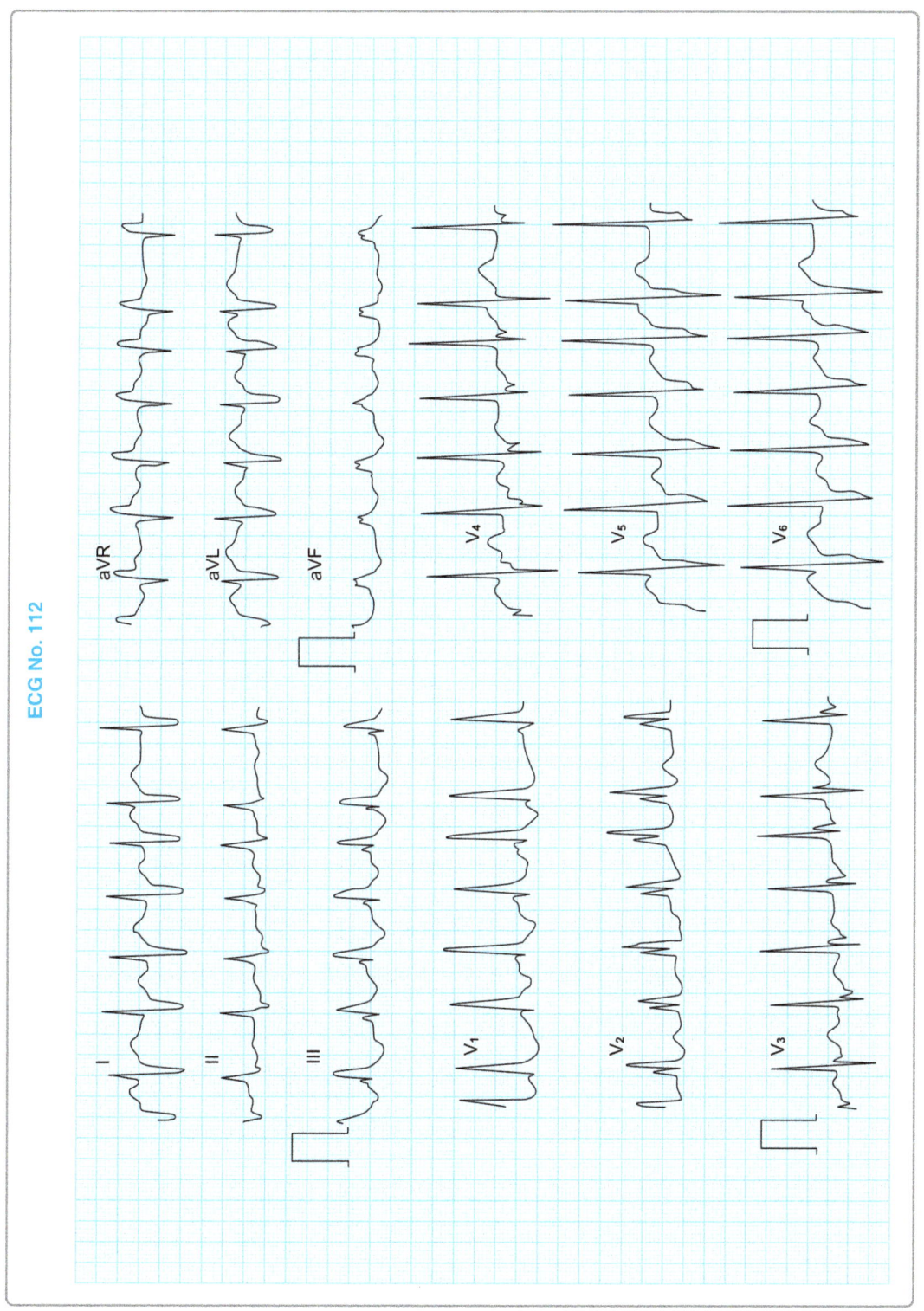

ECG in Medical Practice

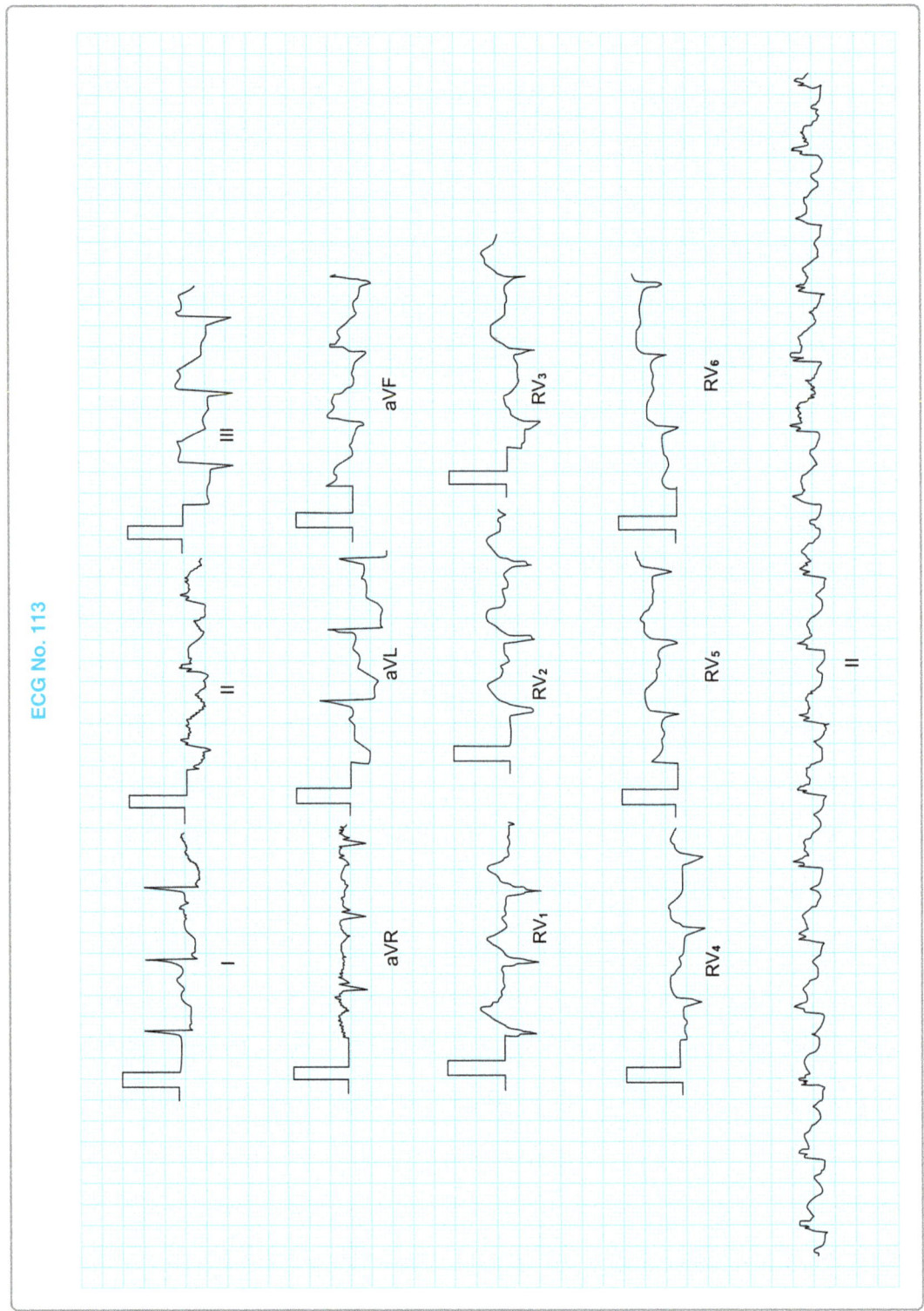

ECG No. 113

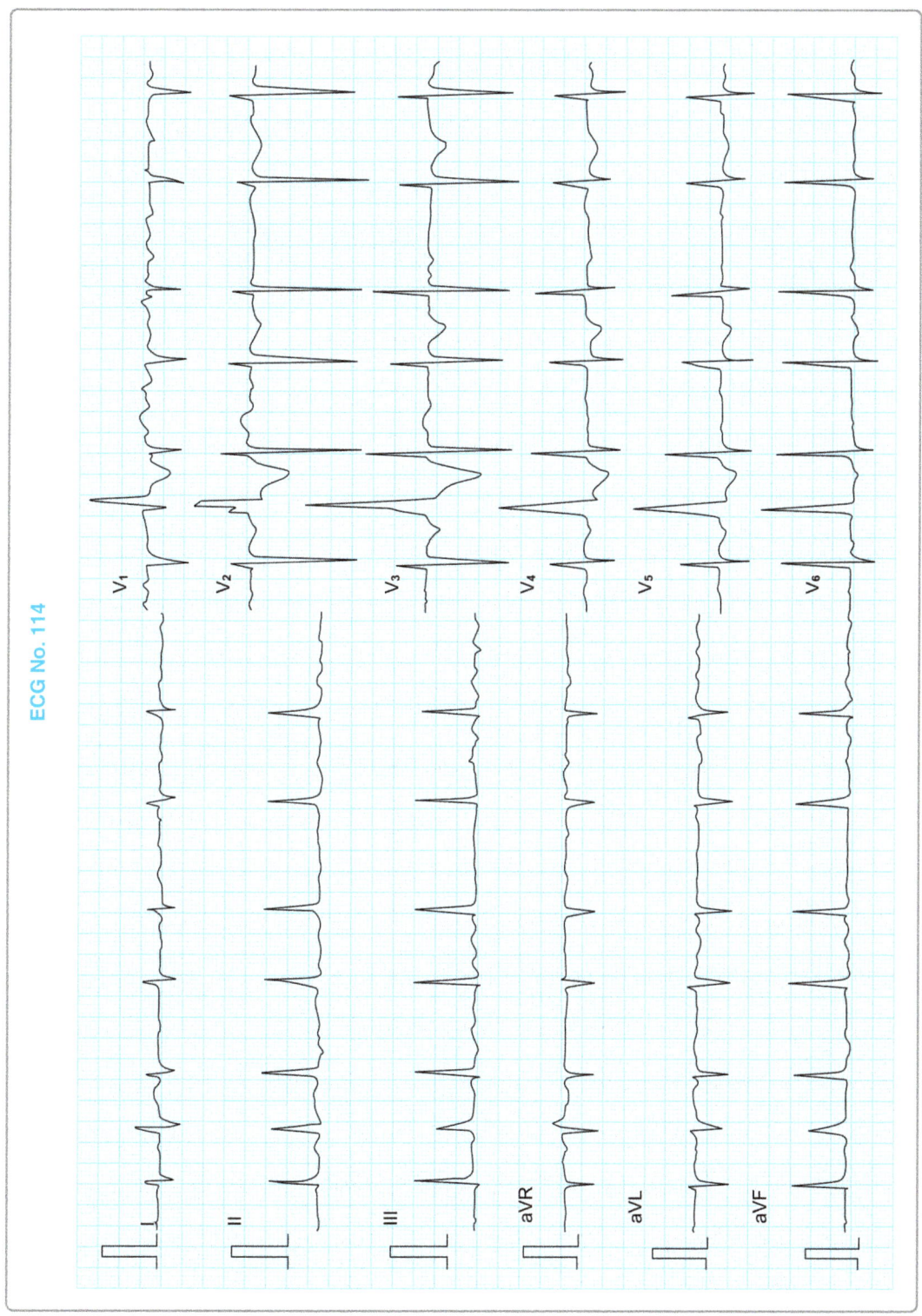

ECG in Medical Practice

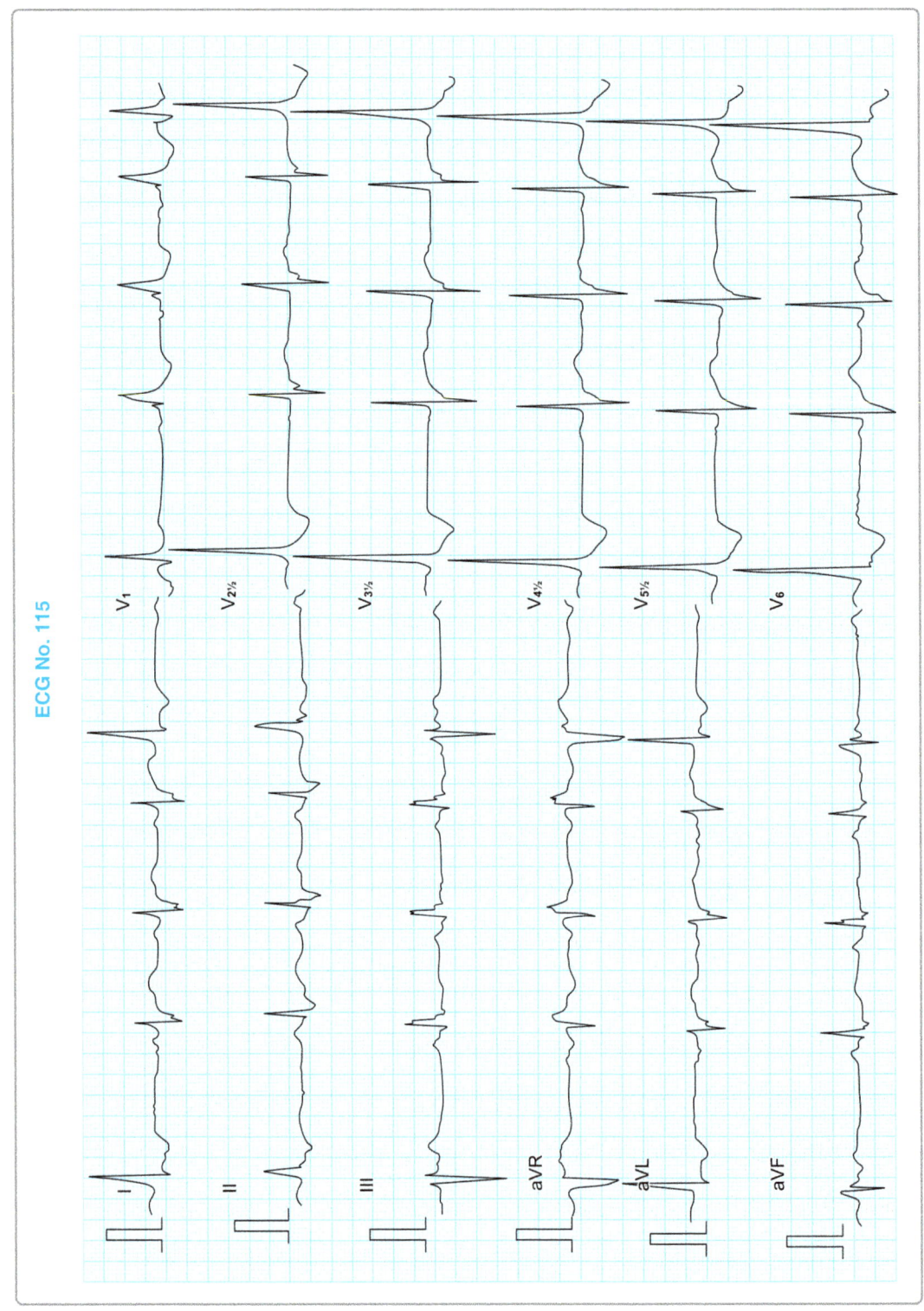

ECG No. 115

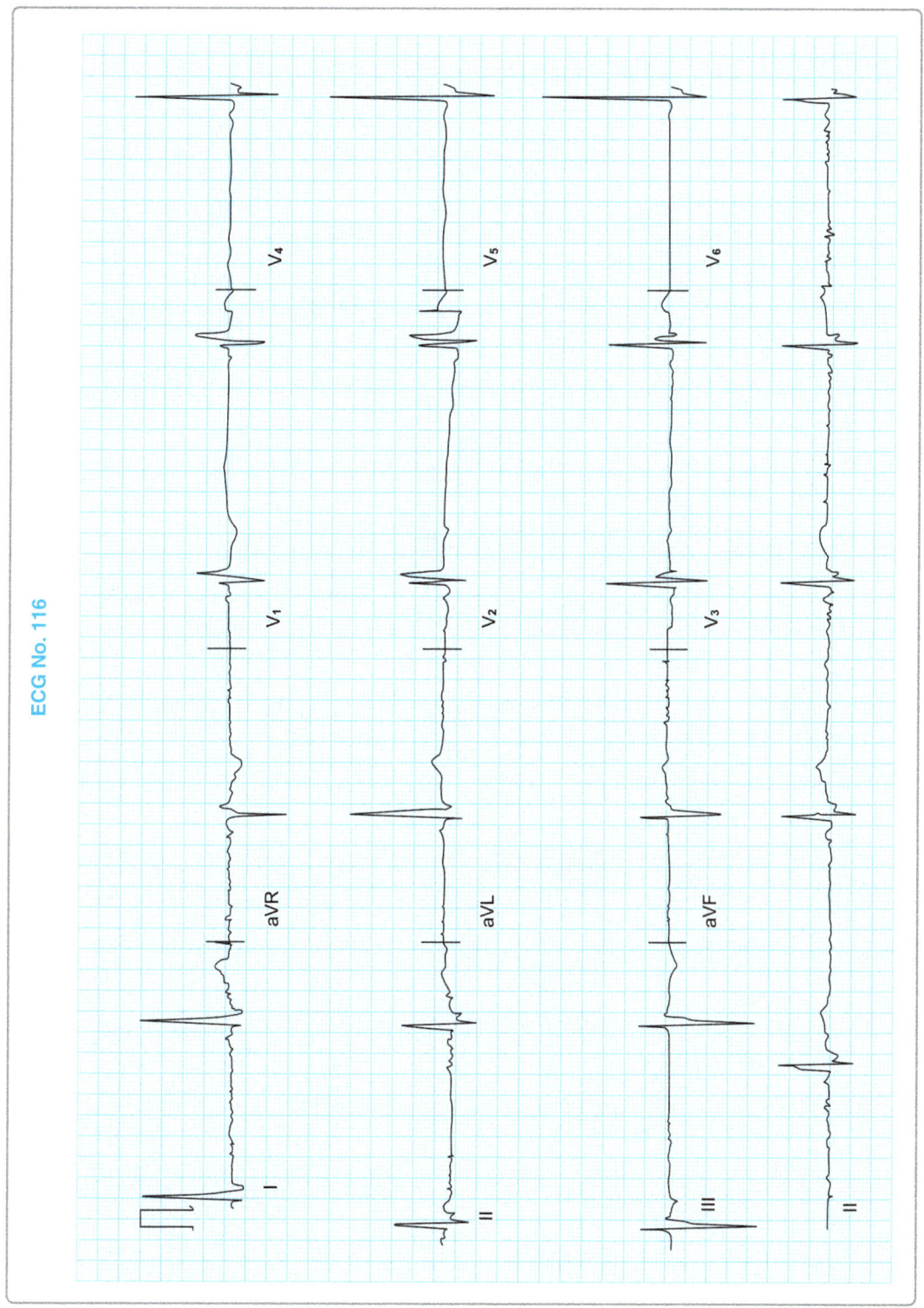

ECG in Medical Practice

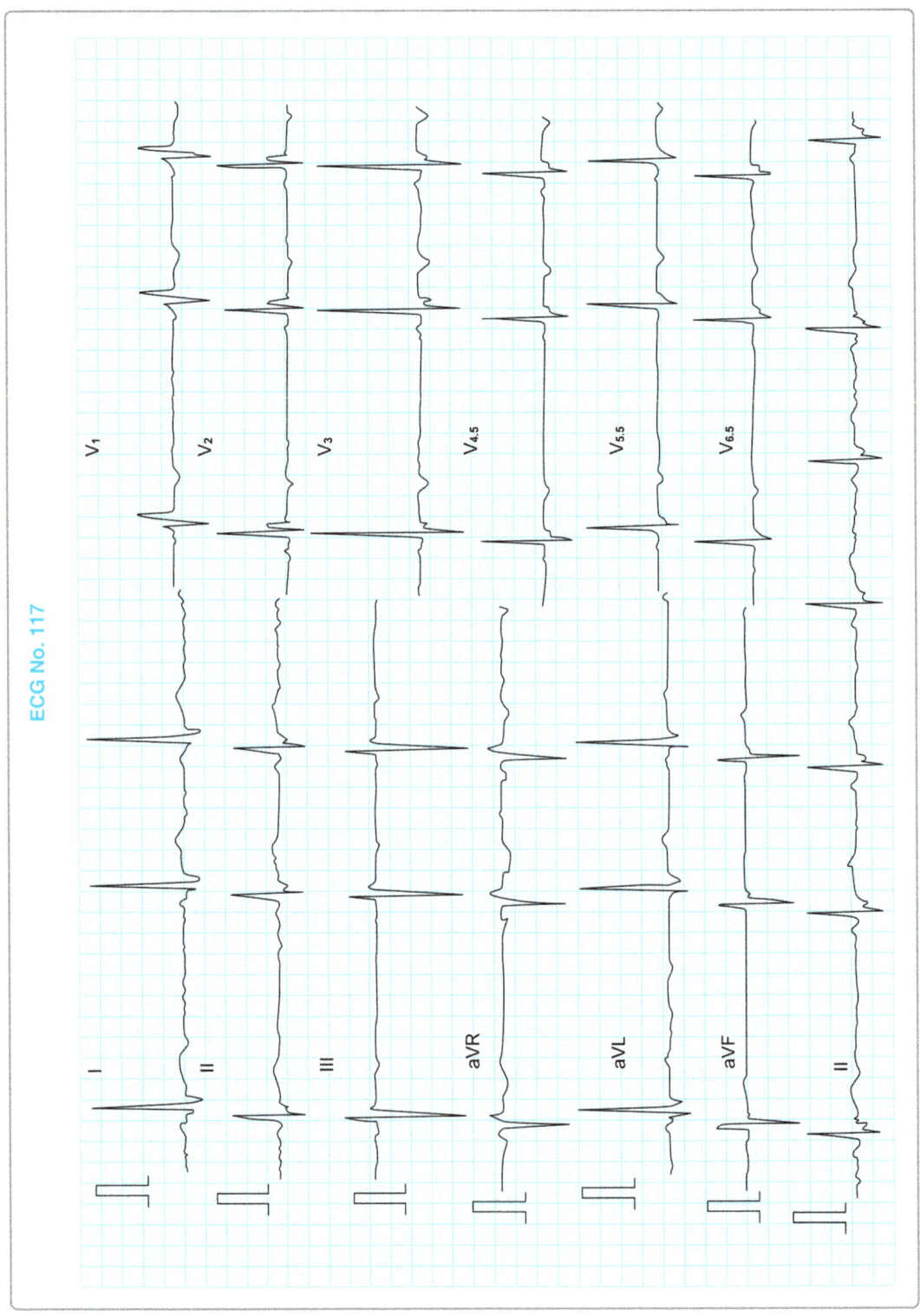

ECG No. 117

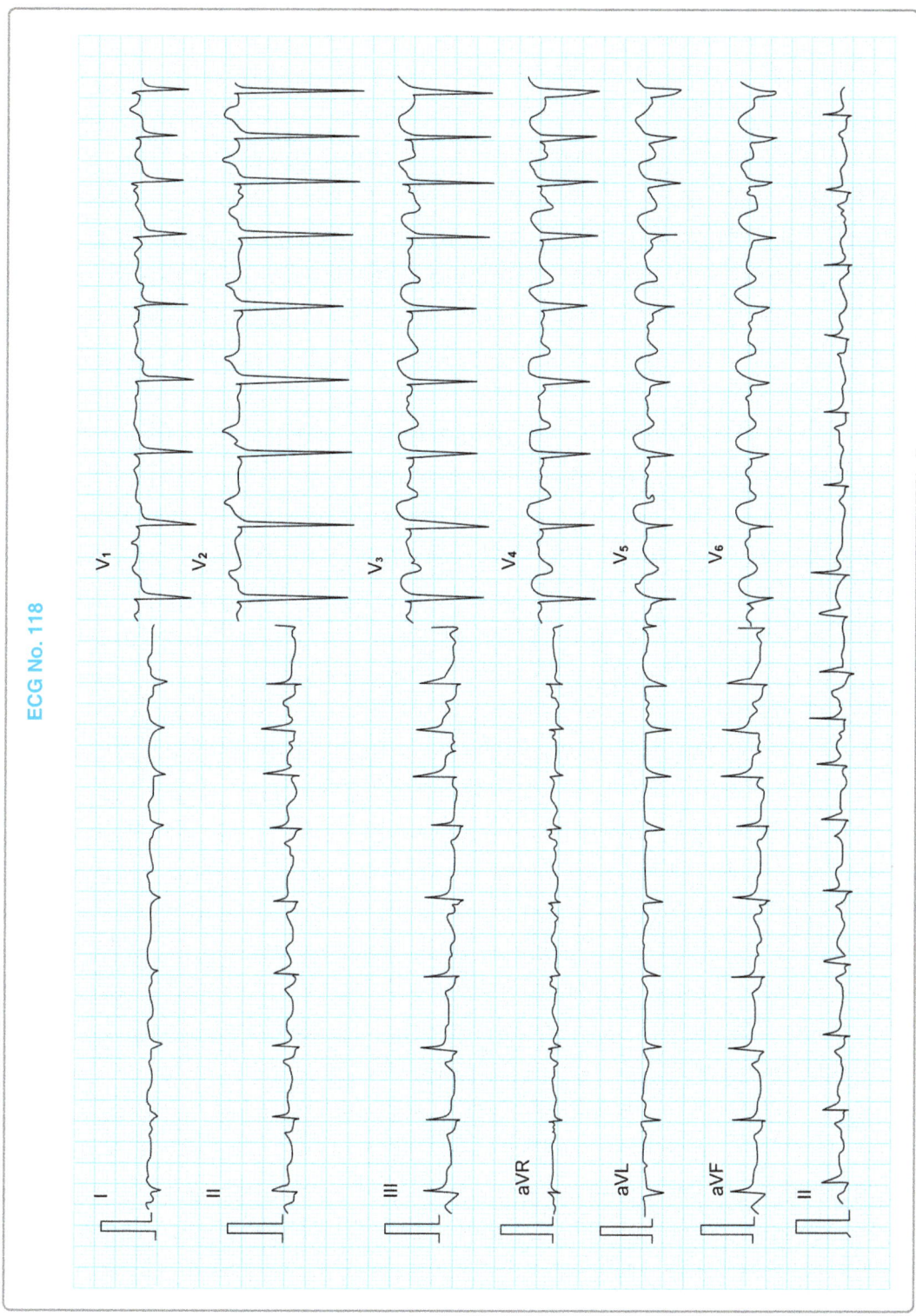

ECG No. 119

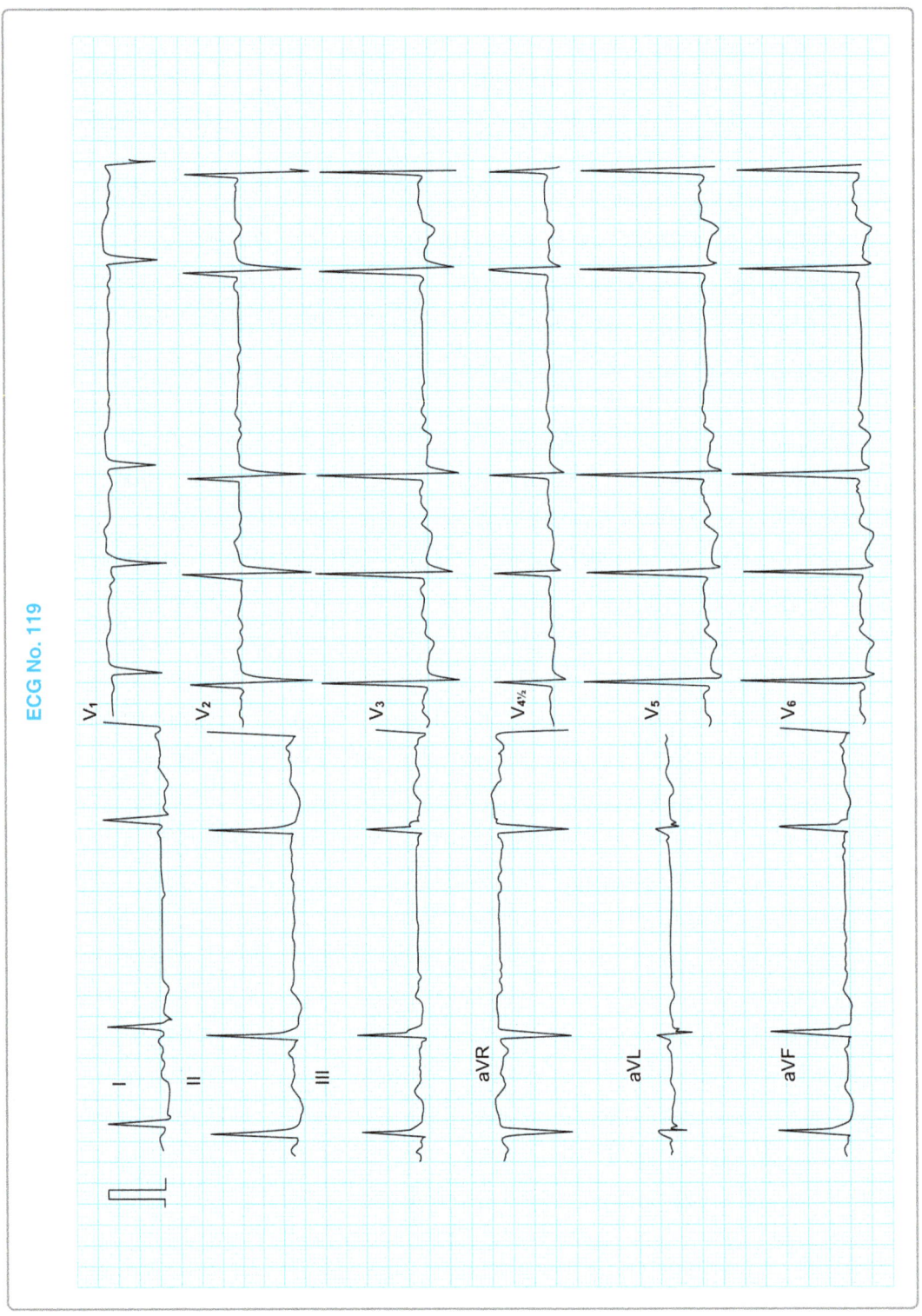

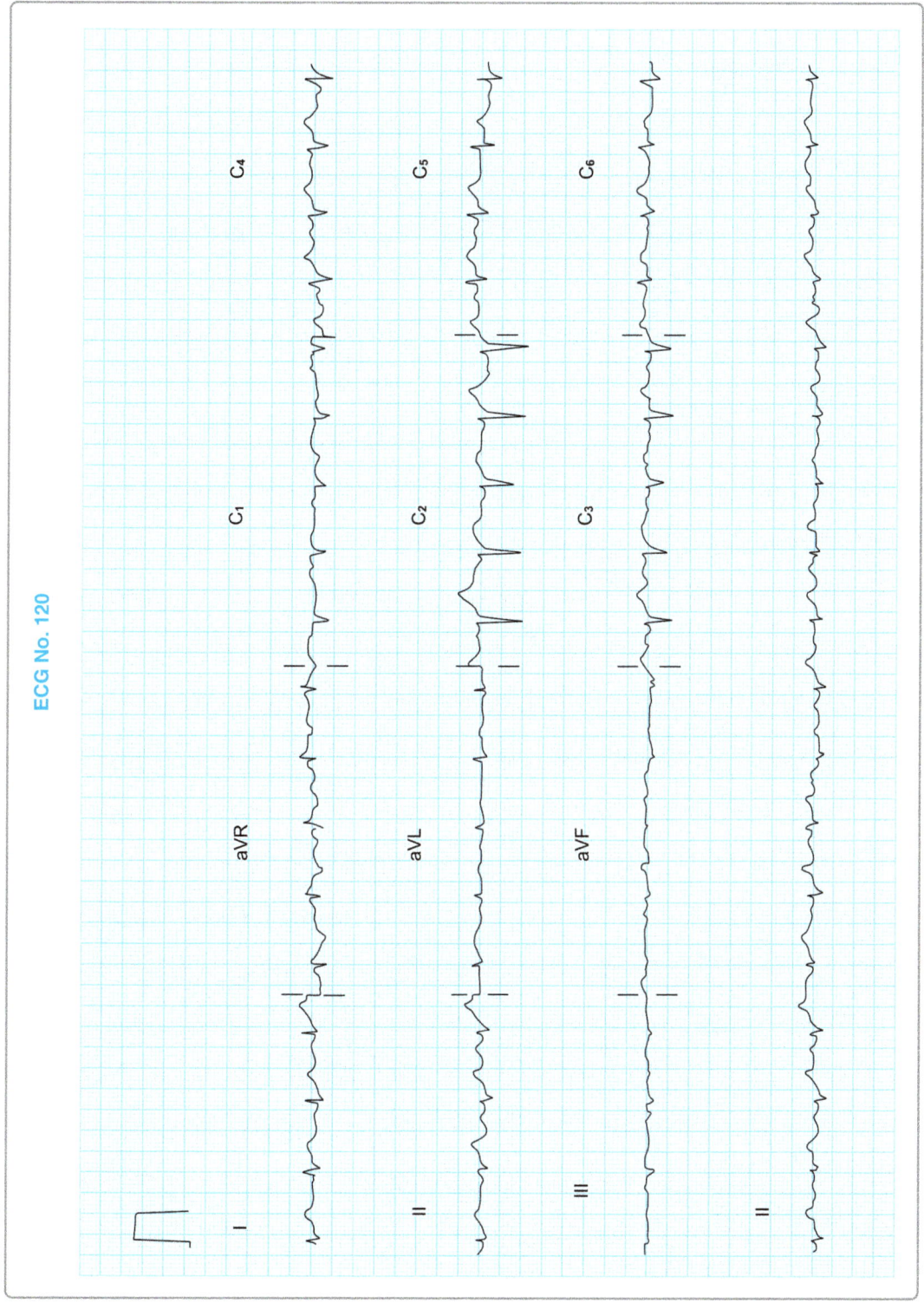

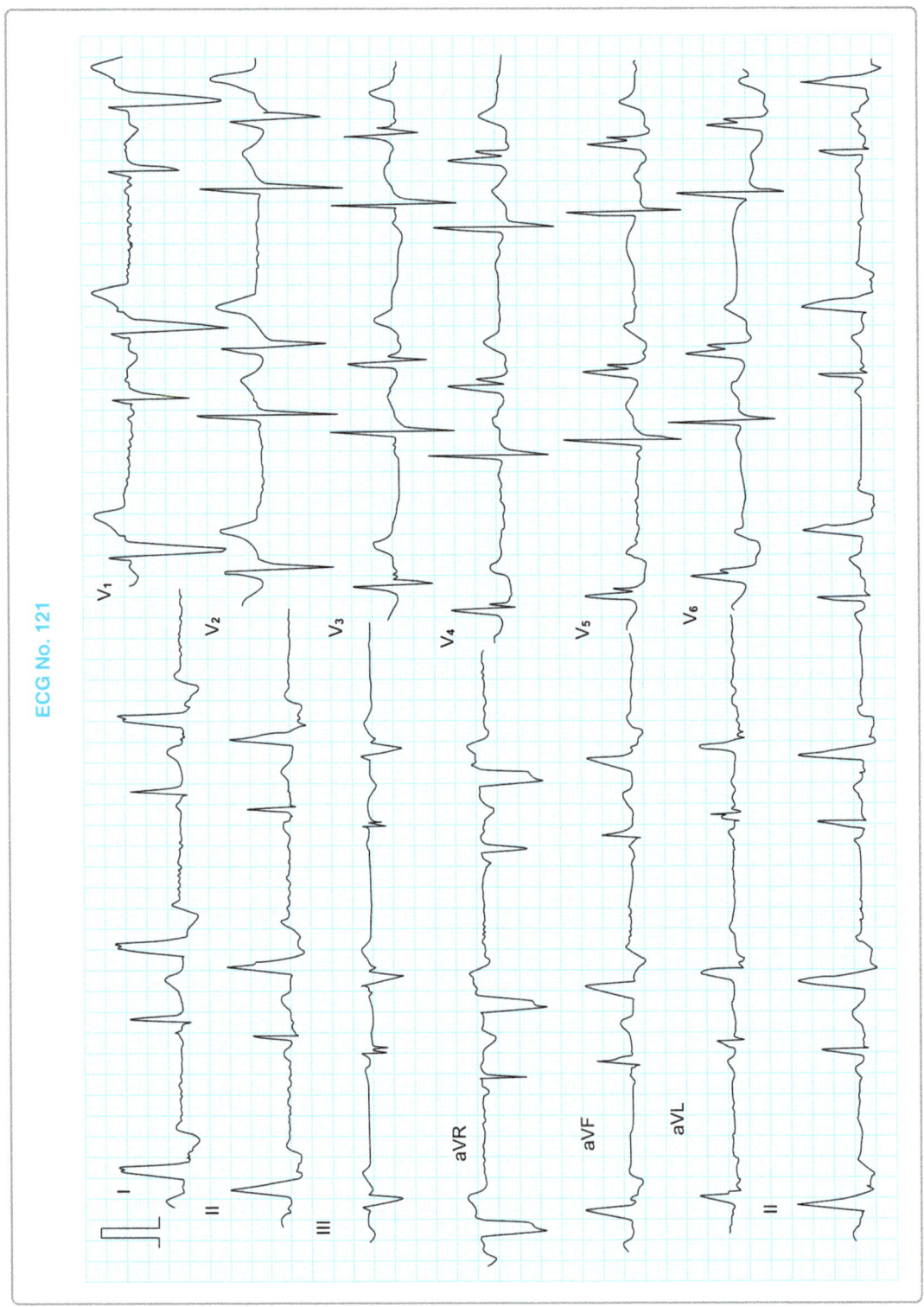

ECG No. 121

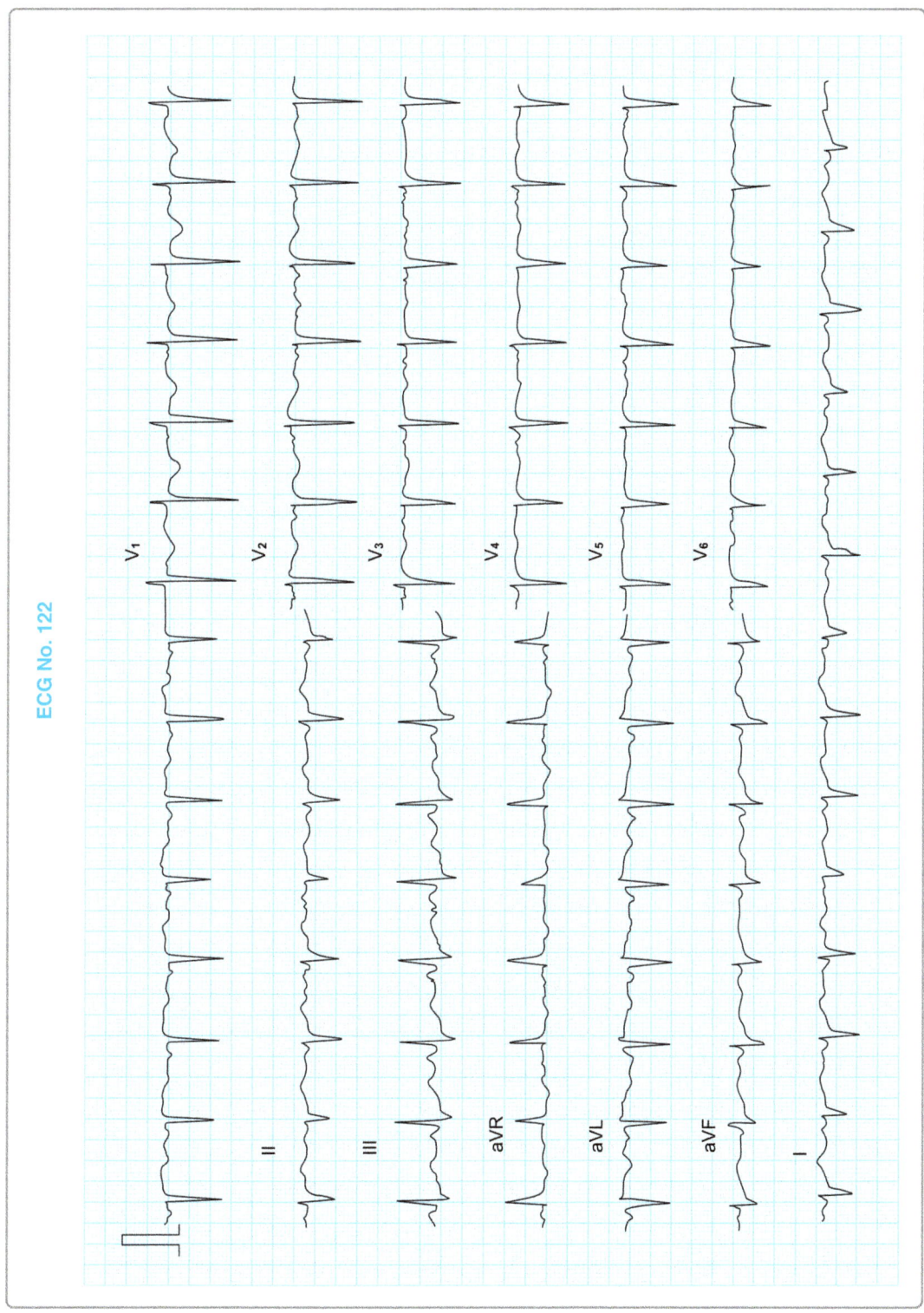

ECG in Medical Practice

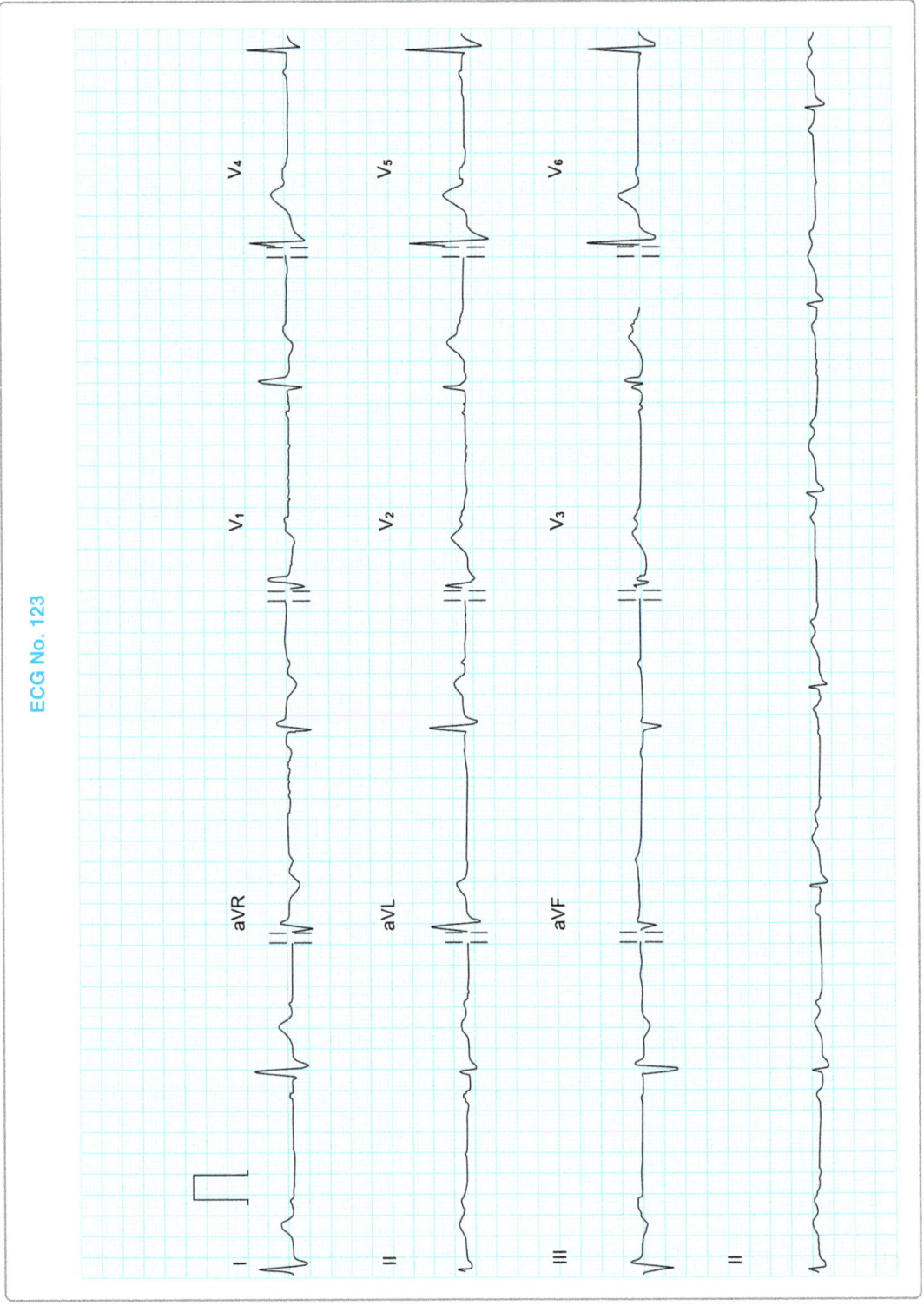

ECG No. 123

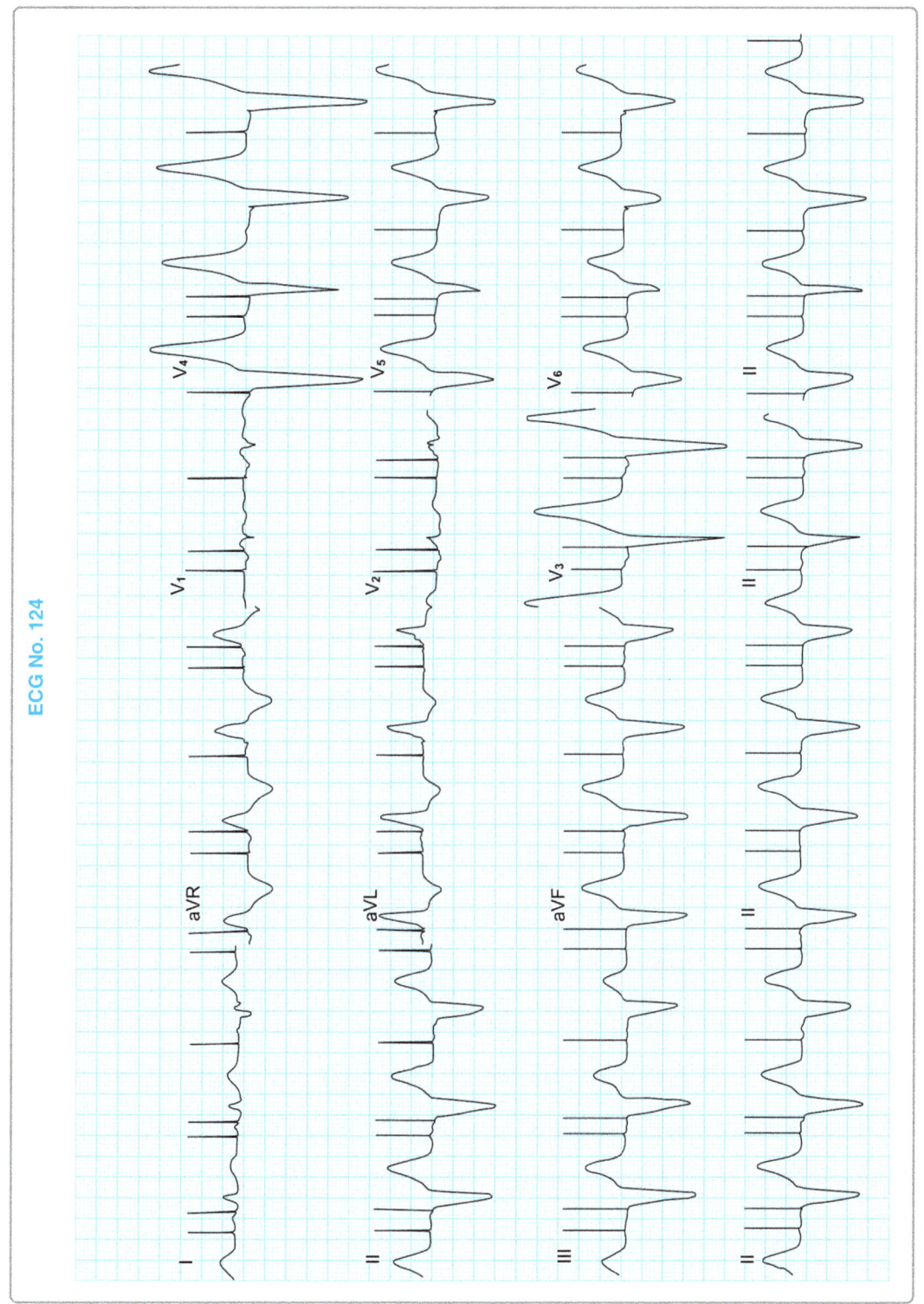

ECG No. 124

ECG in Medical Practice

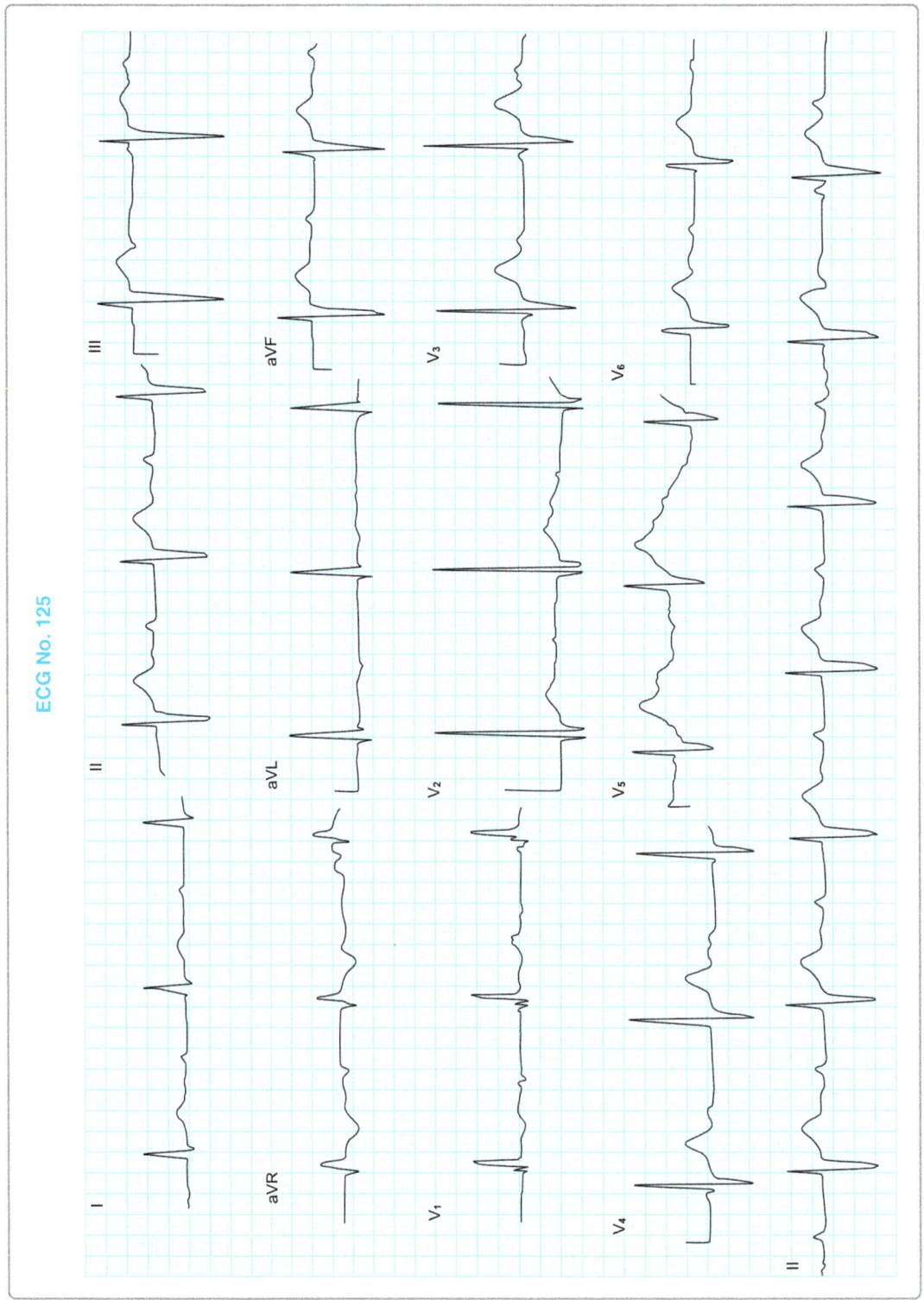

ECG No. 125

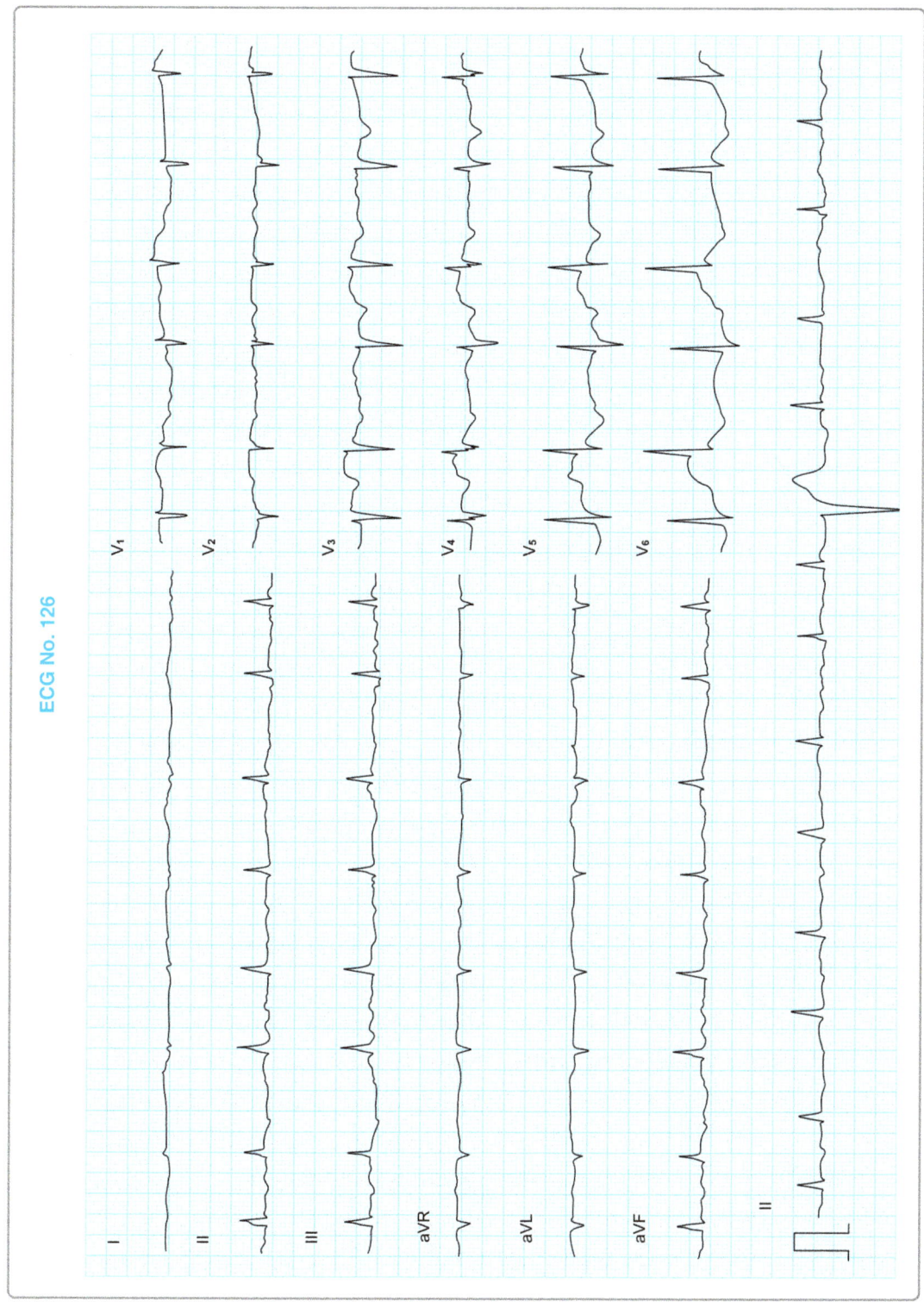

ECG in Medical Practice

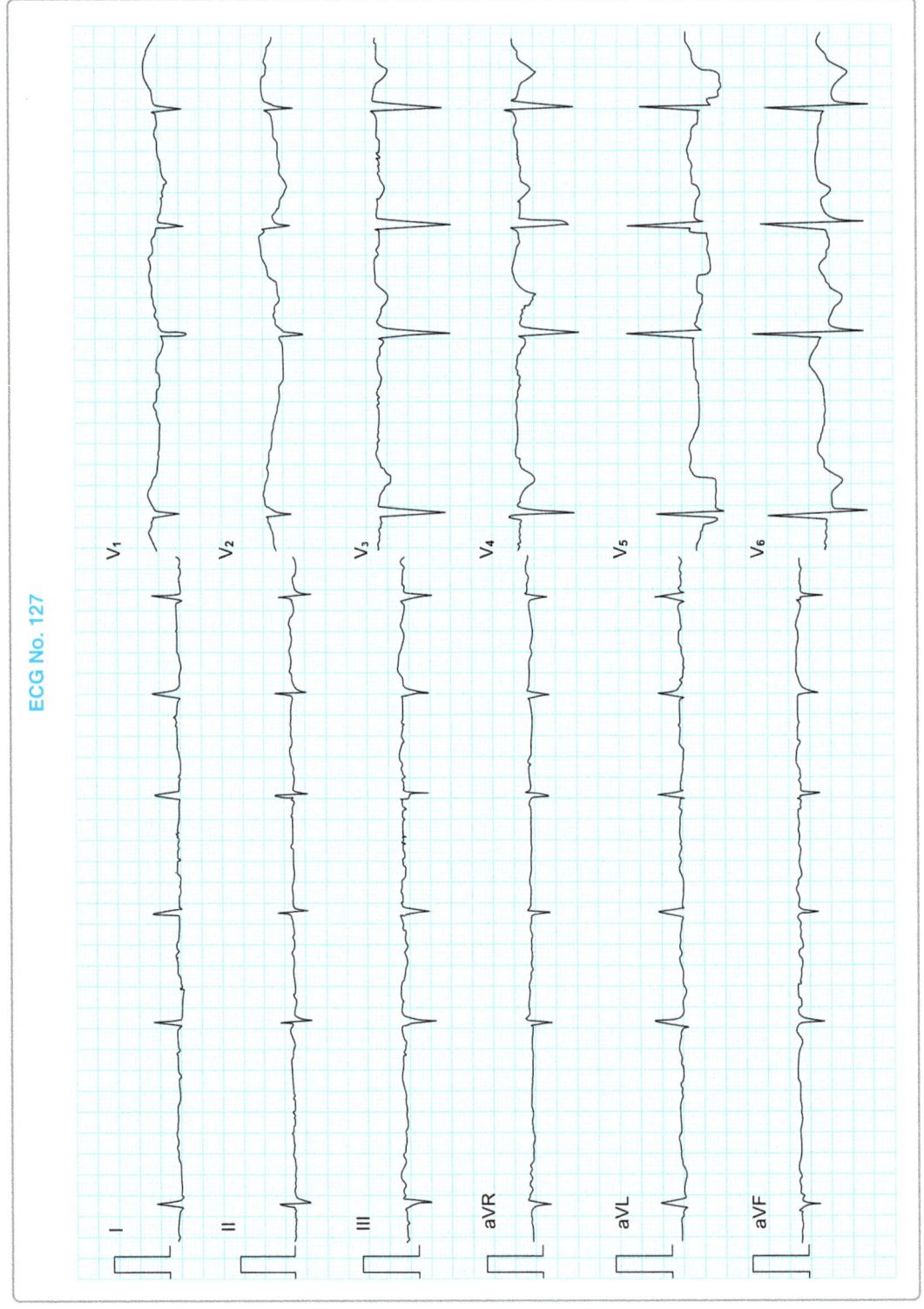

ECG No. 127

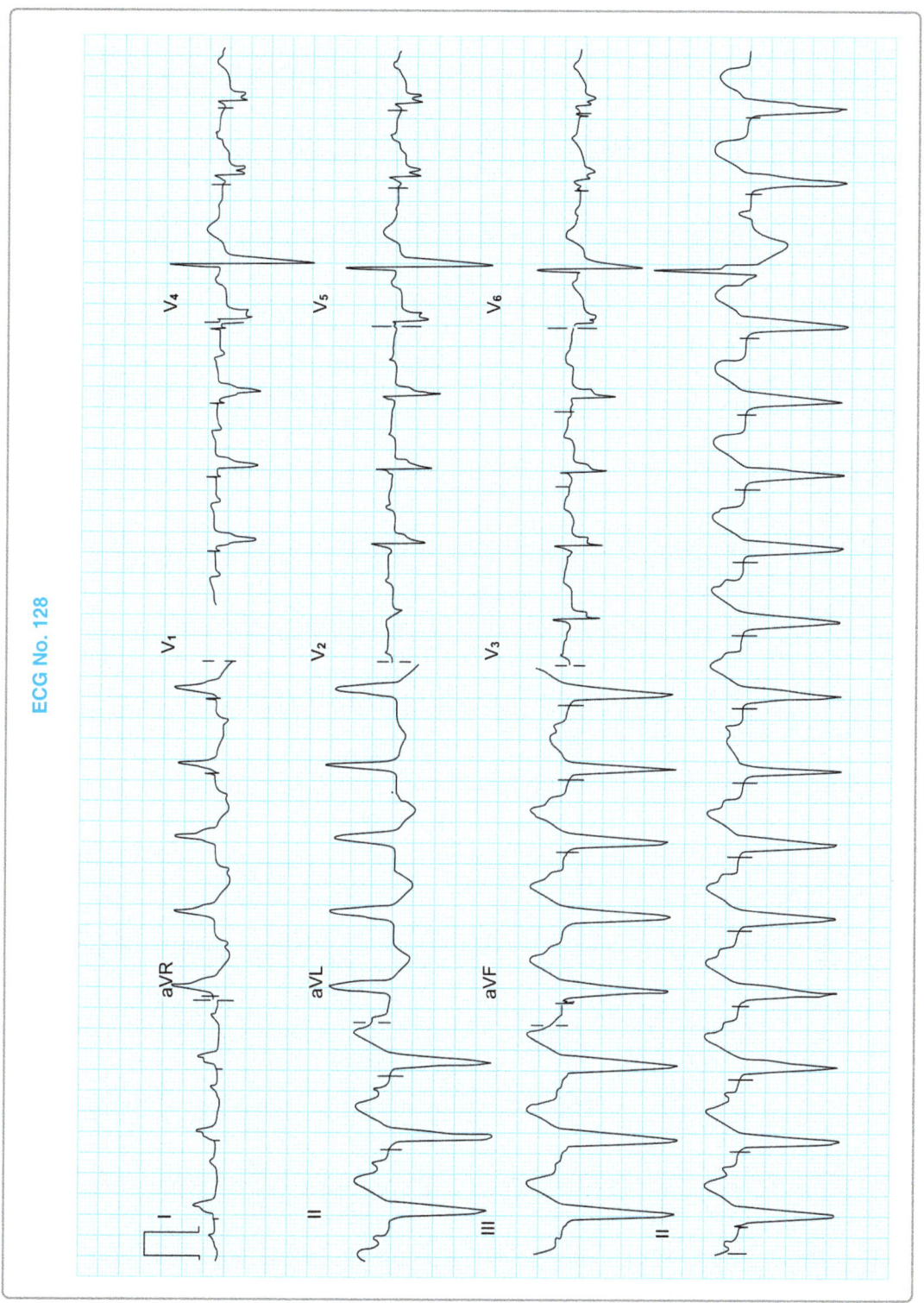

ECG in Medical Practice

ECG No. 129

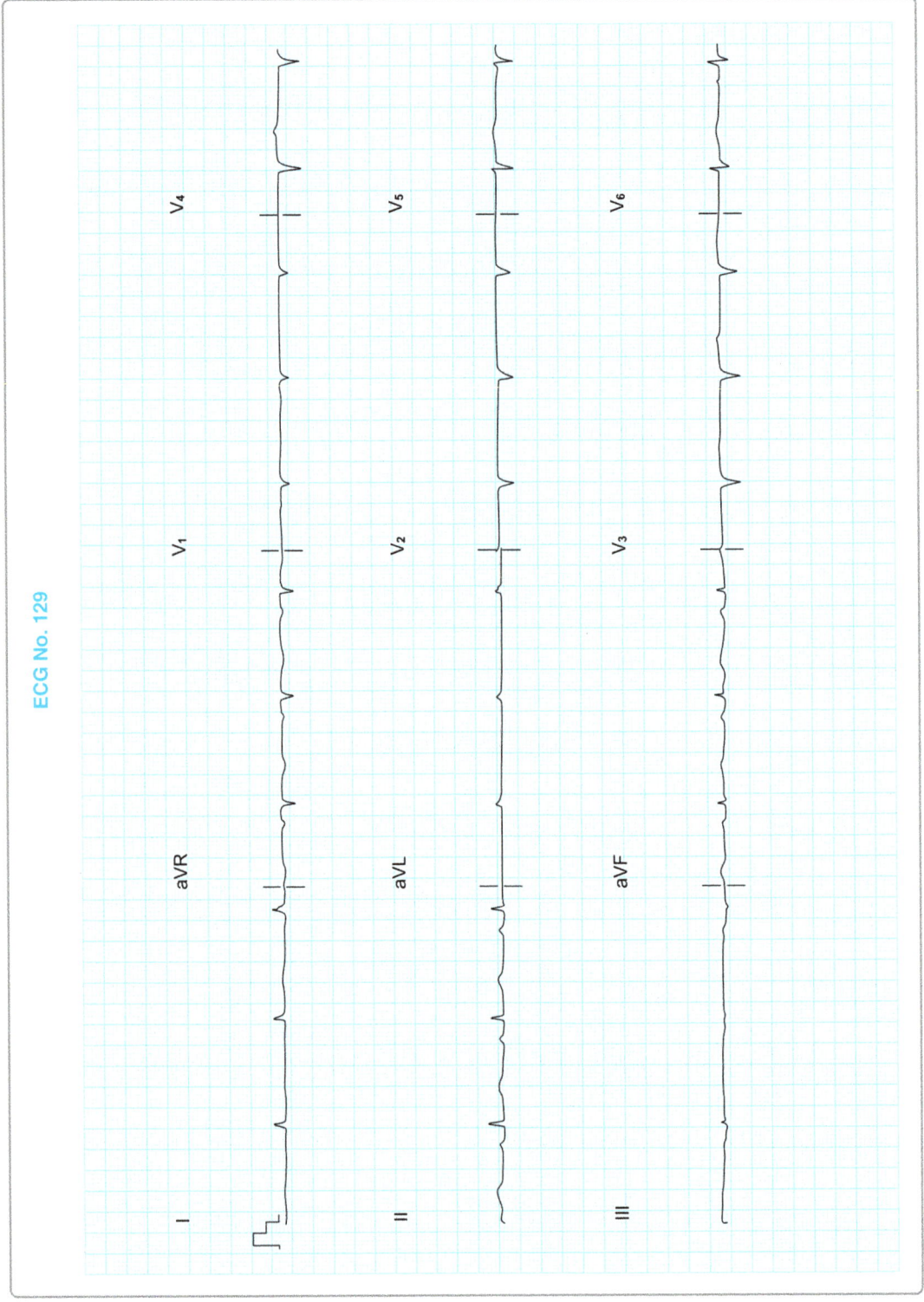

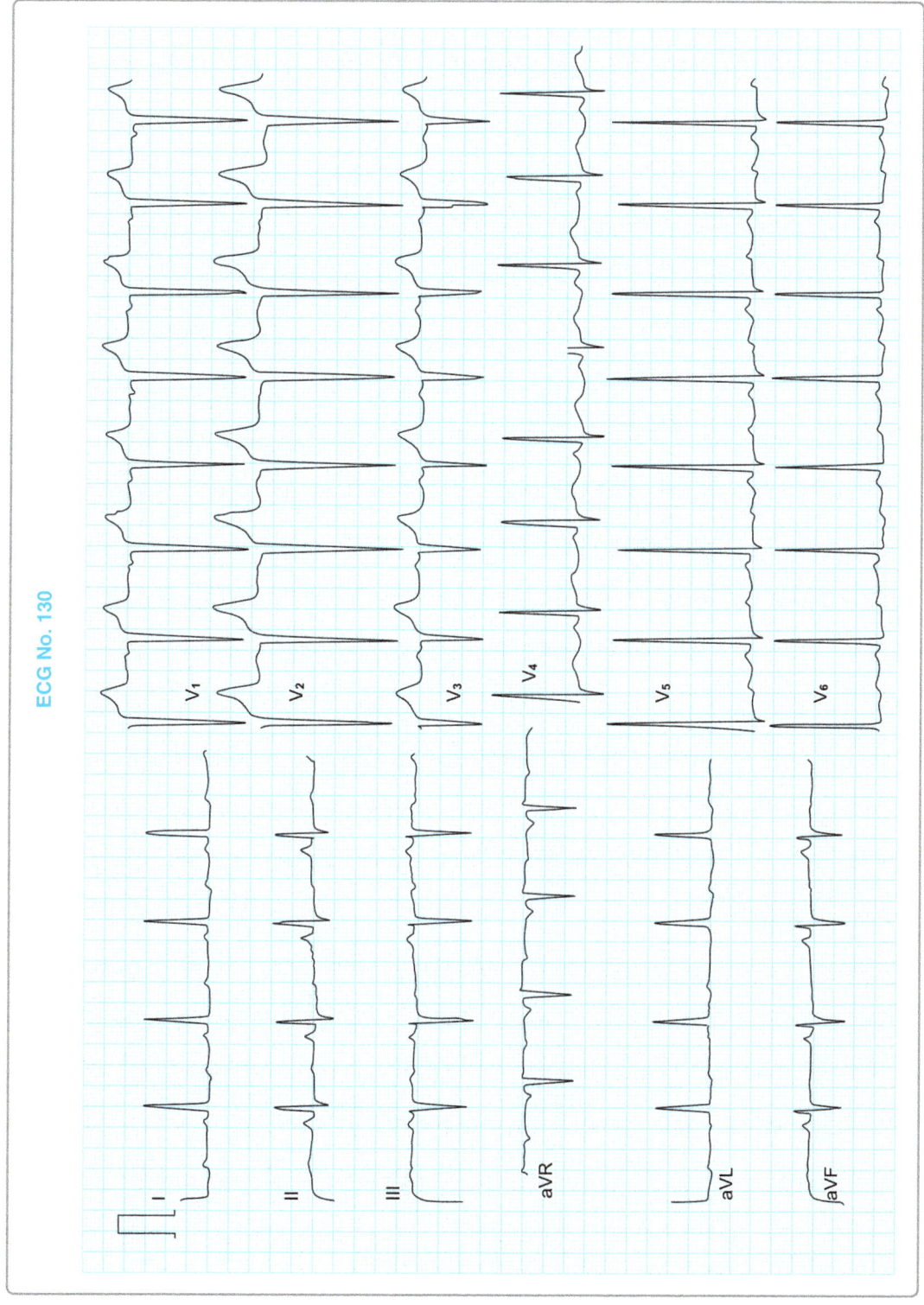

ECG in Medical Practice

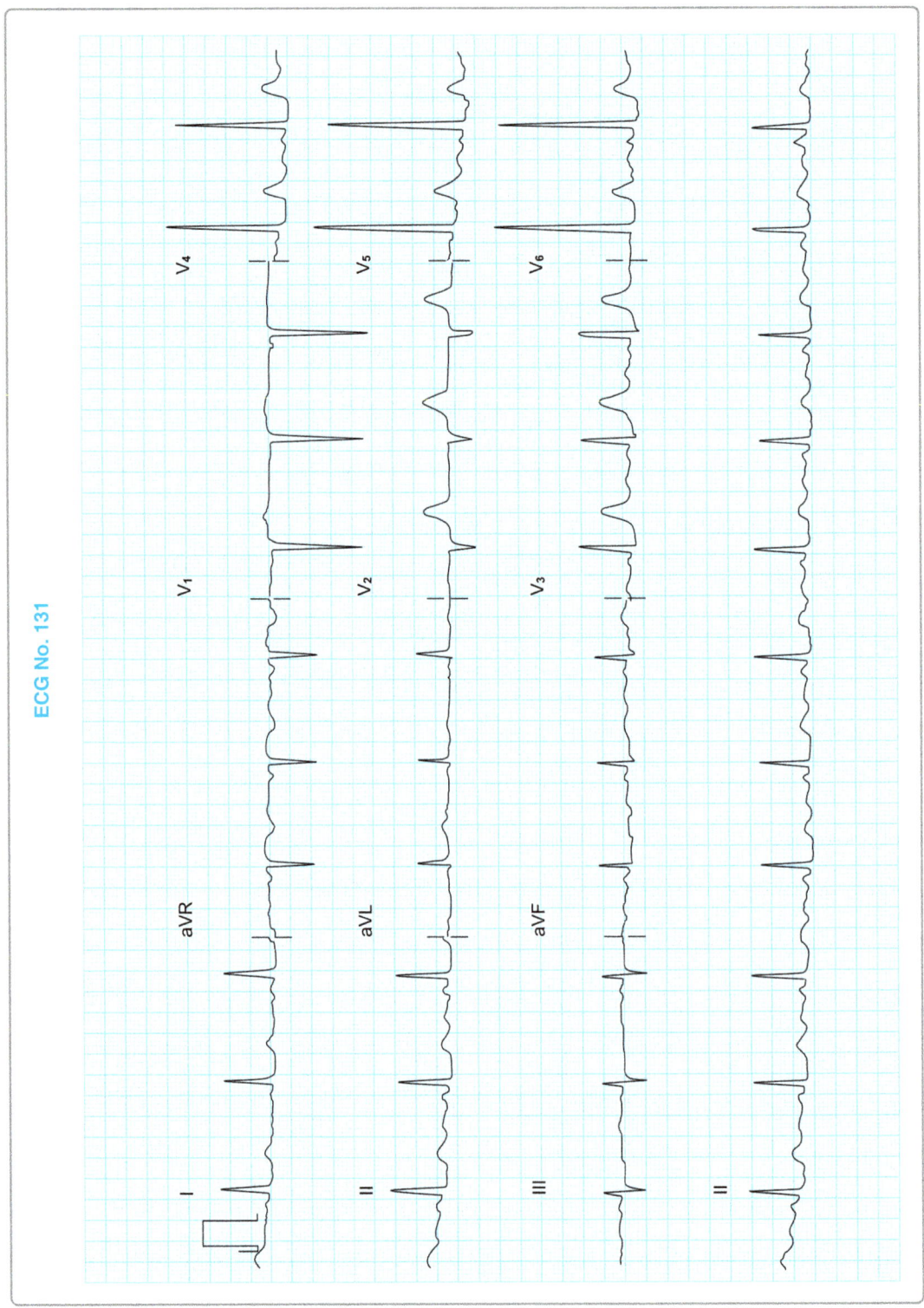

ECG No. 131

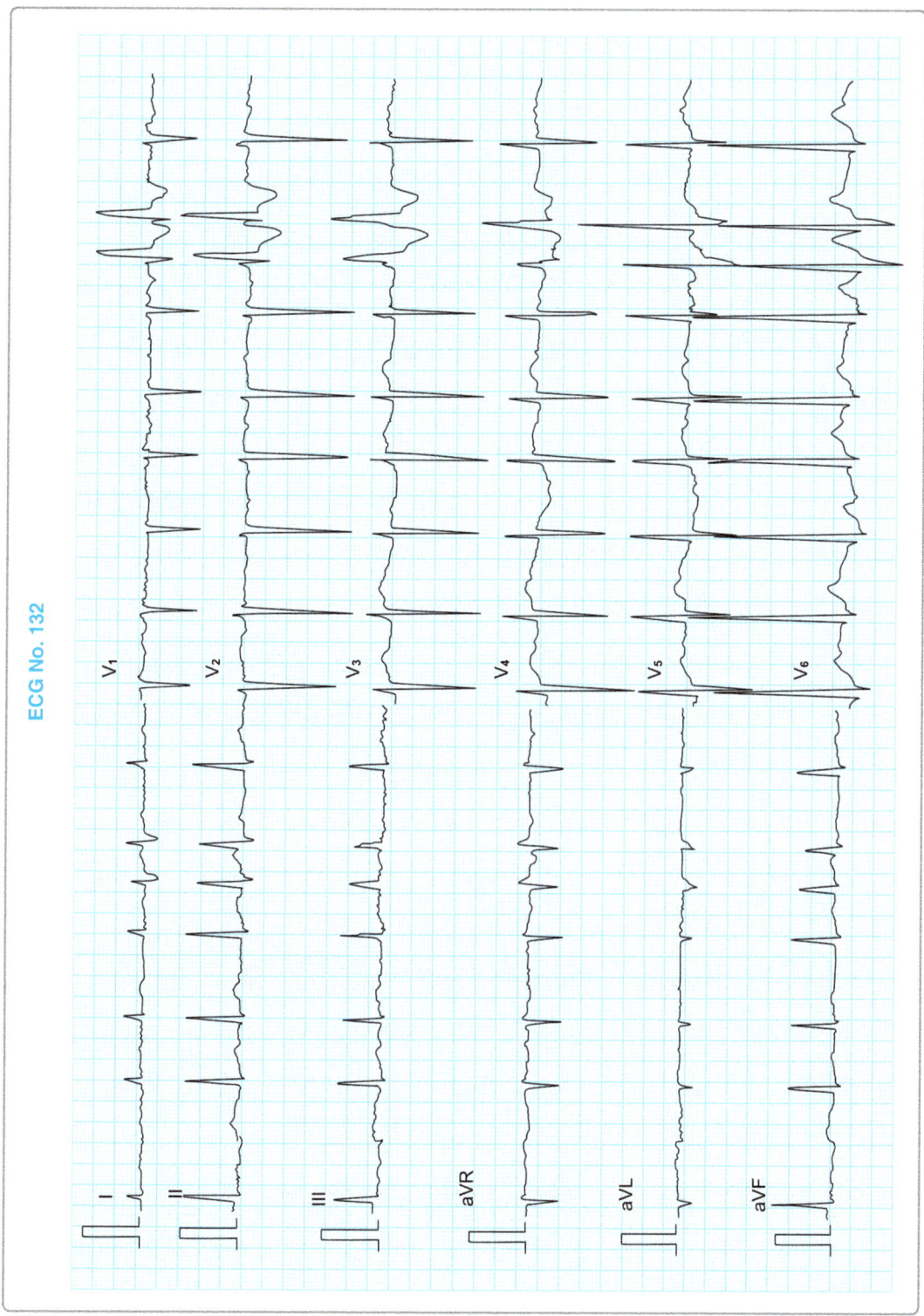

ECG No. 132

ECG in Medical Practice

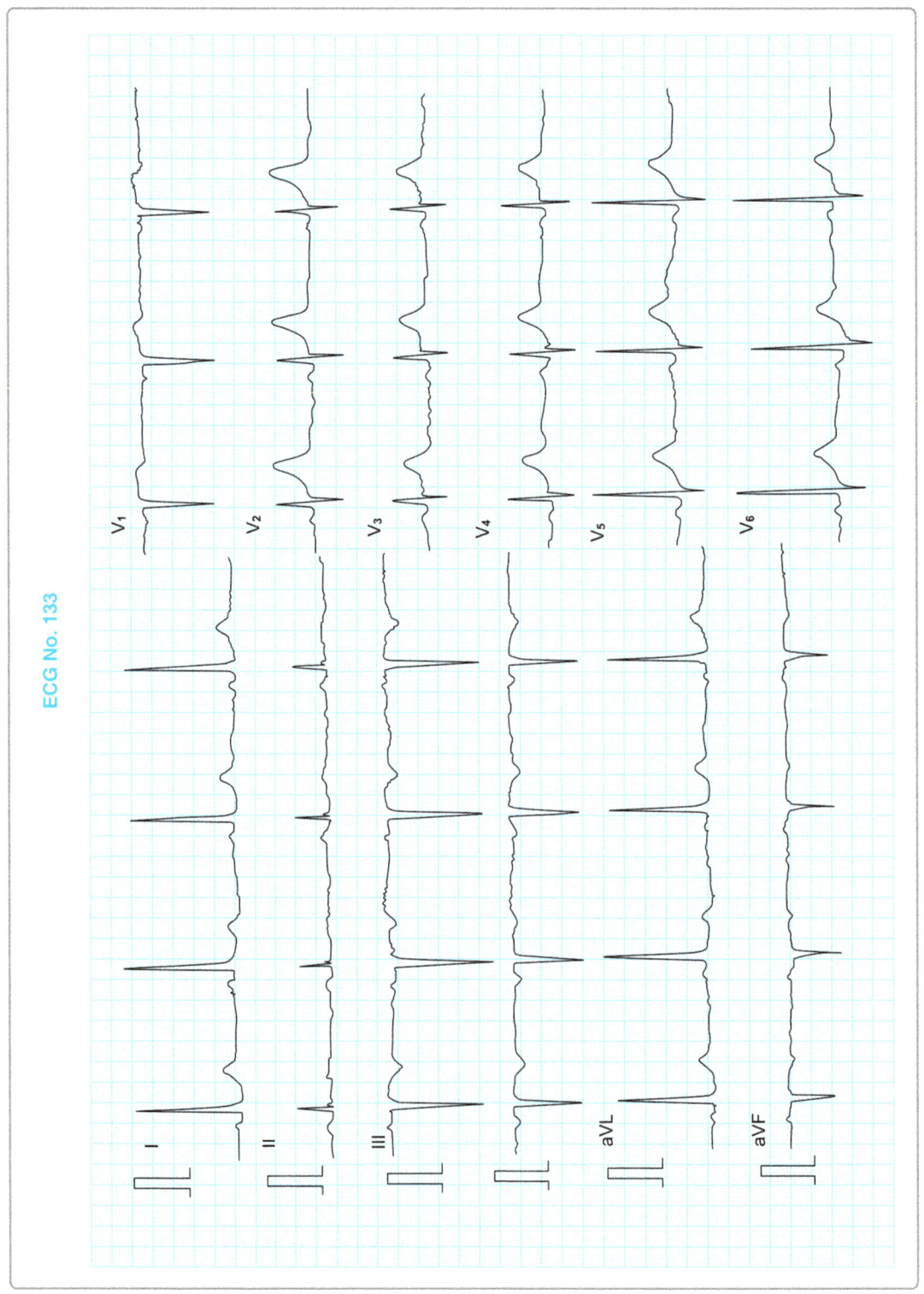

ECG No. 133

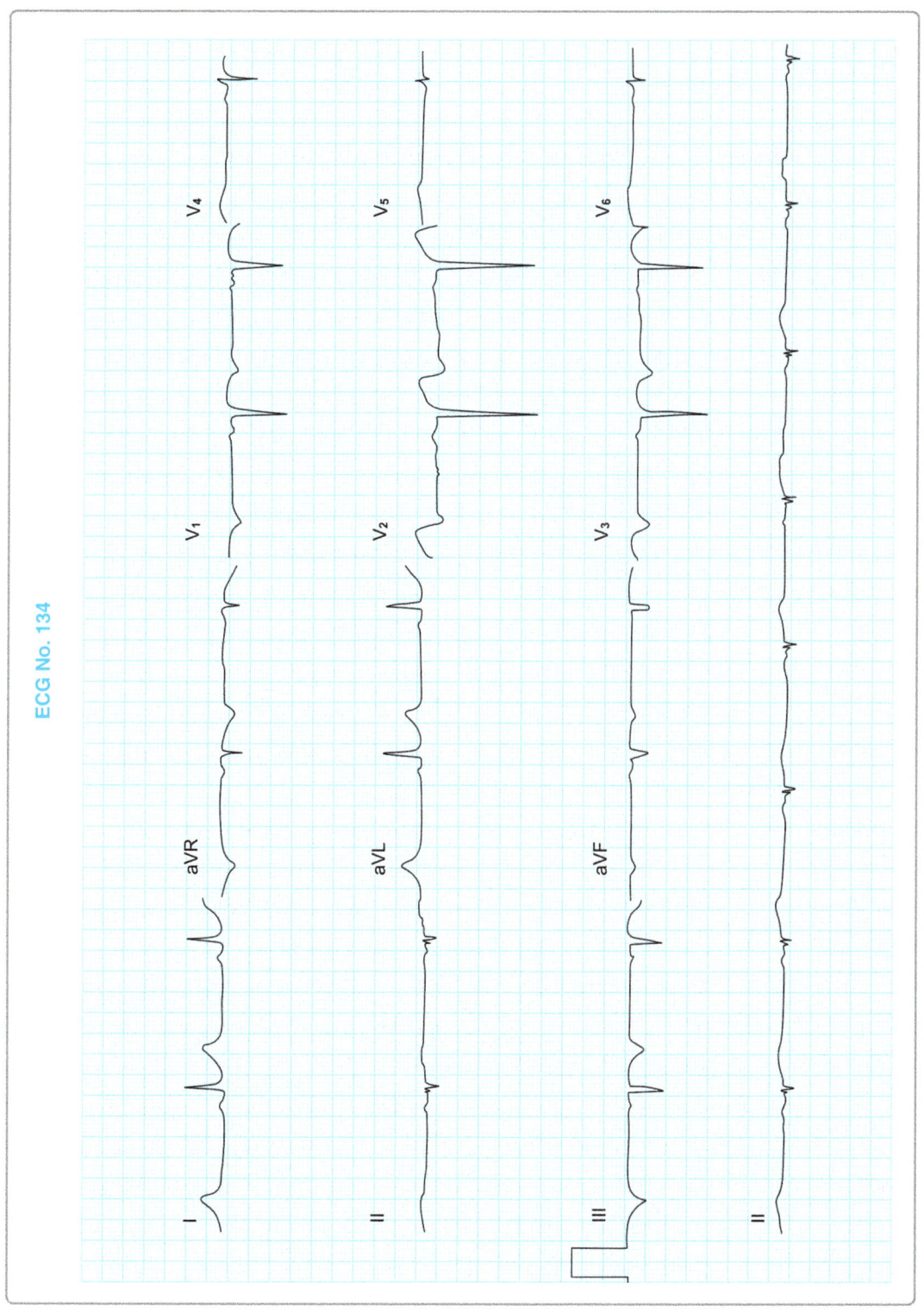

ECG in Medical Practice

ECG No. 135

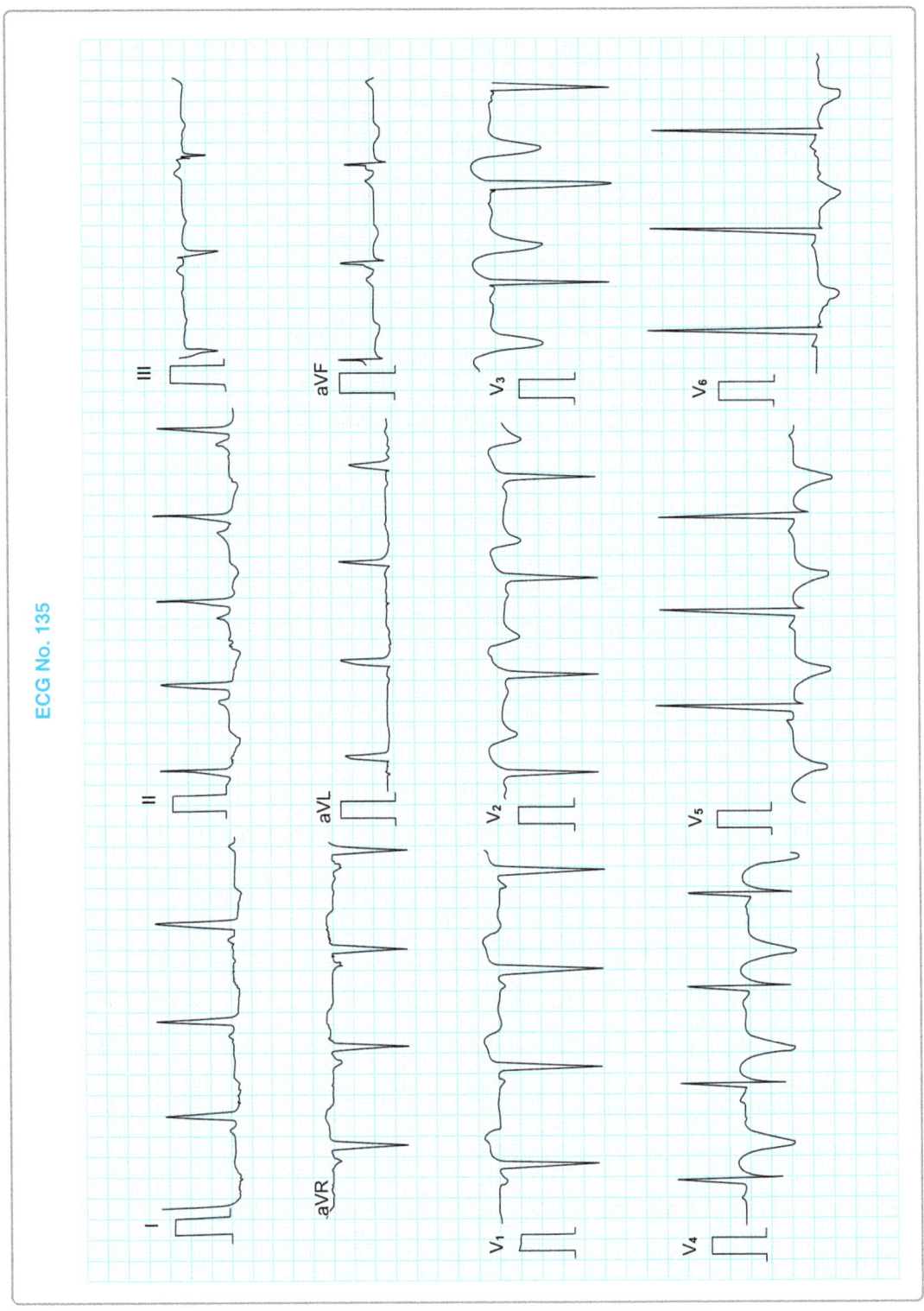

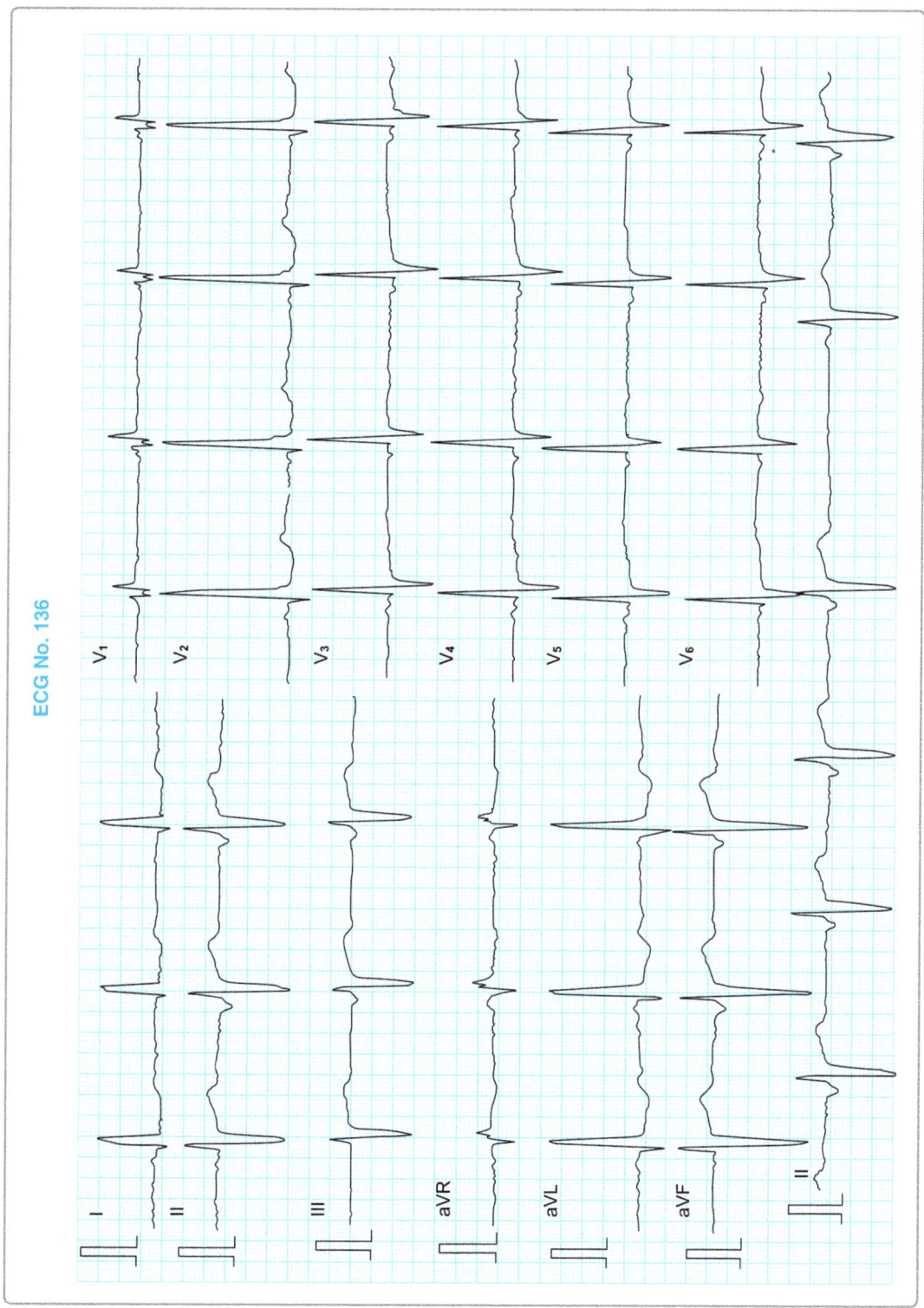

ECG in Medical Practice

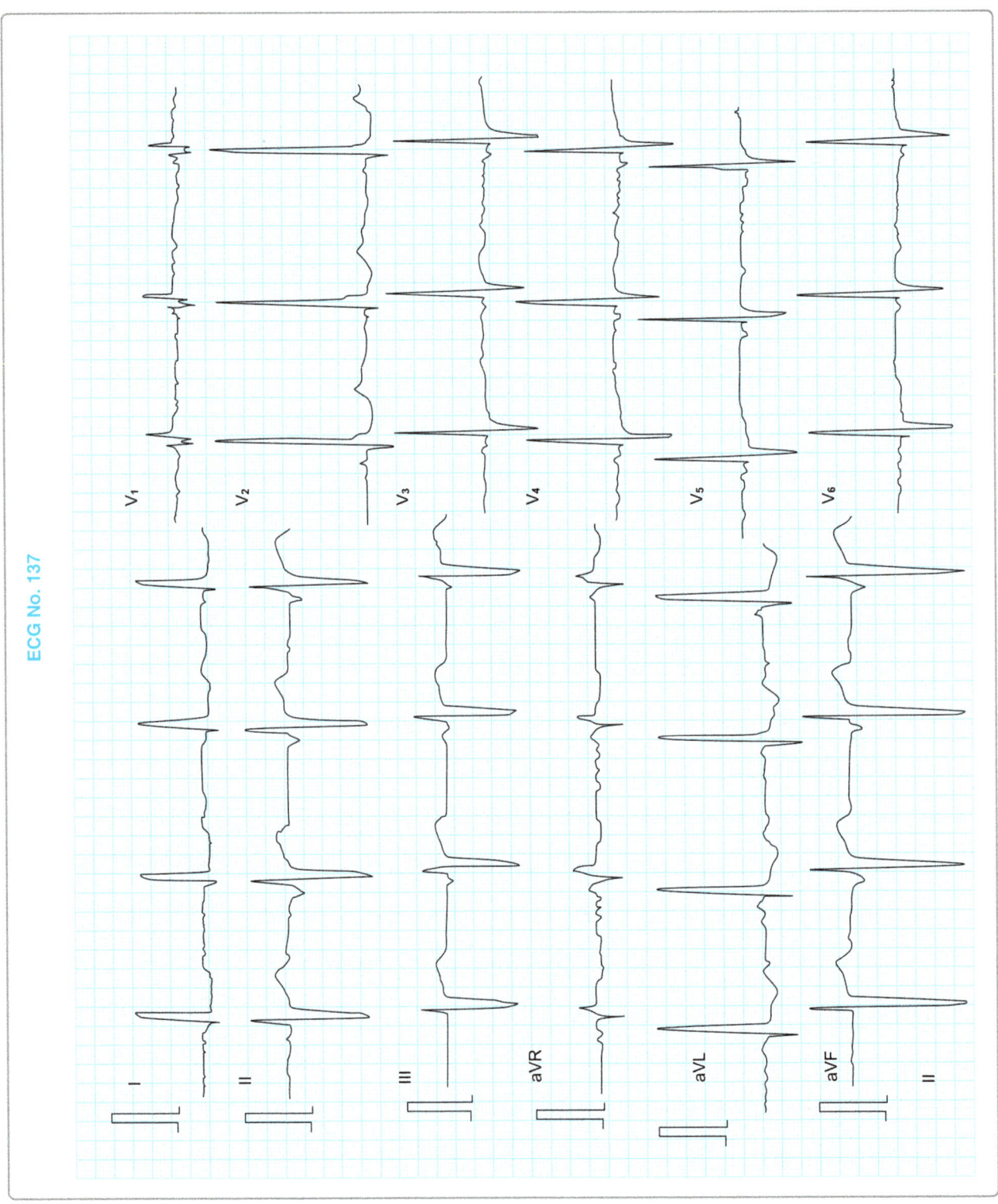

ECG No. 137

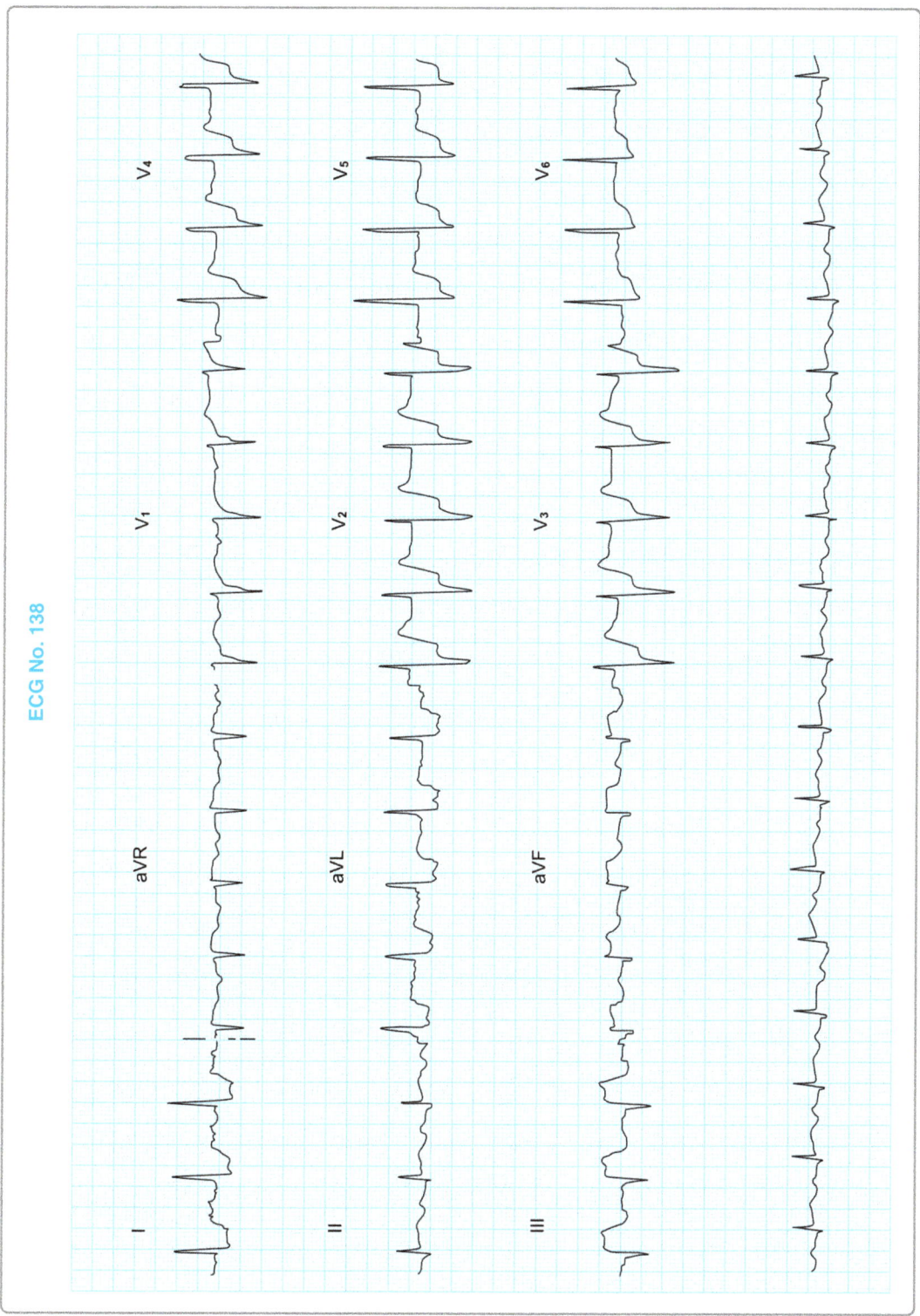

ECG No. 138

ECG in Medical Practice

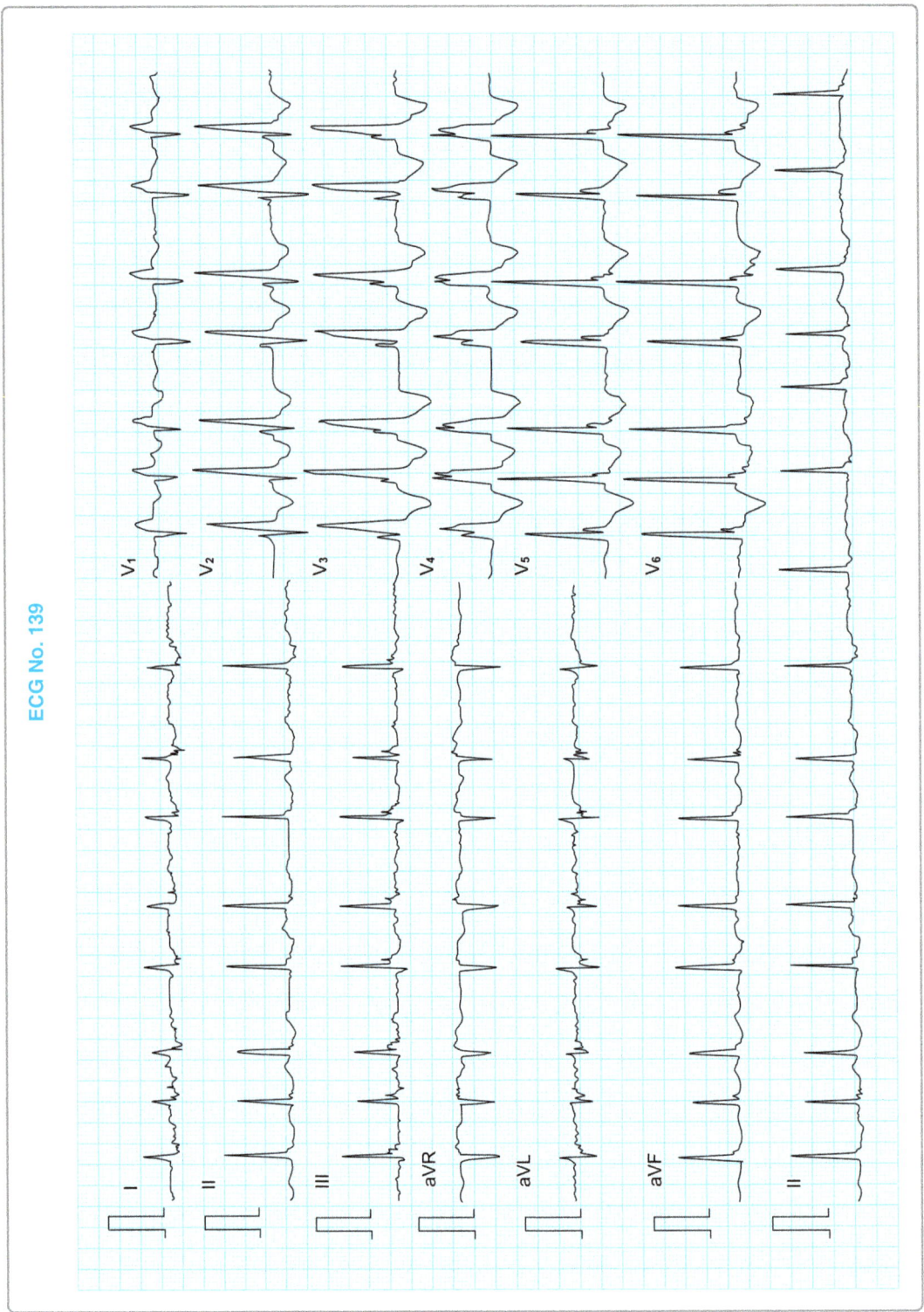

ECG No. 139

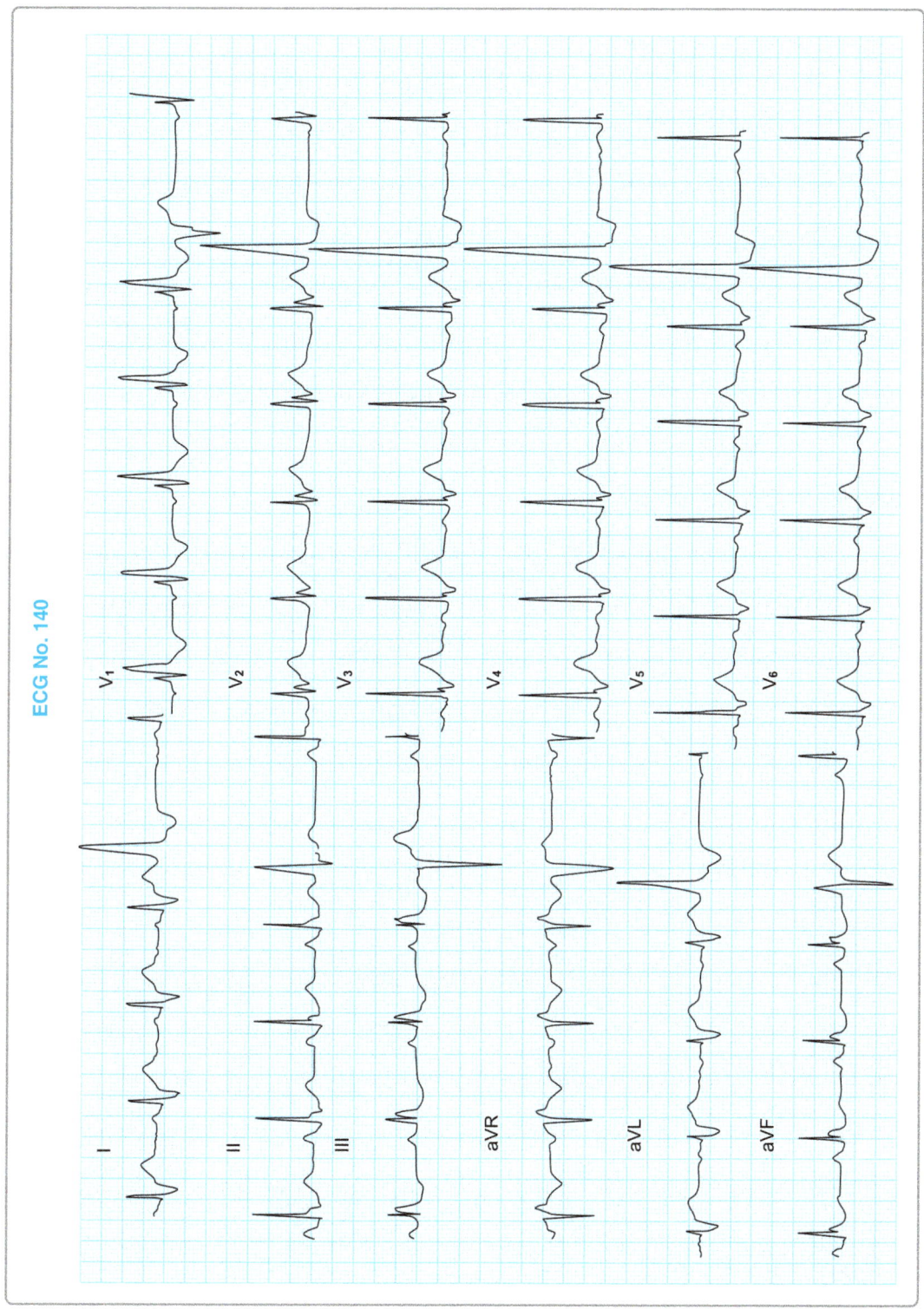

ECG No. 140

ECG in Medical Practice

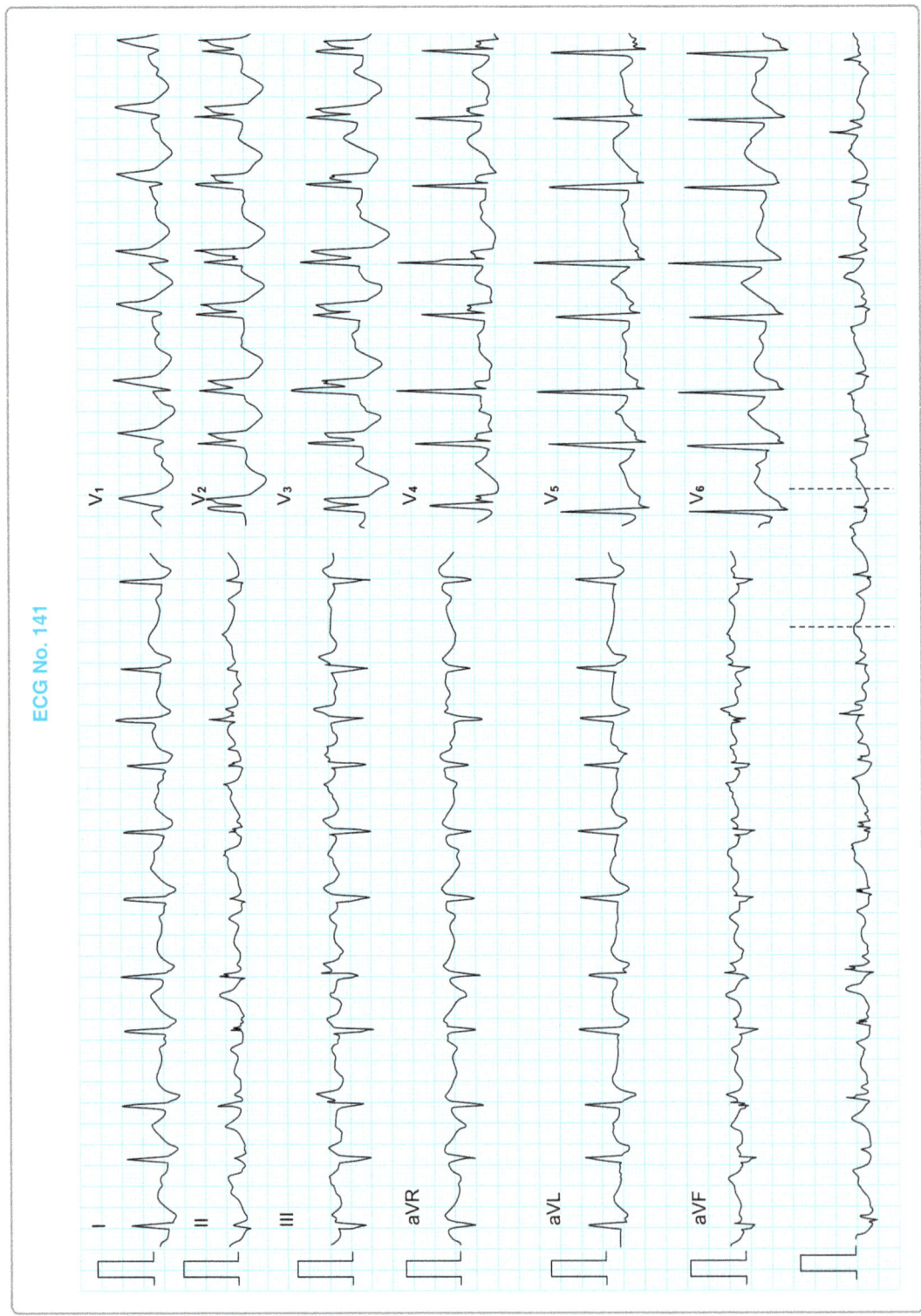

ECG No. 141

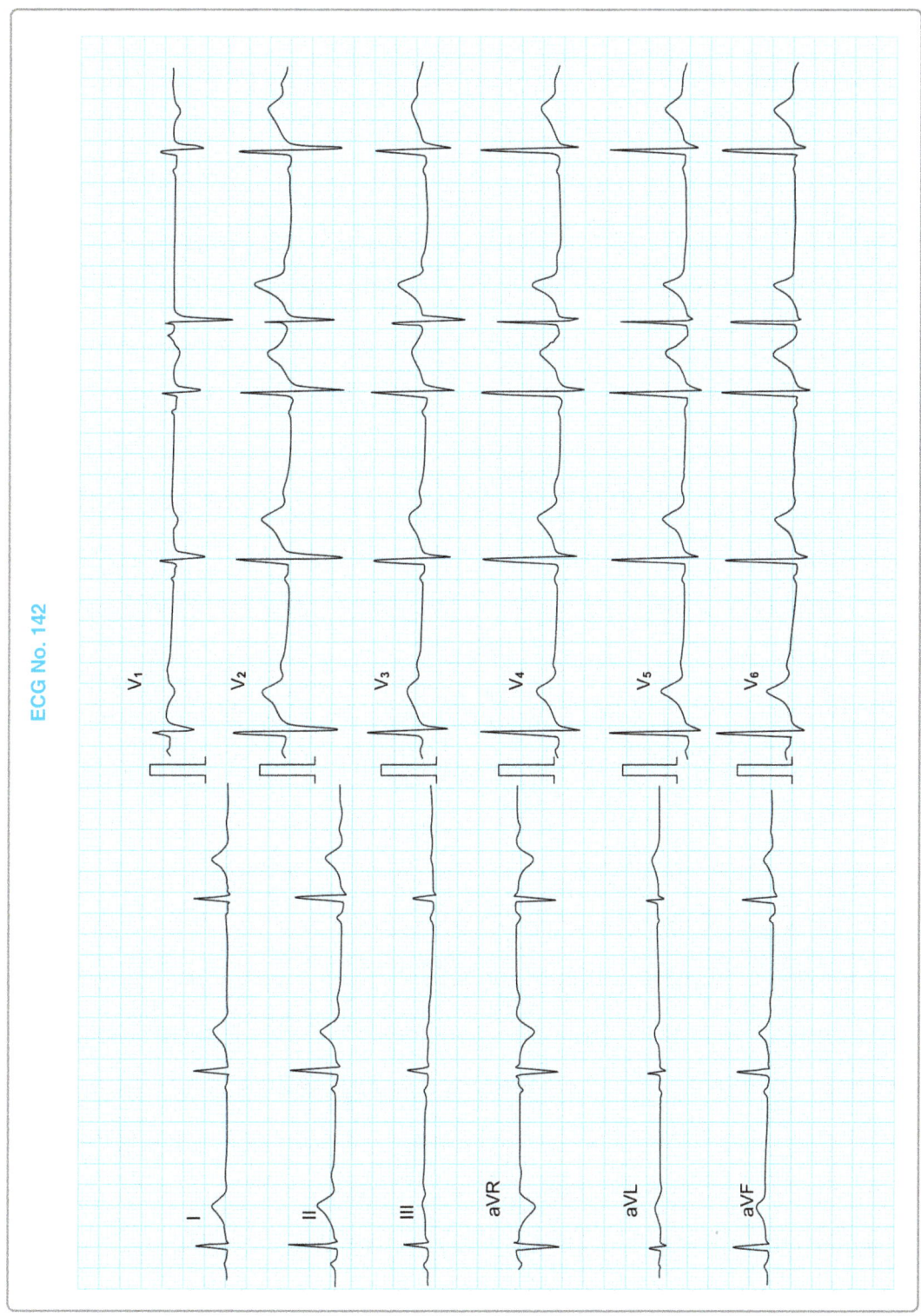

ECG in Medical Practice

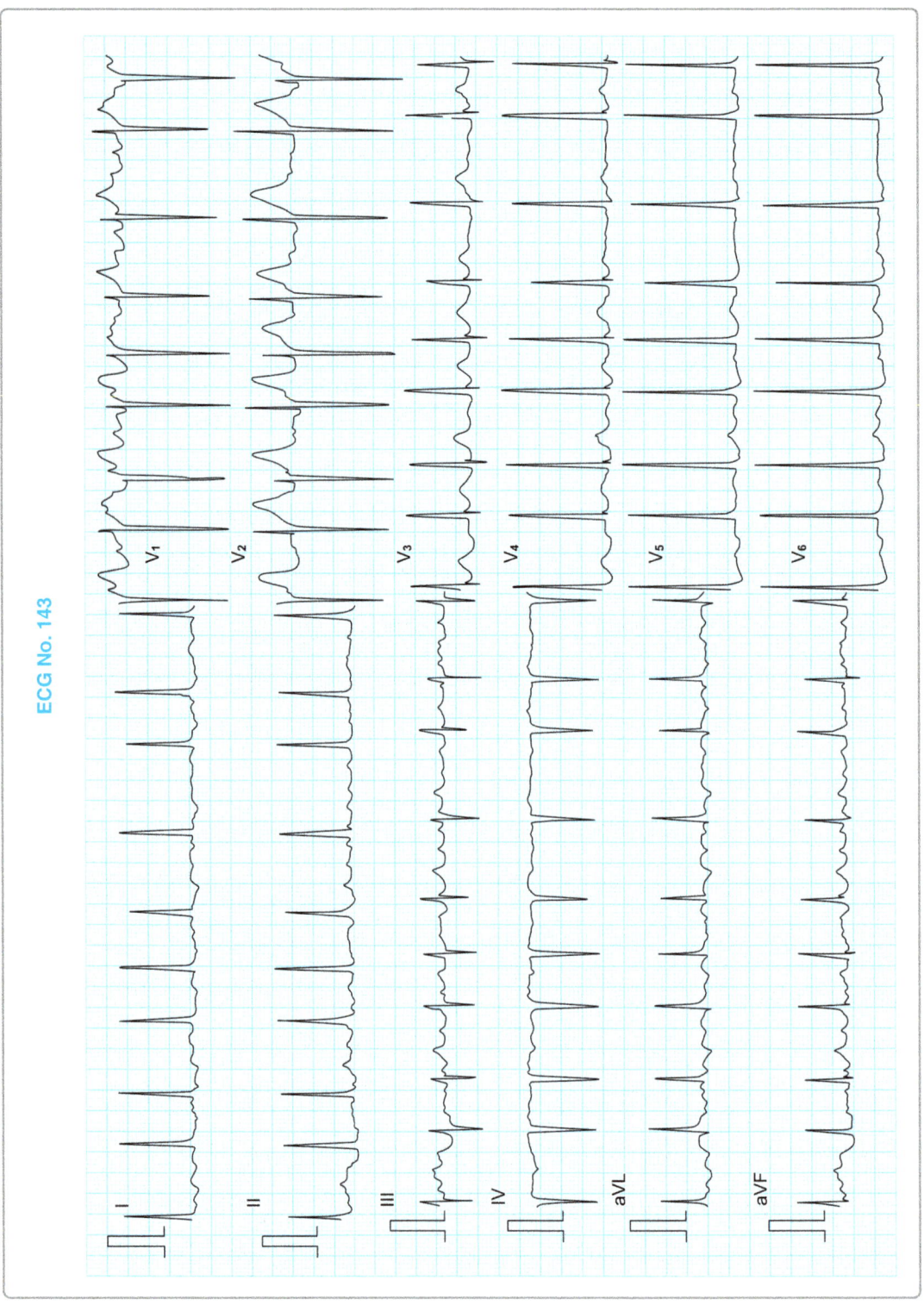

ECG No. 143

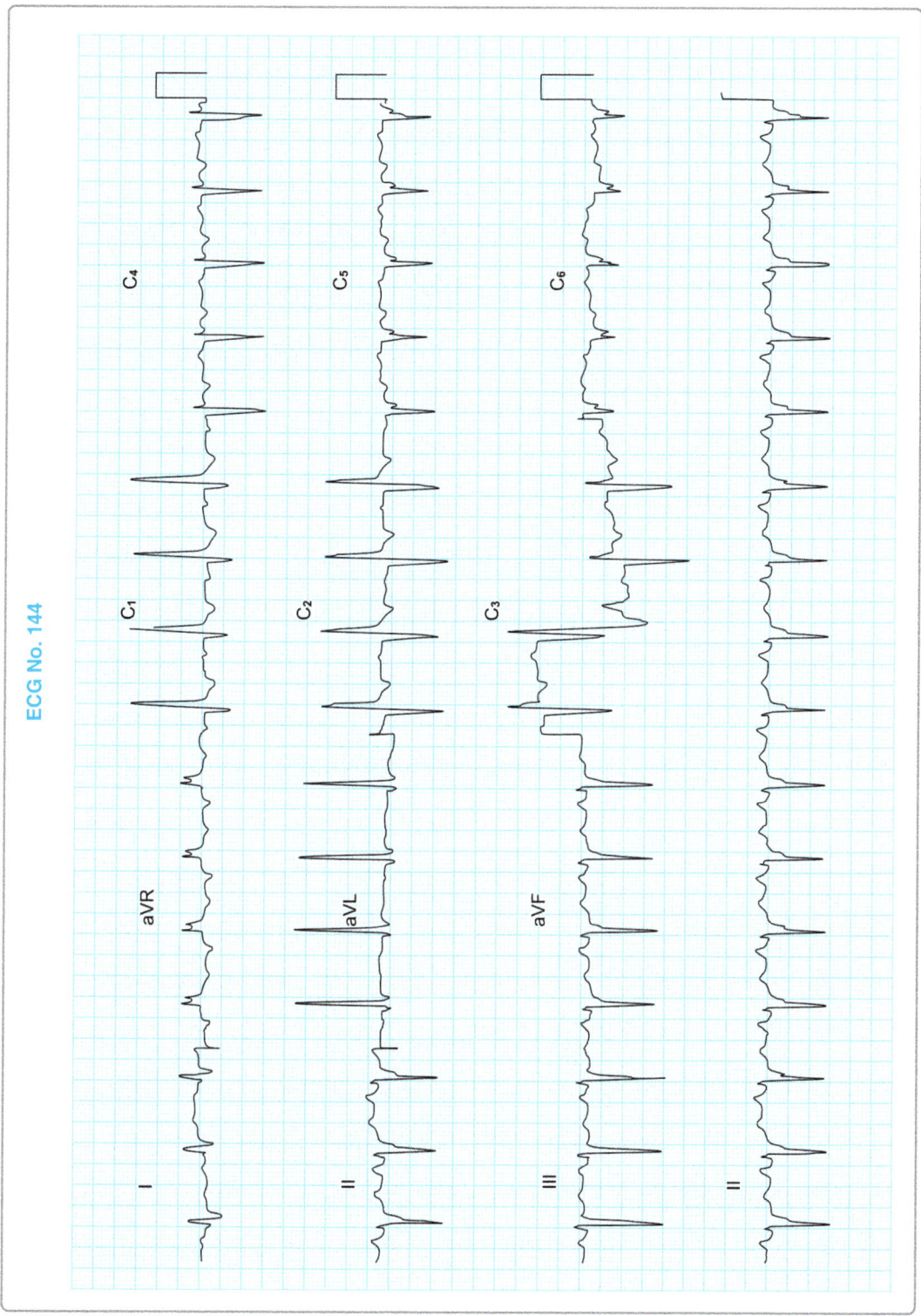

ECG in Medical Practice

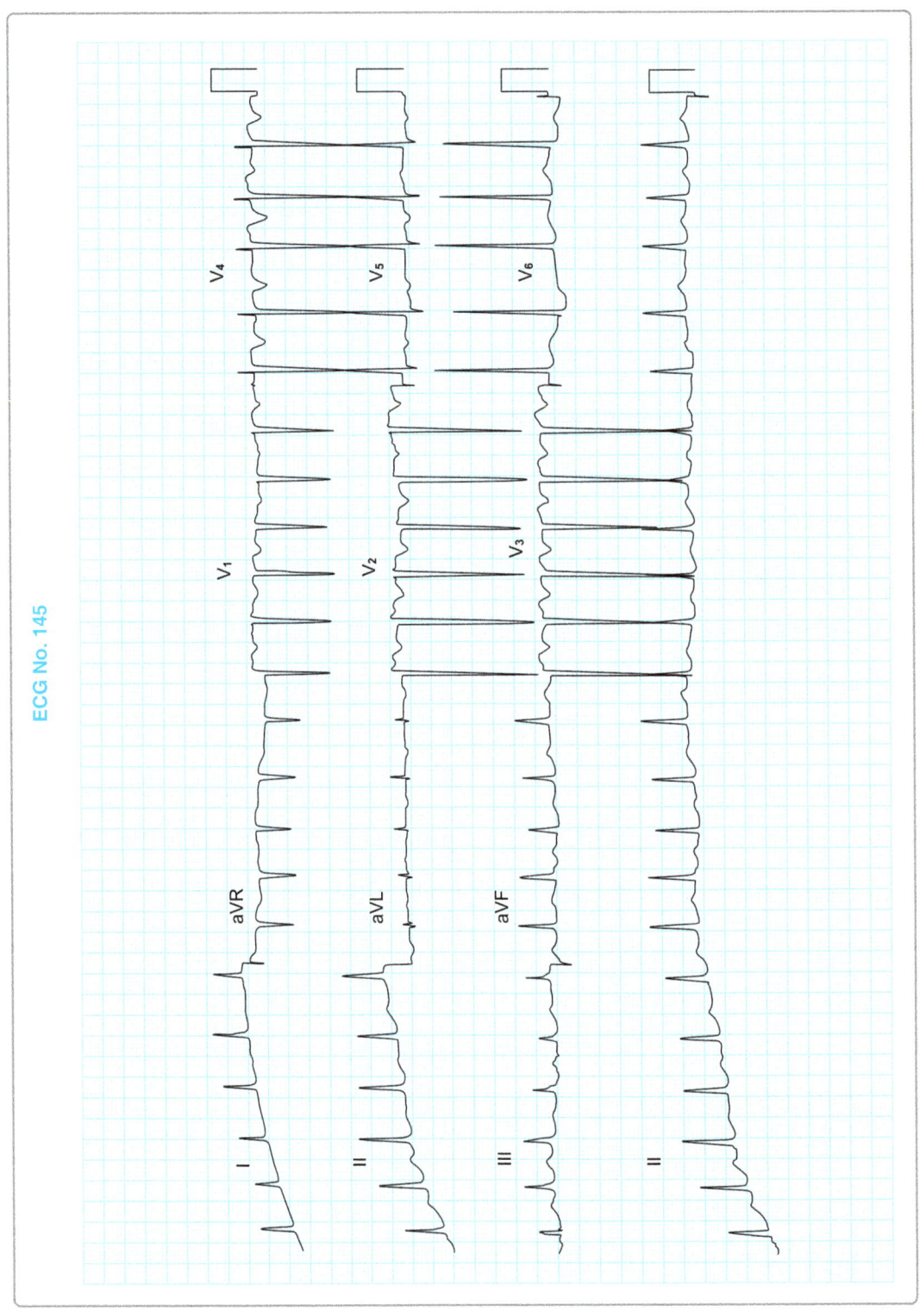

ECG No. 145

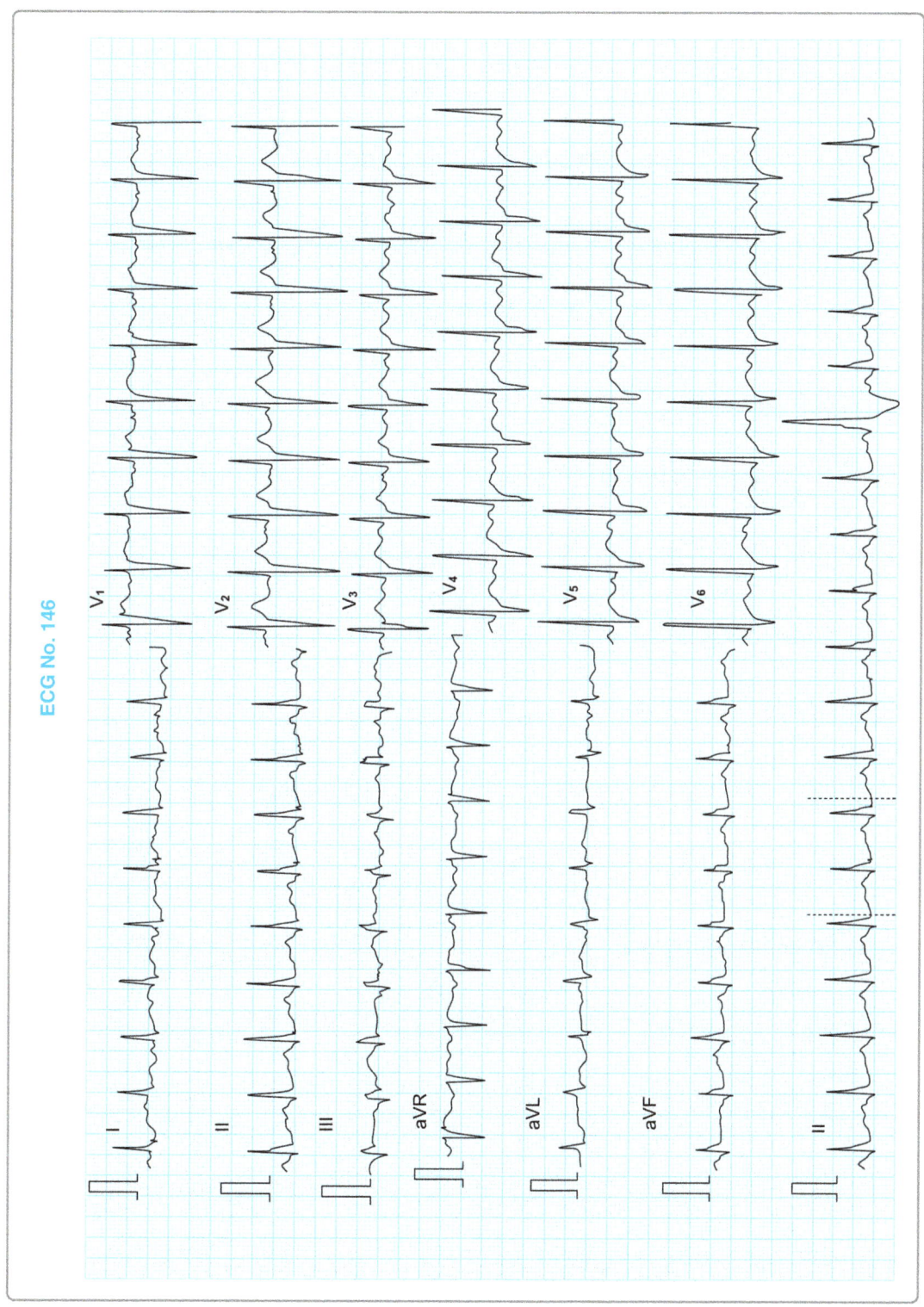

ECG in Medical Practice

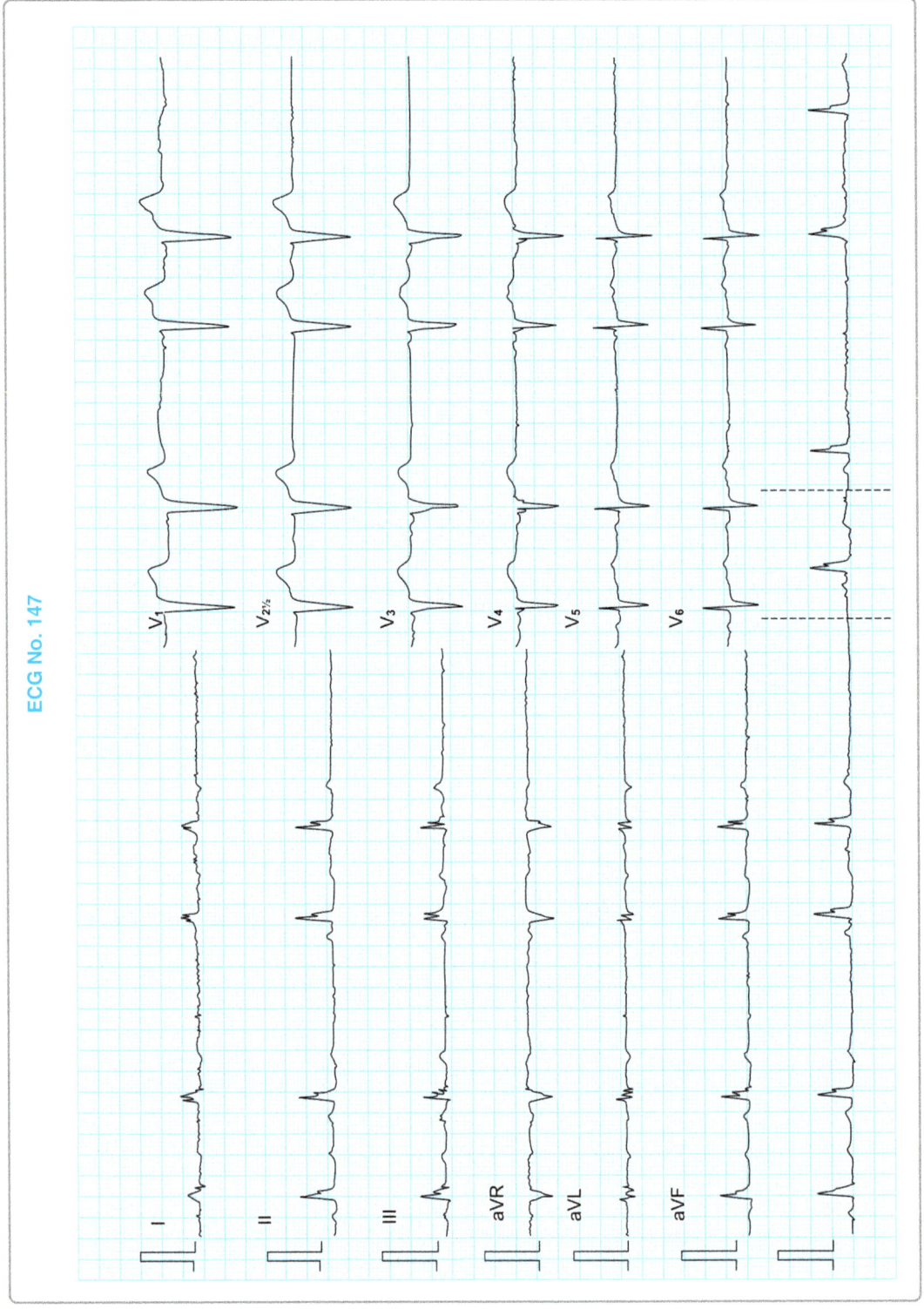

ECG No. 147

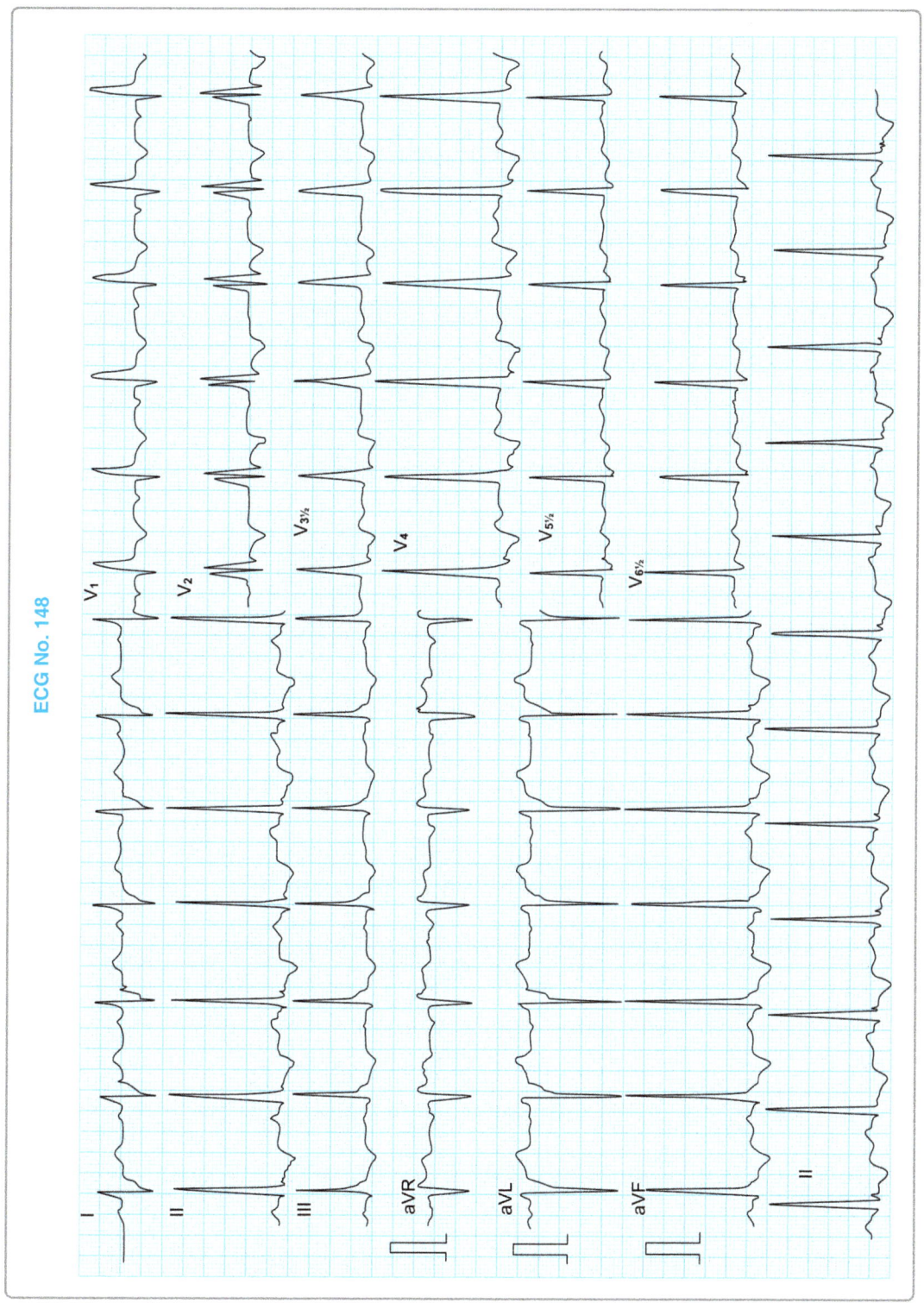

ECG No. 148

ECG in Medical Practice

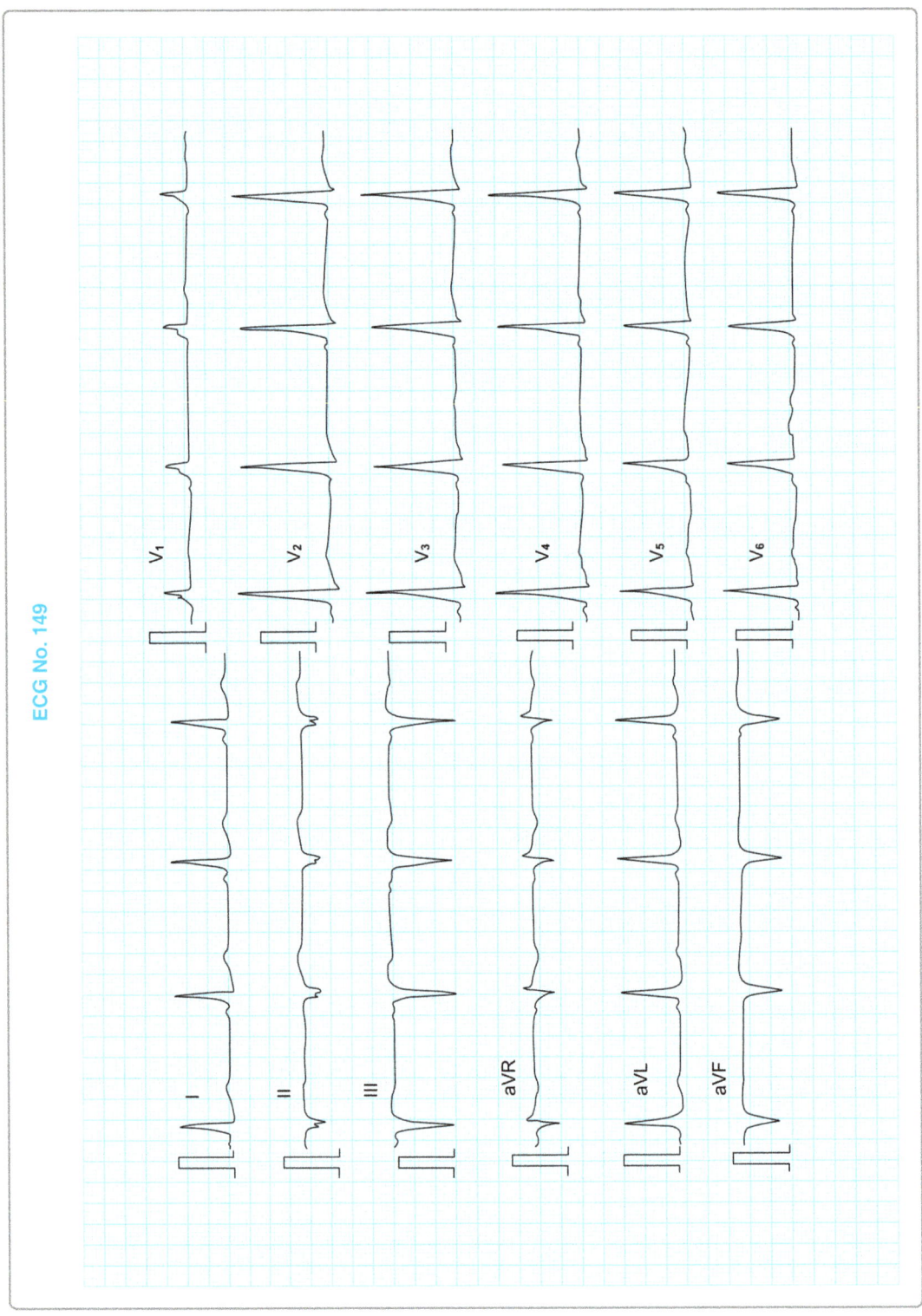

ECG No. 149

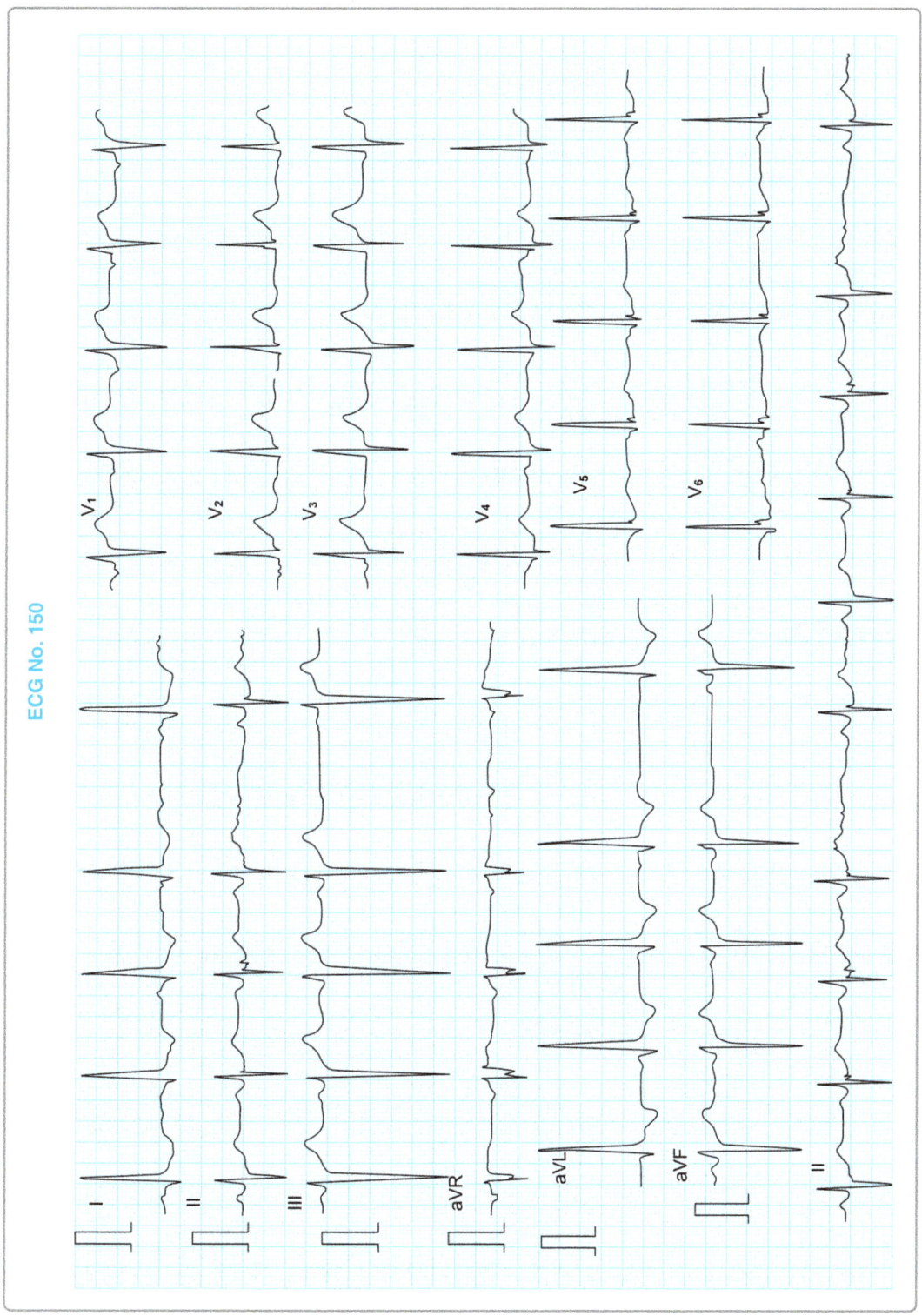

ECG No. 150

ECG in Medical Practice

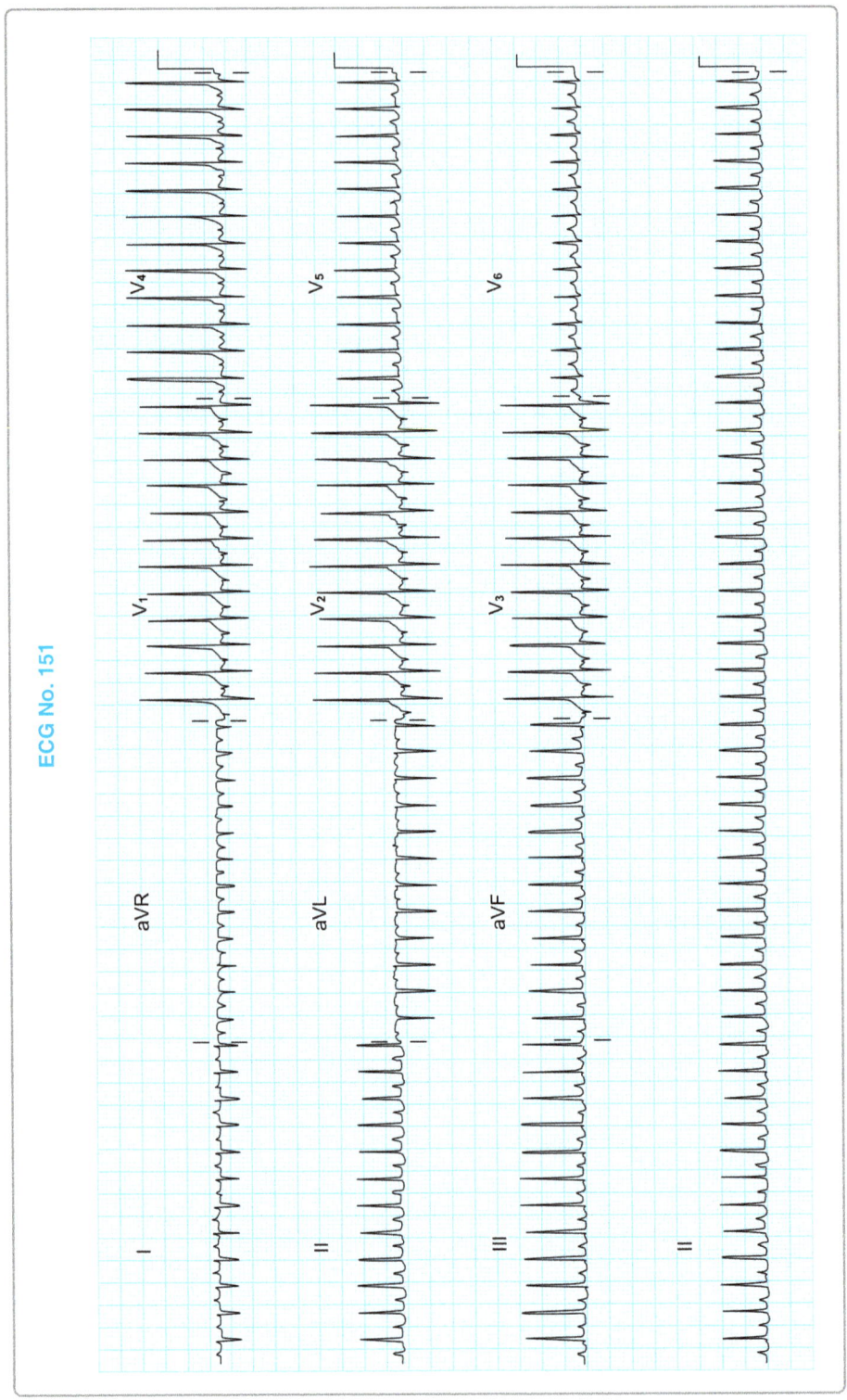

ECG No. 151

FINDINGS OF ECG TRACINGS

1. This electrocardiogram (ECG) shows:
   - Atrial rate—75/min
   - Ventricular rate—50/min
   - There is complete dissociation between P and QRS

   Diagnosis: Complete heart block.

2. This ECG shows:
   - P wave—absent
   - RR interval—irregular (rhythm irregular)
   - Heart rate >100 beats/min

   Diagnosis: Fast atrial fibrillation (atrial fibrillation with rapid ventricular response).

3. This ECG shows:
   - Pacemaker spike followed by QRS
   - In some leads, there are no spikes which indicate demand pacemaker

   Diagnosis: Single chamber demand ventricular pacemaker.

4. This ECG shows:
   - Pathological Q in lead III and aVF
   - Tall R in lead I and deep S in aVF (indicates left axis deviation)
   - Tall R (19 mm) in aVL (left ventricular hypertrophy)
   - U wave in V_4 and V_5

   Diagnosis: Old inferior myocardial infarction, left ventricular hypertrophy with hypokalemia.

5. This ECG shows:
   - $SV_1 + RV_6 > 35$ (here 48)
   - T inversion in lead I, aVL, V_2-V_6

   Diagnosis: Left ventricular hypertrophy with strain.

   Ques. Is there any other criteria of left ventricular hypertrophy in this ECG?
   Ans. Yes. There is tall R (33 mm) in V_5 (R >25 in V_5 indicates left ventricular hypertrophy).
   Ques. What is the differential diagnosis in this type of ECG?
   Ans. Hypertrophic cardiomyopathy (echocardiogram should be done to confirm the diagnosis).

6. This ECG shows:
   - Heart rate—150 beats/min
   - P, QRS, and T—normal
   - Rhythm—regular

   Diagnosis: Sinus tachycardia.

7. This ECG shows:
   - Heart rate—124 beats/min
   - Pathological Q in lead II, III and aVF, also in V_1-V_5
   - ST elevation in V_2-V_5

   Diagnosis: Acute anterior and old inferior myocardial infarction with sinus tachycardia.

8. This ECG shows:
   - Tall P in lead II and III (P pulmonale)
   - Q wave in lead II, III and aVF
   - Tall R in V_1
   - Poor R wave progression in V_5 and V_6

   Diagnosis: Right atrial hypertrophy (P pulmonale) with right ventricular hypertrophy with old inferior myocardial infarction.

9. This ECG shows:
    - Short PR interval (0.08 second)
    - Delta wave in lead I, aVL, V_2-V_6
    - Deep S in V_1
    - Q in lead III and aVF—confuses with old inferior myocardial infarction

    Diagnosis: Wolff–Parkinson–White (WPW) syndrome type B.

10. This ECG shows:
    - P wave—absent
    - Rhythm is irregular (RR interval is irregular)
    - ST depression in lead I, II, V_4-V_6 (thumb impression or reversed tick appearance)
    - Heart rate is 160 beats/min

    Diagnosis: Fast atrial fibrillation with digoxin effect.

11. This ECG shows:
    - Pathological Q in V_1-V_4
    - ST elevation in V_2-V_4
    - T inversion in lead I, aVL, V_2-V_6

    Diagnosis: Acute anteroseptal myocardial infarction.

12. This ECG shows:
    - Pathological Q in V_1-V_6
    - ST elevation in V_2-V_6

    Diagnosis: Acute extensive anterior myocardial infarction.

13. This ECG shows:
    - Tall R in lead I and deep S in lead aVF (indicates left axis deviation)
    - Deep T inversion in lead I, II, aVL, V_2-V_6

    Diagnosis: Subendocardial myocardial infarction or non-ST-elevation myocardial infarction (non-STEMI).

    Differential diagnosis: Hypertrophic cardiomyopathy.

14. This ECG shows:
    - Pacemaker spike in V_4-V_6 followed by QRS
    - No spike in other leads

    Diagnosis: Single chamber ventricular pacemaker.

15. This ECG shows:
    - Pacemaker spike in almost all the leads followed by QRS

    Diagnosis: Single chamber ventricular pacemaker.

16. This ECG shows:
    - P wave—absent
    - Flutter wave in V_1-V_3
    - Rhythm—irregular
    - Ventricular ectopic (in some leads)

    Diagnosis: Atrial flutter fibrillation with multiple ventricular ectopics.

17. This ECG shows:
    - P wave—absent
    - QRS normal and narrow
    - Rhythm—irregular (RR irregular)
    - Heart rate—160 beats/min

    Diagnosis: Fast atrial fibrillation.

    Differential diagnosis: Supraventricular tachycardia with variable block.

18. This ECG shows:
    - M pattern (RSR' pattern) in V_5-V_6
    - QRS—wide (0.16 second)
    - Pathological Q in V_1-V_3 (may be old anteroseptal myocardial infarction)

    Diagnosis: Left bundle branch block.

19. This ECG shows:
    - M pattern (RSR' pattern) in V_5-V_6
    - QRS—wide (0.16 second)
    - Pathological Q in V_1-V_2 (may be old myocardial infarction)

    Diagnosis: Left bundle branch block.

20. This ECG shows:
    - Multiple ventricular ectopics
    - Ventricular bigeminy pattern (every normal beat followed by an ectopic)
    - Pathological Q in lead II, III, aVF and in V_1-V_3

    Diagnosis: Old inferior and anteroseptal myocardial infarction with multiple ventricular ectopics (bigeminy pattern).

21. This ECG shows:
    - PP interval—120/min, regular
    - RR interval—58/min, regular
    - There is dissociation between P and QRS

    Diagnosis: Complete heart block.

22. This ECG shows:
    - ST elevation in V_1-V_6 with upward convexity
    - P wave is absent and rhythm is irregular

    Diagnosis: Acute anterior myocardial infarction with atrial fibrillation.

23. This ECG shows:
    - Tall P in lead II (indicates right atrial hypertrophy)
    - Tall R in V_1 and V_2
    - Multiple ventricular ectopics

    Diagnosis: Right ventricular hypertrophy with right atrial hypertrophy with multiple ventricular ectopics.

24. This ECG shows:
    - Pathological Q in lead II, III and aVF
    - Tall R in V_1
    - Wide QRS (0.16 second) and M (RSR' pattern) in pattern in V_2
    - Ventricular ectopics
    - Poor R wave progression in V_5 and V_6

    Diagnosis: Old inferior myocardial infarction with right bundle branch block with ventricular ectopics (unifocal).

25. This ECG shows:
    - Pathological Q in lead II, III and aVF with ST elevation in lead III and aVF
    - Atrial rate (PP interval)—100/min
    - Ventricular rate (RR interval)—50/min
    - Complete dissociation between P and QRS

    Diagnosis: Acute inferior myocardial infarction with complete heart block.

26. This ECG shows:
    - Wide P (P mitrale) in lead II
    - P wave is absent in some leads
    - Rhythm is irregular
    - Multiple ventricular ectopics

    Diagnosis: Left atrial hypertrophy (mitral stenosis) with atrial fibrillation with multiple ventricular ectopics.

27. This ECG shows:
    - Low voltage tracing
    - P wave is absent
    - There are some fibrillary f waves in lead I and II
    - Rhythm—irregular
    - Pathological Q in V_1-V_3

Diagnosis: Old anteroseptal myocardial infarction with fast atrial fibrillation with low voltage tracing.

28. This ECG shows:
    - Multiple ventricular ectopics
    - Tall R in lead I and deep S in lead aVF (indicates left axis deviation)
    - RSR'/M pattern in V_1-V_3 and QRS >0.12 (>3 small squares)

Diagnosis: Right bundle branch block with left anterior hemiblock (bifascicular block) with multiple ventricular ectopics.

29. This ECG shows:
    - P wave is absent, some fibrillary f waves in lead III
    - Rhythm is irregular
    - Few flutter waves in V_1
    - R in V_6 is 36. (Voltage is half in V_2-V_6)

Diagnosis: Atrial flutter fibrillation with left ventricular hypertrophy.

30. This ECG shows:
    - Pathological Q and ST elevation in V_1-V_3

Diagnosis: Acute anteroseptal myocardial infarction.

31. This ECG shows:
    - ST elevation in lead III and aVF
    - RSR'/M pattern in V_1 and V_2 with wide QRS (0.16 second)
    - P wave is absent
    - Rhythm is irregular
    - Deep S in lead I and tall R in lead aVF (indicates right axis deviation)

Diagnosis: Acute inferior myocardial infarction with fast atrial fibrillation with right bundle branch block with left posterior hemiblock.

32. This ECG shows:
    - Multiple atrial ectopics with bigeminy pattern in lead II
    - RSR' in V_1 and V_2 with QRS—0.12 second
    - T inverted in V_2-V_6

Diagnosis: Atrial ectopics with bigeminy with partial right bundle branch block with anterior ischemia.

33. This ECG shows:
    - P wave is absent
    - Rhythm is irregular
    - Pathological Q in lead II, III, aVF and V_1-V_4
    - RSR' (M pattern) in V_5 and V_6

Diagnosis: Old inferior and anteroseptal myocardial infarction with atrial fibrillation with left bundle branch block.

34. This ECG shows:
    - P wave is absent in V_2-V_6
    - Rhythm—irregular in V_2-V_6
    - P, QRS, T normal in other leads

Diagnosis: Paroxysmal atrial fibrillation.

35. This ECG shows:
    - Heart rate—180 beats/min
    - P wave is absent.
    - QRS is normal and narrow
    - Rhythm—regular

    Diagnosis: Supraventricular tachycardia.

36. This ECG shows:
    - Tall R in lead I and deep S in lead aVF (indicates left axis deviation)
    - Tall R in aVL (>11 mm, here it is 22)
    - Tall R in V_6 (>25 mm, here it is 29)
    - $SV_1 + RV_6$ >35 mm (here it is 38 mm)

    Diagnosis: Left ventricular hypertrophy.

37. This ECG shows:
    - Multiple ventricular ectopics with bigeminy pattern in rhythm lead (L_{II})
    - P wave is absent
    - Rhythm—irregular

    Diagnosis: Multiple ventricular ectopics with bigeminy with atrial fibrillation.

38. This ECG shows:
    - QRS—wide in all leads mainly V_5 and V_6 (0.16)
    - rSr' in V_5.

    Diagnosis: Left bundle branch block.

39. This ECG shows:
    - Pathological Q in lead II, III and aVF
    - Tall R in V_1 with wide QRS (0.20)
    - Deep S in V_5 and V_6 with poor R wave progression

    Diagnosis: Old inferior myocardial infarction with right bundle branch block.

40. This ECG shows:
    - Heart rate is 150 beats/min
    - P wave is absent
    - Rhythm is regular
    - QRS—normal
    - Pathological Q with ST elevation in V_2-V_4
    - Deep S in V_5 and V_6 with poor R wave progression

    Diagnosis: Acute anteroseptal myocardial infarction with supraventricular tachycardia.

41. This ECG shows:
    - $SV_1 + RV_6$ >35 mm (here it is 50)
    - Tall peaked T wave in V_4-V_6
    - There is also tall R in V_5 (35 mm)

    Diagnosis: Left ventricular hypertrophy with hyperkalemia (tall peak T).

42. This ECG shows:
    - ST elevation in lead II, III and aVF
    - Also ST elevation in V_5 and V_6

    Diagnosis: Acute inferior and lateral myocardial infarction.

43. This ECG shows:
    - Heart rate—38 beats/min with regular rhythm
    - Pathological Q with ST elevation in I, II, III, aVF

- Also Q in V_2-V_6 with ST elevation
- P wave is absent

Diagnosis: Acute inferior and anterior myocardial infarction with nodal rhythm with bradycardia.

44. This ECG shows:
    - Pathological Q in lead III and aVF
    - RSR' (M pattern) in V_1 and V_2
    - QRS wide (0.28 second)

Diagnosis: Old inferior myocardial infarction with right bundle branch block.

45. This ECG shows:
    - Pathological Q with ST elevation in lead II, III and aVF
    - P—absent
    - Rhythm is irregular
    - Occasional ventricular ectopics

Diagnosis: Acute inferior myocardial infarction with atrial fibrillation with ventricular ectopics.

46. This ECG shows:
    - P—absent
    - Rhythm—irregular
    - Heart rate—140 beats/min

Diagnosis: Fast atrial fibrillation.

47. This ECG shows:
    - P—absent
    - Flutter wave in lead II, III, aVR, aVL and aVF
    - Rhythm—irregular
    - Occasional ventricular ectopics

Diagnosis: Atrial flutter with fibrillation with ventricular ectopics.

48. This ECG shows:
    - Atrial rate (PP interval)—76/min
    - Ventricular rate (RR interval)—40/min
    - Complete dissociation between atria and ventricle

Diagnosis: Complete heart block.

49. This ECG shows:
    - Deep S in lead I and tall R in lead aVF (indicates right axis deviation)
    - Wide notched P wave in lead II and aVF (P mitrale)
    - Bifid P in V_1 with deeper downward deflection
    - Tall R in V_1 and V_2

Diagnosis: Left atrial hypertrophy (mitral stenosis) with right ventricular hypertrophy.

50. This ECG shows:
    - P—absent
    - Rhythm—irregular
    - Pathological Q in V_1-V_3
    - Heart rate is 150 beats/min

Diagnosis: Old anteroseptal myocardial infarction with fast atrial fibrillation.

51. This ECG shows:
    - P—absent
    - Rhythm—irregular

- ST depression with T inversion in lead I, aVL, V_5 and V6.
- $SV_1 + RV_6 > 35$ (Here it is 47 mm. Note R here is 1/2 voltage in V_4-V_6)
- Also R in aVL is 25 mm

Diagnosis: Atrial fibrillation with left ventricular hypertrophy with strain.

52. This ECG shows:
    - Pathological Q with ST elevation in lead II, III and aVF
    - Pathological Q in V_1-V_4
    - Tall R in aVL (>13 mm)

Diagnosis: Acute inferior and old anteroseptal myocardial infarction with left ventricular hypertrophy.

53. This ECG shows:
    - Pathological Q with ST elevation in lead II, III and aVF
    - T inversion in lead II, III and aVF

Diagnosis: Acute inferior myocardial infarction.

54. This ECG shows:
    - P—absent
    - Rhythm—(RR interval) irregular
    - Pathological Q in V_1-V_3.

Diagnosis: Atrial fibrillation with old anteroseptal myocardial infarction.

55. This ECG shows:
    - Heart rate—130 beats/min
    - P, QRS, T—normal
    - Rhythm—regular
    - $SV_1 + RV_6 > 35$ mm (here it is 48)

Diagnosis: Sinus tachycardia with left ventricular hypertrophy.

56. This ECG shows:
    - ST elevation with upward concavity in lead II, III, aVF
    - Also ST elevation with upward concavity V_4-V_6

Diagnosis: Acute pericarditis (It may be confused with acute myocardial infarction. However, in acute myocardial infarction, ST is elevated with upward convexity).

57. This ECG shows:
    - Pathological Q in lead II, III and aVF
    - Tall R in V_1 and V_2, QRS is 0.12 mm
    - Poor R wave progression

Diagnosis: Old inferior myocardial infarction with right ventricular hypertrophy.

58. This ECG shows:
    - Heart rate—56 beats/min
    - P, QRS, T—normal
    - J wave in V_3-V_6

Diagnosis: Sinus bradycardia.

59. This ECG shows:
    - $SV_1 + RV_6 > 35$ mm (here it is 48)
    - U wave in V_2-V_6

Diagnosis: Left ventricular hypertrophy with hypokalemia.

ECG in Medical Practice

60. This ECG shows:
    - P inverted in lead I
    - Deep S in V_4-V_6

Diagnosis: Dextrocardia.

Differential diagnosis: Arm leads reversed. See also **ECG No. 110.**

61. This ECG shows:
    - Heart rate—150 beats/min
    - P is absent, but QRS, T—normal
    - Rhythm—regular (RR interval)

Diagnosis: Supraventricular tachycardia.

62. This ECG shows:
    - P—absent
    - QRS, T—normal
    - Heart rate—98 beats/min
    - Rhythm—regular

Diagnosis: Nodal tachycardia.

63. This ECG shows:
    - PR interval—short (0.08 second)
    - Delta wave in V_4-V_6
    - Pathological Q wave lead III and aVF
    - Deep S in V_1

Diagnosis: WPW syndrome type B (deep S in V_1).

64. This ECG shows:
    - Ectopic beats in all leads, P is inverted with short PR interval
    - QRS complex—0.10 mm

Diagnosis: Atrial ectopics (low atrial).

Differential diagnosis: High nodal ectopics.

65. This ECG shows:
    - In the upper tracing—in the begging, there is ventricular ectopics. Later part of the ECG shows runs of ectopics (ventricular tachycardia)
    - In the middle tracing—ventricular tachycardia
    - In the lower tracing—in the begging, there is Torsades de pointes. Later part of the ECG shows ventricular fibrillation

66. This ECG shows:
    - SV_1 + RV_6 >35 mm (here it is 64 mm)
    - T inversion in lead I, aVL, V_4-V_6

Diagnosis: Left ventricular hypertrophy with strain.

Differential diagnosis: Hypertrophic cardiomyopathy.

67. This ECG shows:
    - Pathological Q in lead III and aVF
    - Multiple ventricular ectopics
    - Every three normal beat is followed by a ventricular ectopic

Diagnosis: Old inferior myocardial infarction with ventricular quadrigeminy.

68. This ECG shows:
    - Multiple ventricular ectopics
    - In L_{II}, every normal beat is followed by a ventricular ectopic

Diagnosis: Ventricular bigeminy.

69. This ECG shows:
    - Multiple ventricular ectopics
    - In L_{II}, every two normal beat is followed by a ventricular ectopic

    Diagnosis: Ventricular trigeminy.

70. This ECG shows:
    - First tracing shows prolonged PR interval (here it is 0.20 mm). Diagnosis: first-degree atrioventricular (AV) block
    - Second tracing shows progressive lengthening of the PR interval followed by a drop. Diagnosis: Mobitz type I second-degree AV block (Wenckebach's phenomenon)
    - Third tracing shows every three P, QRS, T is followed by a drop beat. Diagnosis: Mobitz type II second-degree AV block (3:1)
    - Fourth tracing shows complete dissociation between P and QRS. Diagnosis: Complete heart block (PP interval is 76, RR interval is 34 mm)

71. This ECG shows:
    - P—absent
    - Rhythm—irregular (RR interval is irregular)
    - ST depression with thumb impression appearance (in V_5 and V_6, also in L_{II})

    Diagnosis: Atrial fibrillation with digoxin effect.

72. This ECG shows:
    - Tall R in lead I and deep S in lead aVF (indicates left axis deviation)
    - Tall R in V_1 and V_2 (indicates right ventricular hypertrophy)
    - Tall R in aVL (here it is 17 mm)—indicates left ventricular hypertrophy

    Diagnosis: Biventricular hypertrophy.

73. This ECG shows:
    - Tall R in lead I and deep S in lead aVF (indicates left axis deviation)
    - RSR' (M pattern) with wide QRS in V_1 (0.16 mm)
    - Tall R in aVL (here it is 18 mm)—indicates left ventricular hypertrophy

    Diagnosis: Right bundle branch block with left anterior hemiblock (bifascicular block) with left ventricular hypertrophy.

74. This ECG shows:
    - Deep S in lead I and tall R in lead aVF (indicates right axis deviation)
    - Tall R in V_1 and V_2 with T inversion (indicates right ventricular hypertrophy)
    - Also T inversion in lead II, lead III and aVF

    Diagnosis: Right ventricular hypertrophy with strain with left posterior hemiblock with inferior ischemia.

75. This ECG shows:
    - Tall R in lead I and deep S in lead aVF (indicates left axis deviation)
    - RSR' (M pattern) in V_1 with wide QRS (0.16 mm)

    Diagnosis: Right bundle branch block with left anterior hemiblock (bifascicular block).

76. This ECG shows:
    - Pathological Q in lead II, III, aVF
    - Also pathological Q in V_1-V_3

    Diagnosis: Old inferior and anteroseptal myocardial infarction.

77. This ECG shows:
    - Deep S in lead I and tall R in lead aVF (indicates right axis deviation)
    - Tall P in lead II (here it is 4 mm, indicates P pulmonale)
    - Bifid P in V_1 with tall upward deflection
    - Tall R in V_1-V_3 with T inversion in V_1-V_4

    Diagnosis: Right ventricular hypertrophy with strain with right atrial hypertrophy.

78. This ECG shows:
    - Pathological Q in lead II, III and aVF

    Diagnosis: Old inferior myocardial infarction.

79. This ECG shows:
    - RSR' in V_1
    - QRS is normal (0.08 second)
    - Heart rate is 104 beats/min

    Diagnosis: Partial right bundle branch block with sinus tachycardia.

80. This ECG shows:
    - Tall P in lead II (here it is 5 mm, indicates P pulmonale, due to right atrial hypertrophy)
    - Bifid P in V_1 (with tall upward deflection)
    - Wide notched P in V_2-V_4 (indicates P mitrale due to left atrial hypertrophy)

    Diagnosis: Biatrial hypertrophy.

81. This ECG shows:
    - Low voltage tracing
    - Occasional ventricular ectopics
    - PR interval—prolonged (0.24 second)

    Diagnosis: First-degree heart block with ventricular ectopics with low voltage tracing.

82. This ECG shows:
    - Deep S in lead I
    - Deep Q and T inversion in lead III

    Diagnosis: Pulmonary embolism (typical $S_I Q_{III} T_{III}$ pattern).

83. This ECG shows:
    - P—absent
    - Rhythm is irregular (RR interval is irregular)
    - Pathological Q in lead II, III, aVF and also in V_1-V_4
    - QRS—0.12 second
    - RSR'/M pattern in lead I, aVL, V_5 and V_6

    Diagnosis: Old inferior and anteroseptal myocardial infarction with atrial fibrillation with partial left bundle branch block.

84. This ECG shows:
    - P—absent
    - Rhythm is irregular (RR interval is irregular)
    - Heart rate—110 beats/min

    Diagnosis: Fast atrial fibrillation.

85. This ECG shows:
    - Pathological Q in lead II, III and aVF
    - Tall R in V_1 and V_2, QRS is 0.12 second

    Diagnosis: Old inferior myocardial infarction with right ventricular hypertrophy.

86. This ECG shows:
    - PR interval is prolonged (0.24 second)
    - Pathological Q in lead II, III and aVF, also in V_1-V_3
    - Tall R in V_1
    - QRS—wide (0.16 second)

    Diagnosis: Old inferior and anteroseptal myocardial infarction with first-degree heart block with right bundle branch block.

87. This ECG shows:
    - Tall R in lead I and deep S in lead aVF (indicates left axis deviation)
    - Tall P in lead II (here it is 3 mm, indicates right atrial hypertrophy)
    - Bifid P with deeper downward deflection in V_1 (indicates left atrial hypertrophy)
    - $SV_1 + RV_6 > 35$ mm (here it is 40 mm), also tall R in aVL (>11 mm, here it is 17 mm)
    - T inversion in lead I, aVL, V_5 and V_6

    Diagnosis: Left ventricular hypertrophy with strain and right atrial hypertrophy with left atrial hypertrophy (biatrial).

88. This ECG shows:
    - Complete dissociation between P and QRS (PP is 100 and RR is 60)
    - Pathological Q with ST elevation in V_1-V_3

    Diagnosis: Acute anteroseptal myocardial infarction with complete heart block.

89. This ECG shows:
    - PR interval is prolonged (0.24 second)
    - Pathological Q in lead III and aVF
    - Symmetrical T inversion in V_1-V_6
    - Tall R in aVL (here it is 17 mm)

    Diagnosis: Old inferior myocardial infarction with subendocardial myocardial infarction or non-STEMI with first-degree heart block with left ventricular hypertrophy.

90. This ECG shows:
    - P—absent
    - Rhythm—irregular (RR interval is irregular)
    - Pathological Q in lead II, III, aVF and also in V_1-V_4
    - Heart rate—110 beats/min

    Diagnosis: Old inferior and anteroseptal myocardial infarction with fast atrial fibrillation.

91. This ECG shows:
    - Pathological Q and ST elevation in V_1-V_4
    - RSR'/M pattern in V_5 and V_6
    - QRS is 0.12 second
    - Heart rate—102 beats/min

    Diagnosis: Acute anteroseptal myocardial infarction with partial left bundle branch block with sinus tachycardia.

92. This ECG shows:
    - P—absent and sawtooth appearance in V_1
    - Rhythm is irregular (RR interval is irregular)
    - RSR'/M pattern in V_6
    - QRS—0.12 second

    Diagnosis: Atrial flutter with fibrillation with partial left bundle branch block.

93. This ECG shows:
    - P wave is absent
    - Multiple ventricular ectopics
    - Rhythm is irregular (RR interval is irregular)

    Diagnosis: Atrial fibrillation with multiple ventricular ectopics.

94. This ECG shows:
    - Every two P wave is followed by absent QRS complex

    Diagnosis: Mobitz type II, second-degree AV block (2:1).

95. This ECG shows:
    - ST elevation with pathological Q in V_2-V_5
    - Multiple ventricular ectopics
    - QRS wide (0.20 second) in V_1 with RSR' (M pattern)
    - Prolonged absence of P, QRS and T in rhythm strip

Diagnosis: Acute anterior myocardial infarction with right bundle branch block with multiple ventricular ectopics with sinus arrest.

96. This ECG shows:
    - Heart rate—150 beats/min
    - Pathological Q with ST elevation in lead II, III and aVF
    - RSR' (M pattern) in V_1 with wide QRS (0.16 second)

Diagnosis: Acute inferior myocardial infarction with right bundle branch block with sinus tachycardia.

97. This ECG shows:
    - P—absent
    - Rhythm—irregular (RR interval is irregular)
    - Multiple ventricular ectopics
    - Pathological Q in V_1-V_4

Diagnosis: Atrial fibrillation with multiple ventricular ectopics with old anteroseptal myocardial infarction.

98. This ECG shows:
    - Pathological Q in lead III and aVF
    - $SV_1 + RV_6 > 35$ mm (here it is 40 mm)
    - Tall R in aVL (here it is 18 mm) with T inversion in lead I, aVL and V_6

Diagnosis: Old inferior myocardial infarction with left ventricular hypertrophy with strain.

99. This ECG shows:
    - Pathological Q in lead III and aVF
    - ST elevation and pathological Q in V_1-V_3
    - Tall R in V_1 and V_2 with wide QRS (0.26 second)
    - Heart rate—140 beats/min

Diagnosis: Old inferior and acute anteroseptal myocardial infarction with right bundle branch block sinus tachycardia.

100. This ECG shows:
    - Progressive lengthening of PR interval followed by drop beat
    - RSR' in V_1 with QRS 0.12 second

Diagnosis: Wenckebach's phenomenon (Mobitz type I) with partial right bundle branch block.

101. This ECG shows:
    - P wave—absent
    - Rhythm—irregular (RR interval irregular)
    - QRS—wide >0.12 (here it is 0.16)
    - Delta wave in V_4, V_5 and V_6
    - Heart rate is 280 beats/min

Diagnosis: WPW syndrome with fast atrial fibrillation.

102. This ECG shows:
    - ST elevation and pathological Q in lead II, III and aVF
    - Pathological Q in V_4, V_5 and V_6

Diagnosis: Acute inferior and old lateral myocardial infarction.

103. This ECG shows:
    - P—absent
    - Rhythm—irregular (RR interval is irregular)
    - RSR' (M pattern) in V_5 and V_6
    - QRS—wide >0.12 second (here it is 0.16)

Diagnosis: Left bundle branch block with atrial fibrillation.

104. This ECG shows:
    - PR interval—0.22 second
    - Pathological Q in lead II, III and aVF
    - RSR' (M pattern) in V_1 and V_2
    - QRS—wide >0.12 second (here it is 0.16)

Diagnosis: Old inferior myocardial infarction with first-degree heart block with right bundle branch block (bifascicular block).

105. This ECG shows:
    - P—bifid and wide (here it is 0.12)
    - Tall R in V_1
    - Tall R in V_5 (32. See voltage here is 5 mm in the beginning of ECG)

Diagnosis: Biventricular hypertrophy with left atrial hypertrophy (or enlargement).

106. This ECG shows:
    - Multiple unifocal ventricular ectopic
    - Pathological Q in C_1, C_2 and C_3

Diagnosis: Old anteroseptal myocardial infarction with ventricular ectopics.

107. This ECG shows:
    - Pacemaker spike
    - One spike before P wave
    - Also another spike before QRS

Diagnosis: Dual chamber pacing.

108. This ECG shows:
    - P—absent
    - Rhythm—irregular (RR interval is irregular)
    - ST—depression in lead II, III, aVF, V_1-V_6
    - RSR' (M pattern) in V_1 and V_2 with QRS 0.12 second

Diagnosis: Fast atrial fibrillation with digoxin effect with partial right bundle branch block.

109. This ECG shows:
    - Tall R in lead I and deep S in aVF (indicates left axis deviation)
    - Tall R in aVL (18 mm)
    - RSR' (M pattern) in V_5 and V_6 with QRS 0.10 second
    - T inversion in lead I, aVL, V_3-V_6

Diagnosis: Left ventricular hypertrophy with strain with partial left bundle branch block.

110. This ECG shows:
    - P inverted in lead I
    - QRS in chest leads—normal

Diagnosis: Arms leads reversed or incorrectly placed arms lead (technical dextrocardia, see also **ECG No. 60**).

ECG in Medical Practice

111. This ECG shows:
    - Tall R in lead I and deep S in aVF (indicates left axis deviation)
    - Tall R in aVL (17 mm)
    - RSR'/M pattern in V_1 and V_2 with QRS 0.16 second
    - Tall R in V_5 (30 mm) with T inversion in V_5 and V_6

    Diagnosis: Left ventricular hypertrophy with strain with right bundle branch block with left anterior hemiblock.

112. This ECG shows:
    - P wave—absent
    - Rhythm—irregular (RR interval is irregular)
    - ST—depression in lead II, III, aVF, V_1-V_6
    - RSR'/M pattern in V_1 and V_2 with QRS 0.16 second
    - Heart rate—150 beats/ min

    Diagnosis: Fast atrial fibrillation with right bundle branch block.

113. This ECG shows:
    - ST elevation and pathological Q in lead II, III and aVF
    - ST elevation in V_1-V_6 (right side)

    Diagnosis: Acute inferior and right ventricular infarction (right ventricular infarction is associated with inferior myocardial infarction, seen in V_1, also RV_3 and RV_4).

114. This ECG shows:
    - P—absent
    - Rhythm—irregular (RR interval is irregular)
    - Unifocal ventricular ectopics in V_1-V_5
    - Flutter wave in V_1

    Diagnosis: Atrial flutter fibrillation with ventricular ectopics.

115. This ECG shows:
    - Tall R in lead I and deep S in aVF (indicates left axis deviation)
    - Unifocal ventricular ectopics in V_1-V_6
    - Absent of PQRST in lead I to V_6
    - Tall R in V_1-V_2 with QRS 0.12

    Diagnosis: Right ventricular hypertrophy with ventricular ectopics with sinoatrial (SA) block.

116. This ECG shows:
    - Heart rate—28 beats/min
    - Tall R in lead I and deep S in aVF (indicates left axis deviation)
    - Tall R in aVL (15 mm)
    - RSR'/M pattern in V_1 and V_2 with QRS 0.16

    Diagnosis: Sinus bradycardia with left ventricular hypertrophy with right bundle branch block.

117. This ECG shows:
    - Tall R in lead I and deep S in aVF (indicates left axis deviation)
    - Tall R in aVL (16 mm)
    - Absent QRS in some leads
    - RSR'/M pattern in V_1 and V_2 with QRS 0.16

    Diagnosis: Left ventricular hypertrophy with right bundle branch block with SA block.

118. This ECG shows:
    - ST elevation in lead III and aVF, also V_3-V_6
    - Pathological Q in lead I, aVL, V_5 and V_6
    - Few supraventricular ectopic in L_{II}

    Diagnosis: Acute inferior and anterolateral myocardial infarction with supraventricular ectopic.

119. This ECG shows:
    - Absent of PQRST in some leads
    - T inversion in lead I and V_3-V_6

Diagnosis: Sinus arrest with lateral ischemia.

120. This ECG shows:
    - Heart rate—130 beats/min
    - Low voltage tracing (R <5 mm in limb leads and <10 mm in chest leads)

Diagnosis: Low voltage tracing with sinus tachycardia.

121. This ECG shows:
    - Multiple unifocal ventricular ectopics
    - Every one normal beat is followed by an ectopic beat

Diagnosis: Ventricular ectopics with bigeminy pattern.

122. This ECG shows:
    - P inverted in lead I
    - Deep S in V_2-V_6

Diagnosis: Dextrocardia.

Differential diagnosis: Arms leads reversed, see **page 334 and 339**.

123. This ECG shows:
    - Every two P, QRS, T is followed by a drop beat—Mobitz type II second-degree AV block (2:1)

124. This ECG shows:
    - Two consecutive pacemaker spikes followed by QRS

Diagnosis: Dual chamber pacemaker.

125. This ECG shows:
    - Atrial rate—100/min (PP is 100/min)
    - Ventricular rate—50/min (RR is 50/min)
    - Complete dissociation between P and QRS

Diagnosis: Complete heart block.

126. This ECG shows:
    - P—absent
    - Rhythm—irregular (RR interval is irregular)
    - Pathological Q in V_1-V_3
    - One ventricular ectopic beat

Diagnosis: Old anteroseptal myocardial infarction with atrial fibrillation with ventricular ectopic beat.

127. This ECG shows:
    - P—absent
    - Rhythm—irregular
    - Pathological Q in III and aVF, also in V_1-V_3

Diagnosis: Old inferior and anteroseptal myocardial infarction with atrial fibrillation.

128. This ECG shows:
    - Pacemaker spike followed by QRS
    - One ventricular ectopic beat

Diagnosis: Ventricular pacemaker with ventricular ectopic.

129. This ECG shows:
    - Low voltage tracing (R <5 mm in limb leads and <10 mm in chest leads)
    - Pathological Q in V_1-V_4

Diagnosis: Old anteroseptal myocardial infarction with low voltage tracing.

130. This ECG shows:
    - Pathological Q in V_1-V_3
    - Tall R in lead I and deep S in aVF (indicates left axis deviation)

    Diagnosis: Old anteroseptal myocardial infarction (with probable left ventricular hypertrophy).

131. This ECG shows:
    - $SV_1 + RV_6 > 35$ mm
    - U wave in V_3-V_6

    Diagnosis: Left ventricular hypertrophy with hypokalemia.

132. This ECG shows:
    - P—absent
    - Rhythm—irregular (RR interval is irregular)
    - Ventricular ectopics in V_1-V_6

    Diagnosis: Atrial fibrillation with ventricular ectopics (confuses with Ashman phenomenon).

133. This ECG shows:
    - Pathological Q in lead III and aVF
    - Heart rate—58 beats/min
    - P, QRS, T—normal

    Diagnosis: Sinus bradycardia with old inferior myocardial infarction.

134. This ECG shows:
    - Heart rate—58 beats/min
    - Pathological Q in lead III and aVF
    - Pathological Q with ST elevation in V_1-V_6

    Diagnosis: Old inferior and acute anterior myocardial infarction with sinus bradycardia.

135. This ECG shows:
    - Pathological Q with ST elevation in V_1-V_3
    - Tall R in V_6 (>25, here it is 30 mm)
    - T inversion in V_2-V_6

    Diagnosis: Acute anteroseptal myocardial infarction with left ventricular hypertrophy with strain.

136. This ECG shows:
    - Tall R in lead I and deep S in aVF (indicates left axis deviation)
    - RSR' (M pattern) with wide QRS in V_1
    - Tall R in V_1 and V_2
    - Tall R in aVL (>11, here it is 17 mm)
    - One complex (PQRST) is absent in rhythm lead (indicates sinus arrest)
    - Heart rate is 50 beats/min

    Diagnosis: Right bundle branch block with left anterior hemiblock (bifascicular block) with left ventricular hypertrophy with sinus arrest with sinus bradycardia.

137. This ECG shows:
    - Short PR interval
    - Tall R in lead I and deep S in aVF (indicates left axis deviation)
    - RSR' (M pattern) with wide QRS in V_1
    - Tall R in V_1
    - Tall R in aVL (>11)

    Diagnosis: Right bundle branch block with left anterior hemiblock (bifascicular block) with left ventricular hypertrophy with short PR interval.

138. This ECG shows:
   - Pathological Q with ST elevation in lead III and aVF
   - ST depression in lead I, aVL, V_2-V_6
   - Heart rate is 104 beats/min

Diagnosis: Acute inferior myocardial infarction with anterolateral ischemia with sinus tachycardia.

139. This ECG shows:
   - P—absent
   - Rhythm is irregular (RR interval is irregular)
   - RSR' (M pattern) with wide QRS (0.16) in V_1-V_4
   - ST depression in V_2-V_6 (thumb impression or reversed tick appearance)

Diagnosis: Atrial fibrillation with digoxin effect with right bundle branch block.

140. This ECG shows:
   - Ventricular ectopics in lead I, aVL, aVF, V_1-V_6
   - Atrial ectopics in lead II, III
   - RSR' (M pattern) with wide QRS (0.16) in V_1 and V_2

Diagnosis: Ventricular ectopics with atrial ectopics with right bundle branch block.

141. This ECG shows:
   - P—absent
   - Rhythm is irregular (RR interval is irregular)
   - Pathological Q in lead III and aVF
   - RSR'/M pattern with wide QRS (0.16) in V_1-V_3

Diagnosis: Old inferior myocardial infarction with atrial fibrillation with right bundle branch block.

142. This ECG shows:
   - Heart rate—50 beats/min
   - P, QRS, T—normal
   - Supraventricular ectopics in V_1-V_6

Diagnosis: Sinus bradycardia with supraventricular ectopics.

143. This ECG shows:
   - P wave is absent, some fibrillary f waves in lead III
   - Rhythm is irregular (RR interval is irregular)
   - Few flutter waves in II, III and aVF
   - $SV_1 + RV_6 > 35$ (here it is 42 mm)
   - Heart rate—120 beats/min

Diagnosis: Fast atrial flutter fibrillation with left ventricular hypertrophy.

144. This ECG shows:
   - Tall R in lead I and deep S in aVF (indicates left axis deviation)
   - Tall R in C_1 and C_2 (right ventricular hypertrophy)
   - Tall R in aVL (here it is 15 mm, indicates left ventricular hypertrophy)
   - Pathological Q in C_1-C_6
   - Heart rate—106 beats/min

Diagnosis: Biventricular hypertrophy with old extensive anterior myocardial infarction with sinus tachycardia.

145. This ECG shows:
   - P—absent
   - Rhythm is irregular (RR interval is irregular).

- Pathological Q in V_1-V_3
- Heart rate—120 beats/min

Diagnosis: Fast atrial flutter fibrillation with old anteroseptal myocardial infarction.

146. This ECG shows:
    - ST elevation lead III and aVF
    - One ventricular ectopic in lead II
    - Heart rate—130 beats/min

Diagnosis: Acute inferior myocardial infarction with ventricular ectopic with sinus tachycardia.

147. This ECG shows:
    - Pathological Q in V_1-V_4
    - Absent of PQRST in all leads

Diagnosis: Old anteroseptal myocardial infarction with SA block.

148. This ECG shows:
    - Deep S in L_1 and tall R in aVF (indicates right axis deviation)
    - RSR′ (M pattern) in V_1-V_2 (QRS >0.12)
    - Tall R in V_6 (see the voltage is half)
    - T inversion in lead II, III and aVF, also in V_1-V_6

Diagnosis: Right bundle branch block with left posterior hemiblock with left ventricular hypertrophy with strain.

149. This ECG shows:
    - PR interval—short (0.08 second)
    - Delta wave in V_1-V_6 with tall R in V_1
    - Pathological Q in II, III and aVF (confuses with old inferior myocardial infarction)

Diagnosis: WPW syndrome type A.

150. This ECG shows:
    - Tall R in lead I and deep S in aVF (indicates left axis deviation)
    - Tall R in aVL (here it is 18 mm)
    - One PQRST complex is absent in some leads, also in rhythm lead

Diagnosis: Left ventricular hypertrophy with SA block.

151. This ECG shows:
    - Heart rate is >300 beats/min
    - No P wave
    - Deep S in L_1 and tall R in aVF (indicates right axis deviation)
    - Tall R in V_1

Diagnosis: Narrow-complex supraventricular tachycardia with right ventricular hypertrophy.

Suggested Reading

1. Luthra A. **ECG Made Easy**, 6th edition. New Delhi: Jaypee Brothers Medical Publishers (P) Ltd.; 2020.
2. Hampton J, Hampton J. **The ECG Made Easy**, 9th edition. Elsevier Ltd.; 2019.
3. Hampton J, Adlam D. **The ECG Made Practical**, 7th edition. Elsevier Ltd.; 2019.
4. Hampton J, Adlam D, Hampton J. **150 ECG cases**, 5th edition. Elsevier Ltd. 2019.
5. Chakraborty B. **Textbook of Basic and advanced electrocardiography**, 1st edition. New Delhi: Jaypee Brothers Medical Publishers (P) Ltd.; 2020.
6. Goldberger AL, Goldberger E. **Clinical Electrocardiography: A Simplified Approach**, 8th edition. Elsevier Ltd.; 2012.
7. Goldman MJ. **Principles of Clinical Electrocardiography**, 12th edition. Lange Medical Publications; 1986.
8. Leo S. **An Introduction to Electrocardiography**, 8th edition (adapted edition). Wiley Ltd. 2018.
9. Chowdhury AB, Chowdhury A. **Practical Electrocardiography**, 3rd edition. New Maitri Printers, Anderkilla, Chittagong.
10. Raiston SH, Penman ID, Mark WJ Strachan, Hobson RP. **Davidson's Principles and Practice of Medicine**, 23rd edition. Elsevier Ltd.; 2018.
11. Kumar P, Clark M. **Kumar & Clark's Clinical Medicine**, 9th edition. London: Elsevier Ltd.; 2017.
12. Kasper DL, Fauci AS, Hauser SL, Longo DL, Jameson JL, Loscalzo J, et al. **Harrison's Principles of Internal Medicine**, 20th edition. McGraw Hill; 2018.

Index

A

Acidosis 153
   correction of 153
Acute coronary syndrome 130
Addison's disease 159
Adenosine
   intravenous 61
   mode of action of 62
   therapy, contraindications of 62
Adrenaline 55
Alkalosis 157
Amiloride 152
Amiodarone 31, 102, 104, 106
Amyloidosis 100, 104, 106
Aneurysm, aortic 136
Angina
   pectoris 128, 129
   types of 128
Anorexia 27, 147
Anticoagulant 132
   role of 73, 126
Anxiety 27
Aortic valve
   disease 115
   stenosis 38
Arm leads, reversing of 15
Arrhythmia 3, 10, 32, 124, 153, 161, 171
   documentation of 40
   ventricular 157
Artery
   coronary 5
   posterior descending 5
Ashman beats 74
Ashman phenomenon 74
Aspirin 132
Atherosclerosis 170
Atrial beat 14
Atrial dilatation 19
Atrial ectopic 79, 334
   causes of 79
   electrocardiogram criteria of 79
   high 77
Atrial fibrillation 17, 70, 72, 73, 140, 148, 161, 166, 171, 329, 331-333, 335, 337-339, 342, 343
   causes of 71
   complications of 71
   electrocardiogram criteria of 70
   permanent 143
   persistent 73
   types of 70
Atrial flutter 17, 75, 161, 332, 337
   appearance of wave of 75
   causes of 75
   differential diagnosis of 76
   electrocardiogram criteria of 75
   fibrillation 328, 330, 340
   mechanism of 75
Atrial septal defect 168, 169
   complications of 169
Atrial tachycardia 62, 64
   causes of 64
   electrocardiogram criteria of 64
   mechanism of 64
   multifocal 65
Atrioventricular block 102
   second-degree 103
Atrioventricular dissociation 108
   causes of 108
Atrioventricular node 3
Atropine 55
Attack, acute 61, 129
Automatic cells, number of 4
Axis deviation, types of 34

B

Beta-blocker 106
Biatrial enlargement, causes of 53
Bidirectional ventricular tachycardia 90
Bifascicular block 96, 113, 335, 339
   causes of 113
   complications of 96
   prognosis of 96
Bigeminy, causes of 84
Bipolar limb leads 7
   position 8
Bisphosphonate 157
Biventricular hypertrophy 49, 335, 339, 343
   causes of 49
Bizarre QRS widening 154
Brachial plexus 144
Bradycardia 10, 29, 55, 59, 72, 101, 152, 173, 332
   causes of 59
   symptomatic 68
Breast, carcinoma of 134
Broad-complex tachycardia 56
   causes of 56
Bronchus, carcinoma of 134
Brugada syndrome 92
Bundle branch block 21, 27, 38, 110

C

Calcium
   channel blockers 102, 104
   lowering drugs 160
Camel hump T waves 28
Cannon wave, mechanism of 106
Cardiac arrest 153
Cardiac axis 34, 35
   quick and simple way of determination of 35
Cardiac contraction, stimulus for 7
Cardiac cycle 7
Cardiac failure 124
   congestive 170
   high output 171
Cardiac muscle 6, 7
   fibers 6
   properties of 6
Cardiac plexus 6
Cardiac rhythm 33
Cardiac rupture 172
Cardiac surgery 66, 136
Cardiac tamponade 136, 145, 172
   causes of 136
Cardiomyopathy 27, 64, 84, 88, 114, 115
   dilated 12
   hypertrophic 49, 328, 334
Carditis, acute rheumatic 19, 108
Cells, types of 6
Cerebral injury 31
Chamber enlargement 10
Chest
   leads 2, 8
   pain 125
   wall 8
   thin 20
Cholinergic nerves 6
Chronic obstructive pulmonary disease 17, 52, 167
Circumflex artery 5
Citrate 157

Coccidioidomycosis 134
Complete heart block 105, 106, 109, 329,
    332, 337, 341
  causes of 106
  signs of 106
  sites of 105
Conduction 3
  system 4
Conductive tissue, anatomy of 4
Confusion 147
Conn's syndrome 151
Cor pulmonale, chronic 36
Coronary artery
  disease, severe 115
  normal 5
  right 5
Coronary circulation 5
Coronary vessels 5
Cushing's reflex 173
Cushing's syndrome 151
Cyanosis 161
Cyclizine 125
Cyclosporine 152

D

Deafness, congenital 31
Decubitus angina 128
Delirium 147
Demand pacemaker 144, 145
Depolarization 13
Depression 128, 147
Dextrocardia 36, 164, 334, 339, 341
  differential diagnosis of 164
  electrocardiogram criteria of 164
  prognosis of 165
Diabetic retinopathy 126
Diamorphine 125
Diarrhea 147
Digitalis toxicity 19
Digoxin 27, 30, 72, 88, 100, 106, 169, 343
  effect 147, 148, 328, 335, 339
  effect, electrocardiogram criteria of
      147
  normal value of 149
  poisoning 147, 153
  toxicity 38, 60, 64, 66, 83, 84, 102, 108,
      114, 147-149
Disopyramide 31, 102
Diuretics 169
Dressler syndrome 124, 125
Drowsiness 147
Drug effect 10
Dual chamber pacemaker 143, 341
Dual chamber pacing 145, 339
  electrocardiogram criteria of 143

E

Early repolarization syndrome 37
Echocardiogram 162
Ectopics
  beat 77, 78, 81
    causes of 78
    electrocardiogram criteria of 77
    types of 77
  couplet 81
  multifocal 80
    ventricular 21
  multiple ventricular 38, 328-331, 337
  runs of 81
  supraventricular 343
  unifocal 80
Edema, pulmonary 62
Eisenmenger's syndrome 49, 169
Electrical interference 13
Electricity conducting cells 6
Electrocardiogram 7, 15-17, 37
  ambulatory 40
  basic concepts of 1
  before interpretation of 10
  normal 14
  paper 11
  tracing, normal 14
Electrocardiographic patterns, types
    of 45, 48
Electrolyte
  imbalance 84, 114, 172
  serum 148
Electromechanical dissociation 172
  electrocardiogram criteria of 172
Emphysema 12, 21-23
Endocardial pacing 35
Endocrine disease 152, 159
Endothelin 5
Enzymes 128
Ephedrine 55
Epicardial pacing 36
Escape rhythm 105
Esmolol 62
Exercise 27
  electrocardiogram 38
  testing
    contraindications of 38
    indications of 38
  tolerance test 38

F

False positive exercise test, causes of 38
Fascicular block 112
Fast atrial fibrillation 70, 328, 330, 332,
    336-340, 343, 344

Fenoterol 151
Fibers, parasympathetic preganglionic 6
Fibrinolytic therapy 163
First-degree atrioventricular block 102
  causes of 102
  clinical features of 102
First-degree block, electrocardiogram
    criteria of 102
Flecainide 31
Foscarnet 157
Frozen shoulder 124
Frusemide 150, 151
Functional syncytium 6

G

Gitelman syndrome 151
Gordon syndrome 153
Gynecomastia 147

H

Haemophilus influenzae 134
Hallucination 147
Head injury 31
Heart 6, 7, 111, 153
  block 3, 95, 107
    acute complete 106
    chronic complete 106
    congenital complete 106
    first-degree 37, 97, 102, 339
    partial 19
    second-degree 37, 97
    sites of 95
    types of 95
  disease 7
    chronic ischemic 88
    congenital 36
    hypertensive 29
    ischemic 19, 60, 64, 66, 114, 170
    multiple valvular 49
    organic 83
    rheumatic 64
  failure 54, 151
  lung transplantation 169
  nerve supply of 6
  normal 90
  rate 33
    calculation of 33
    control of 73
  rhythm of 32
  specialized conductive system of 3
  ventricular tachycardia, normal 90
Heartbeat 7
Hemiblock 95, 112
Hemochromatosis 100, 104, 106

Hemolysis 152
Hemorrhage, intracerebral 31
Hepatic failure 166
Hereditary syndrome 31
High-voltage
    electrocardiogram tracing, causes of 12
    QRS, causes of 20
His bundle 3-5
Histoplasmosis 134
Holter monitoring 40
Hormones, systemic 5
Hyocardial infarction, hyperacute 27, 119
Hypercalcemia 10, 30, 159
    cardiac effects in 159
    causes of 159
    clinical features of 160
Hyperkalemia 10, 17, 21, 27, 85, 104, 114, 115, 152, 153, 331
    causes of 152
    effects of 153
    electrocardiogram criteria of 152
    features of 153
    severe 154
Hypermagnesemia 155
    cardiac effects of 155
    causes of 155
    electrocardiogram criteria of 155
Hypertension 115, 171
Hyperthyroidism 29, 171
    cardiac complication of 171
    electrocardiogram criteria of 171
Hypertrophy 19
    biatrial 53, 336
    ventricular 20, 21, 29, 38
Hypoalbuminemia 157
Hypoaldosteronism, hyporeninemic 153
Hypocalcemia 157, 158
    causes of 157
    electrocardiogram criteria of 157
    features of 158
Hypokalemia 10, 19, 27, 29, 38, 58, 79, 84, 85, 88, 102, 114, 150, 172, 333, 342
    causes of 151
    effects of 150, 151
    electrocardiogram criteria of 150
    severe 151
Hypomagnesemia 19, 85, 114, 88, 102, 156
    cardiac effects of 156
    causes of 156
    electrocardiogram criteria of 156
Hypoparathyroidism 157
Hypotension 62, 153

Hypothermia 12, 21, 23, 166, 172
    electrocardiogram criteria of 166
Hypothyroidism 21, 23, 170
    cardiac complication of 170
    electrocardiogram criteria of 170
Hypovolemia 172
Hypoxemia 84
Hypoxia 172

I

Idioventricular rhythm 17, 21
Infarction, right ventricular 123
Infection 145
Infiltrative disease 100, 106
Irregular rhythm, causes of 32
Ischemia
    inferior 335
    lateral 341
    myocardial 10, 27, 128
Isoelectric line 11, 16
Isoprenaline 55
Ivabradine 100

J

James bypass tract 139
Jaundice, obstructive 58
Jervell and Lange-Nielsen syndrome 31
Junctional rhythm 37, 66

K

Kent bundle 139

L

Lactate 157
Large U wave, significance of 30
Lead displacement 145
Left anterior
    descending artery 5
    hemiblock 96, 97, 112, 330, 335, 340
Left atrial hypertrophy 50, 53, 329, 332, 337, 339
    causes of 50
    criteria of 50
Left axis deviation 35, 112, 168
Left bundle branch 3-5
    block 115, 329, 331, 339
        causes of 115
        electrocardiogram criteria of 115
        incomplete 115

Left coronary
    artery 5
    sinus of Valsalva 5
Left posterior hemiblock 36, 96, 113, 335, 344
Left ventricle, inferoposterior aspect of 5
Left ventricular
    hypertrophy 43, 44, 49, 330, 331, 333-335, 337-340, 342-344
    wall 5
Lenègre-Lev disease 115
Leukemia 134, 152
Levocardia 164
Limb leads 7, 8
Lithium 100
    intoxication 159
Liver failure 151
Lone atrial fibrillation 71
Long QT
    interval, causes of 31
    syndrome, congenital 30
Low atrial ectopics 77
Low nodal
    ectopic 78
    rhythm 66
Low voltage tracing 135, 341
Lown classification 83
Lown-Ganong-.Levine syndrome 139, 141
    electrocardiogram criteria of 141
    prognosis of 141
Low-voltage
    electrocardiogram tracing, causes of 12
    QRS, causes of 21
    tracing, criteria of 12
Lung diseases, chronic 52
Lymphoma, carcinoma of 134

M

Mahaim fiber 139
Massive pulmonary embolism 172
Mesocardia 165
Metoprolol 62
Mid-nodal rhythm 66
Milk alkali syndrome 159
Mitral stenosis 329, 332
Mitral valve
    prolapse 38, 88
    repair 104
Mobitz type atrioventricular block 103, 104

Mononucleosis, infectious 152
Morphine 125
Muscles fibers
　contract 6
　ventricular 4
Myocardial cells 6
Myocardial infarction 10, 12, 22, 36, 54, 117, 118, 126, 127, 131
　acute 25, 84, 88, 107, 108, 112, 115, 117, 124, 125, 127, 133
　　anterior 55, 329, 342
　　anteroseptal 328, 330, 331, 337, 338, 342
　　extensive anterior 328
　　inferior 329, 330, 332, 333, 338, 343, 344,
　anterior 131, 332, 343
　anteroseptal 36, 329, 333, 335, 337, 338, 340
　complications of 124
　inferior 123, 140, 332
　lateral 331, 338
　non-Q wave 120, 121
　old anteroseptal 330, 332, 339, 341, 344
　old inferior 119, 331, 333-339, 342, 343
　posterior 140
　sites of 117
　subendocardial 120, 328
　transmural 120
　true posterior 122
Myocardial ischemia, transient 128
Myocarditis 19, 66, 84, 88, 114, 115
　rheumatic 66
Myocardium, ventricular 139
Myxedema 12, 27

N

Narrow-complex supraventricular tachycardia 344
Narrow-complex tachycardia 56
　causes of 56
Nausea 147
Nephrotic syndrome 151
Neuropeptides 5
Nitroglycerin, sublingual 125
Nodal ectopic, high 78, 334
Nodal rhythm 17, 66, 67
　electrocardiogram criteria of 66
　high 66
Nodal tachycardia 334
Nonrespiratory sinus arrhythmia 54
Non-ST-elevation myocardial infarction 328

O

Obesity 12
Oral anticoagulant 163
Ostium
　primum defect 168
　secundum defect 168

P

P mitrale
　causes of 50
　indicate 50
P pulmonale 17, 51, 52
　causes of 52
　transient 52
P wave 17
　abnormalities of 17
　causes of multiple 18
　characters of normal 17
Pacemaker 21, 114, 142, 144
　cells 6
　complications of 145
　malfunction 146
　permanent 143, 144
　syndrome 146
　temporary 144
　ventricular 142, 341
Pacing modes and functions, letter code of 145
Paget's disease 159
Pain 125
　abdominal 147
Pancreatitis, acute 157
Paralysis, hyperkalemic periodic 153
Paralytic ileus 153
Paroxysmal atrial fibrillation 330
　causes of 71
Partial left bundle branch block 337, 339
Partial right bundle branch block 48, 110, 336, 338, 339
Pathological Q wave
　causes of 22
　characters of 22
Pentamidine 31
Pericardial disease 10
Pericardial effusion 12, 21, 23, 125, 135, 136, 170
　electrocardiogram criteria of 135
Pericardial rub 133
Pericarditis 66, 125, 144
　acute 25, 27, 124, 133, 134, 333
　chronic constrictive 12, 21

Phenothiazine 21, 27, 30
Plasma 149
Pleurisy 125
Plural effusion 12
Pneumonitis 125
Pneumothorax 12, 144, 145
Pocket hematoma 145
Polycythaemia 169
Postcardiac surgery 88
Postinfarct angina 124
Postmyocardial infarction
　pericarditis 134
　syndrome 124, 125
Potassium
　serum 151
　sparing diuretics 152
P-R interval 19
　abnormalities of 19
　characters of normal 19
　variable 19
Prinzmetal's angina 25, 27, 128
Procainamide 21, 31, 102
Propantheline 55
Propranolol 62
Pseudo and pseudopseudohypoparathyroidism 157
Pulmonary embolism 36, 161-163, 336
　causes of 162
　electrocardiogram criteria of 161
　types of 162
Pulmonary hypertension 52
　features of 47
　signs of 47
Pulseless electrical activity 172
　causes of 172
Purkinje fibers 3, 4, 139
Pyrexia 125

Q

Q wave 21
　characters of normal 21
QRS complex 20
　abnormalities of 20
　characters of normal 20
　components of 20
QT interval 30
　abnormalities of 31
　characters of normal 30
　prolongation of 31
Quinidine 19, 21, 30, 88, 102

Index

R

R wave 22
   abnormalities of 22
   characters of normal 22
   poor progression of 23
   progression 23
Raised intracranial pressure 173
   electrocardiogram criteria of 173
Recurrent pulmonary embolism 163
Refractory period, absolute 6
Regularly irregular rhythm, causes of 32
Renal diseases 152
Repolarization 13
Respiratory sinus arrhythmia 54
Rhabdomyolysis 153
Rhythm, accelerated idioventricular 89
Right atrial hypertrophy 51, 53, 329, 335, 337
   causes of 51
   electrocardiogram criteria of 51
Right atrium 5
Right axis deviation 34, 36, 113
Right bundle branch block 3-5, 36, 96, 97, 110-113, 168, 330-332, 335, 338-340, 342-344
   causes of 111
   electrocardiogram criteria of complete 110
Right ventricular hypertrophy 46, 47, 49, 329, 332, 333, 335, 336, 340, 344

S

S wave 24
   characters of normal 24
Salbutamol 55, 151
Sarcoidosis 100, 104, 106
Sensory fibers 6
Serum digoxin level 148
Shock, hypovolemic 166
Short PR interval 19
   causes of 141
Short QT interval, causes of 31
Sick sinus syndrome 40, 58, 64, 100, 101
   causes of 100
   electrocardiogram criteria of 100
Single chamber ventricular pacemaker 328
Sinoatrial block 98, 99, 340
   causes of 98
   electrocardiogram criteria of 98
   prognosis of 99
Sinoatrial node 3, 4, 7
Sinus arrest 100, 341
Sinus arrhythmia 32, 37, 54
   types of 54

Sinus bradycardia 5, 37, 58, 59, 80, 166, 170, 333, 340, 342, 343
   causes of 58
   electrocardiogram criteria of 58
Sinus node function 145
Sinus of Valsalva, right coronary 5
Sinus rhythm 32, 146
   characters of 32
Sinus tachycardia 55-57, 61, 161, 171, 173, 333, 336-338, 341, 343, 344
   causes of 55
   electrocardiogram criteria of 55
Situs inversus 164
   clinical importance of 165
   prognosis of 165
Slow atrial fibrillation 70
Small P wave, causes of 18
Small R wave, causes of 23
Small T wave, causes of 27
Sodium ethylenediaminetetraacetic acid 157
Spironolactone 152
ST depression, causes of 26
ST elevation, causes of 25
ST segment 25
   abnormalities of 25
   characters of normal 25
Stable angina 128
   electrocardiogram criteria of 128
Staphylococcus aureus 134, 144
Stenosis
   aortic 49
   pulmonary 49, 52
Stokes-Adams attack 107
   clinical features of 107
Stored blood, transfusion of 153
Streptokinase 126
Stress tests 129
Stroke 166
Subclavian artery injury 144
Subendocardium, infarction of 120
Supraventricular tachycardia 17, 56, 60, 61, 88, 328, 331, 334
   causes of 60
   complications of 61
   types of 62
Syncytium 6
Systolic flow murmur 106

T

T inversion, causes of 26
T wave 26
   abnormalities of 26
   biphasic 27
   characters of normal 26
   flattened 28
   pattern, juvenile 28
Tachycardia 10, 56, 101, 161
   bradycardia syndrome 100, 101
   pacemaker mediated 145, 146
   types of 56
Tachypnea 161
Tall P wave, causes of 17, 27
Tall R wave, causes of 22
Tall T wave 27
Tension pneumothorax 172
Tetralogy of Fallot 36
Theophylline 88
Thiazide 150, 151
   diuretics 159
Thrombocytosis 152
Thromboembolism 124
Thrombolytic therapy, contraindications of 126
Thyrotoxicosis 60, 66, 159
Thyroxine 55
Tissue plasminogen activator 126
Torsades de pointes 21, 91, 157
   causes of 91
   electrocardiogram criteria of 91
   tachycardia 30
Trauma 136
Triamterene 152
Tricuspid
   regurgitation 52
   stenosis 52
Tricyclic antidepressant 21, 31
Trifascicular block 96, 97, 113, 114
   causes of 114
   complications of 114
Tumor lysis syndrome 153

U

U wave 29
   abnormalities of 29
   causes of prominent 29
   characters of normal 29
Unipolar limb leads 8
Unstable angina 128, 130

V

Venesection 169
Ventricular aneurysm 25, 88, 124, 131, 132
   causes of 131
   complications of 132
   electrocardiogram criteria of 131
Ventricular bigeminy 81, 84, 85, 334
   electrocardiogram criteria of 84

Ventricular ectopics 21, 36, 80-83, 124, 148, 161, 329, 332, 339-343
  causes of 82
  electrocardiogram criteria of 80
  runs of 81
  severity for 83
  types of 80
Ventricular fibrillation 21, 93
  causes of 93
  electrocardiogram criteria of 93
Ventricular flutter 94
  electrocardiogram criteria of 94
  prognosis of 94
Ventricular hexageminy 87
  electrocardiogram criteria of 87
Ventricular pacing, electrocardiogram criteria of 142
Ventricular pentageminy 87
  electrocardiogram criteria of 87
Ventricular premature complex 82
Ventricular quadrigeminy 81, 86, 334
  electrocardiogram criteria of 86
Ventricular tachycardia 21, 81, 88-90, 126, 166
  causes of 88
  differential diagnosis of 88
  electrocardiogram criteria of 88
  mechanism of 90
  types of 89
Ventricular trigeminy 81, 86, 335
  electrocardiogram criteria of 86
Vigorous exercise 153
Visual disturbance 147
Vitamin D
  deficiency 157
  therapy 158
Vomiting 147

W

Wandering pacemaker 19, 37, 68
  causes of 68
  electrocardiogram criteria of 68
Wenckebach phenomenon 19, 37, 103, 338
  causes of 103
  prognosis of 104
Wide P wave, causes of 18
Wide QRS, causes of 21
Wide-complex tachycardia, causes of 89
Wolff-Parkinson-White syndrome 20, 21, 36, 38, 40, 60, 63, 137-140, 328, 338, 344
  presence of 139, 140
  prophylactic treatment of 139
  treatment of 138
  types of 138

EU GSPR Authorised Reprsentative
Logos Europe, 9 rue Nicolas Poussin
1700, La Rochelle, France
Phone: +33 (0) 6 67 93 73 78
E-mail: contact@logoseurope.eu

www.ingramcontent.com/pod-product-compliance
Ingram Content Group UK Ltd.
Pitfield, Milton Keynes, MK11 3LW, UK
UKHW050244150426
5217IPUK00005B/126